Springer Tracts in Advanced Robotics

Volume 161

The Springer Tracts in Advanced Robotics (STAR) publish new developments and advances in the fields of robotics research, rapidly and informally but with a high quality. The intent is to cover all the technical contents, applications, and multidisciplinary aspects of robotics, embedded in the fields of Mechanical Engineering, Computer Science, Electrical Engineering, Mechatronics, Control, and Life Sciences, as well as the methodologies behind them. Within the scope of the series are monographs, lecture notes, selected contributions from specialized conferences and workshops, as well as selected PhD theses.

Special offer: For all clients with a print standing order we offer free access to the electronic volumes of the Series published in the current year.

Indexed by SCOPUS, DBLP, EI Compendex, zbMATH, SCImago.

All books published in the series are submitted for consideration in Web of Science.

Paolo Fiorini
Editor

Towards Autonomous Robotic Surgery

Results of the ERC-ADG project ARS

Springer

Editor
Paolo Fiorini
Department of Engineering for Innovation
Medicine
University of Verona
Verona, Italy

ISSN 1610-7438 ISSN 1610-742X (electronic)
Springer Tracts in Advanced Robotics
ISBN 978-3-032-04246-0 ISBN 978-3-032-04247-7 (eBook)
https://doi.org/10.1007/978-3-032-04247-7

This Springer imprint is published by the registered company Springer Nature Switzerland AG
The registered company address is: Gewerbestrasse 11, 6330 Cham, Switzerland

To all my former Students, who became Colleagues, Friends, or went away, who made this project and my academic career possible.

Series Editor's Foreword

At the dawn of the century's third decade, robotics is reaching an elevated level of maturity and continues to benefit from the advances and innovations in its enabling technologies. These all are contributing to an unprecedented effort to bringing robots to human environment in hospitals and homes, factories, and schools; in the field for robots fighting fires, making goods and products, picking fruits, and watering the farmland, saving time and lives. Robots today hold the promise for making a considerable impact in a wide range of real-world applications from industrial manufacturing to healthcare, transportation, and exploration of the deep space and sea. Tomorrow, robots will become pervasive and touch upon many aspects of modern life.

The *Springer Tracts in Advanced Robotics* (STAR) is devoted to bringing to the research community the latest advances in the robotics field on the basis of their significance and quality. Through a wide and timely dissemination of critical research developments in robotics, our objective with this series is to promote more exchanges and collaborations among the researchers in the community and contribute to further advancements in this rapidly growing field.

The volume edited by Paolo Fiorini reports the results of the ERC Advanced Grant project "ARS—Autonomous Robotic Surgery" from 2017 to 2023. The contents are organized in 16 chapters collecting the work of several doctoral dissertations during the life of the projects. The main challenge is to achieve a certain degree of autonomy in robotics surgery with the integration of embodied AI techniques. The contributions are inspired by a strong interdisciplinary collaboration among researchers in engineering, medicine, surgery, philosophy, ethics, communication, regulatory, and entrepreneurship.

A nice blend of original theoretical and practical results in the field of surgical robotics, this volume is a great addition to the STAR series.

Naples, Italy
July 2025

Bruno Siciliano
STAR Editor

Foreword

The field of robotics is an exciting area. It evolves many different technical aspects from lowlevel hardware to intelligent software, for full or partial automation of actions and decisions. In medicine and specially in surgery, it also requires a high level of performance and safety, as well as of integration within human activities. This book, *Towards Autonomous Robotic Surgery*, by Prof. Paolo Fiorini and his colleagues, showcases the outstanding scientific work and intellectual freedom. It gathers together cutting-edge research in robotics, computer science, and medical technology. And I feel so honored to introduce it.

Science emerges through curiosity and the exploration of new territories. This book reflects that spirit, addressing complex problems with innovative solutions that advance the capabilities of surgical robotics. The difficult problems are not avoided, the real right questions are posed and addressed, and the approaches followed to answer these questions are both sound and intelligent. This work is distinguished by its combination of rigorous theory and practical implementation, putting side by side knowledge modeling and data-driven methods. It reflects a holistic unique vision, integrating multiple disciplines effectively, all in a very innovative way. Albert Einstein's words, "Imagination is more important than knowledge," resonate here, as these researchers have dared to pose unconventional questions and explore uncharted paths.

Achieving scientific excellence involves persistent questioning, thought-provoking questions, and a willingness to challenge established norms. The contributors to this book exemplify these qualities through their meticulous research and pioneering insights. Professor Paolo Fiorini employs a mixture of theoretical depth and practical application to tackle the challenges of autonomous robotic surgery. His work provides a robust foundation for the field.

Each following chapter will explore foundational aspects of robotic surgery, offering comprehensive analyses on knowledge extraction, learning from data, surgical planning, sensing, and cognition, involving artificial intelligence, machine learning, computer vision, and biomechanics. The last chapters additionally demonstrate how the theoretical innovations are implemented within practical applications in order to demonstrate performances and added value.

Innovation, particularly in a field as multifaceted as robotic surgery, demands a unique combination of very large knowledge covering all facets, as well as intellectual freedom to navigate through it. This is what you will find here. The book's authors embark us for a journey through diverse investigations within various domains, fostering a multidisciplinary approach that pushes the boundaries of conventional knowledge. There are so many aspects that I deeply like in this incredible amount of work. For instance, they do not hesitate to invoke both usually-considered-opposite approaches of a priori models and deep complex networks and corresponding architectures. This definitely illustrate this rare combination of large amount of knowledge and intellectual freedom. This is this uniqueness that explains why Prof. Fiorini is really considered by the various communities of computer science, robotics, and computer-assisted surgery as a true leader and a model. I won't use the obvious but so true analogy with renaissance men, whose work transcended traditional boundaries to achieve lasting impact.

As autonomous robotic systems advance, ethical and social considerations become increasingly important. This book addresses these concerns thoughtfully, emphasizing the need for ethical guidelines and societal scrutiny. The chapters on the ethical and social aspects of autonomy highlight the complexities of integrating such technologies into healthcare practice. They underscore the importance of patient safety, informed consent, and the broader impact on the medical profession. Once again, this demonstrates the hindsight owned by Prof. Fiorini in his career. Addressing issues beyond technical and innovative aspects are crucial. The future success of robotic surgery also depends on the consideration of such issues. RAS has to be sustainable, useful, efficient, driven by added value to the quality of life of patients, as well as of professionals, while ensuring compatibility with societal challenges, such as ecological, social and ethical.

I had the privilege to collaborate with Prof. Paolo Fiorini, as many of our international colleagues, attracted by the unique spirit of Verona University. I was privileged to have shared this journey with such distinguished colleagues. Their passion, freedom of thought, and commitment to innovation exemplify what it means to be true pioneers. I dream of having undertaken such a groundbreaking project and achieving similar results. Above all, I cherish the friendships and camaraderie cultivated along the way, highlighting the human dimension of scientific endeavors—life is about passion, freedom, collaboration, and respect. It sounds so obvious to say but Prof. Fiorini has this human and social intelligence: curious to different viewpoints, always eager to learn and share, and the passion to debate. But also available to make a pause. I fondly recall enjoying Amarone red wine and dining in a very beautiful small restaurant in a nice village in the Verona's area, where discussions were as enriching as the company.

This book provides a path forward for robotic-assisted surgery, showcasing the potential of autonomous systems to enhance patient care. The innovative methods and insightful analyses represent a significant progress towards fully or partial autonomous surgical interventions. This work will undoubtedly guide future generations of researchers and practitioners, shaping the future landscape of medical robotics.

In conclusion, *Towards Autonomous Robotic Surgery* stands as a testament to the power of curiosity, collaboration, and scientific rigor. Prof. Paolo Fiorini and his team deserve immense respect for their dedication and impactful work. Their efforts underscore the importance of interdisciplinary approaches and ethical considerations in advancing medical robotics.

This is what you will learn in this book, what you will feel and live. Beyond the very interesting and innovative scientific contributions, you will live a journey, you will feel this spirit, this freedom that we, researchers, have the privilege to own and that we should never forget, the privilege to work freely through various disciplines to try to understand our world and make it better.

I wish you a wonderful travel.

Pierre Jannin
LTSI, Inserm UMR 1099
Faculté de Médecine Rennes
Université de Rennes
Rennes, France
https://medicis.univ-rennes1.fr/
http://www.ltsi.univ-rennes.fr/

Preface

In the last few years, we have witnessed the sweeping raise of Artificial Intelligence (AI) as the key technology for the development of future products and the improvement of human life. Public opinion is bombarded with daily announcements of meetings announcing the application of AI to novel fields and of the introduction of new products with intelligent features. However, when this research was proposed in 2016, AI was not yet as accepted by the scientific community as it is today, and the general public was not even aware of its existence and of its potential impact on everyday life and all activities.

Thus, the environment in which the research was conceived and started impacted the initial hypotheses, the formulation of the research questions, and the dissemination of its results. The rapid development and availability of sophisticated AI tools made it necessary and beneficial to update some of the initial plans and framed this research in a much broader context than initially envisioned. Furthermore, the project traversed the years of the COVID-19 pandemics, which forced to slow down some of the activity, but also allowed us to use in the project the latest AI tools.

The research described in this book was funded by the European Research Council Advanced Grant, ERC-ADG N. 742671 from October 1st 2017 to September 30, 2023, for the project ARS (Autonomous Robotic Surgery) addressing the development of methods for adding autonomous features to robotic surgery, and further exploring the challenged of embodied AI.

Because of the pandemic, the research lasted six years, instead of the planned five years, and it was able to demonstrate with realistic experiments different AI technologies and how they can be used to enhance a few surgical tasks. Besides the technical results, the ARS project had many important collateral effects that made its impact even larger than expected. For example, it created strong collaborations with the medical national and international communities, it motivated many meetings with different groups of stakeholders, it raised important ethical and legal questions about AI, and it supported the transfer of some technology into commercial products.

Because of the shifting technical and social landscape in which the ARS project was carried out, the development changed during the years, the underlying philosophy was clarified, and the technical solutions were adapted to the changing tools and the evolving understanding of the field. Thus, the narration presented in the book is the result of this evolution, and strongly benefited by the many discussions with colleagues, students and stakeholders.

The main outcome of the ARS research project was the development of practical methods to merge robotics and AI and to validate them in the challenging field of robot-assisted surgery. Instrumental to achieving the project results was the availability of the da Vinci Research Kit (dVRK), which is an open source laboratory surgical robot consisting of the first generation da Vinci Surgical System, donated by Intuitive Surgical, and of the custom software and electronics developed by the John Hopkins University. This set up permitted to span most of the aspects of robot-assisted surgery, such as knowledge representation, medical image processing, software engineering, robotic control, human-machine interfaces, haptics and tele-robotics. Each topic was the subject of the doctoral dissertation of the contributors to this book, which is briefly summarized in the dedicated chapters.

Then, the main contribution of this book is to put these research results into a unified perspective, which is difficult to see in the single thesis. We merge the results in a single publication, and we state the overall understanding of the technology, as it has matured during the past years. The ARS project motivated a strong interdisciplinary collaboration among researchers in engineering, medicine, surgery, philosophy, ethics, communication, regulatory, and entrepreneurship.

Ultimately, the goal of creating a strong community of researchers focusing of the many aspects of embodied AI was achieved and this goal far exceeds the specific technical results demonstrated by the ARS project, since it will persist in the future times and will continue to foster new ideas and results.

Verona, Italy Paolo Fiorini

Contents

Contributors

Marco Bombieri Department of Computer Science, University of Verona, Verona, Italy;
Department of Information Engineering and Computer Science, University of Trento, Trento, Italy

Andrea Calanca Department of Engineering for Innovation Medicine, University of Verona, Verona, Italy

Zhuoqi Cheng Italian Institute of Technology, Genova, Italy;
University of Southern Denmark, Odense, Denmark

Diego Dall'Alba Department of Engineering for Innovation Medicine, University of Verona, Verona, Italy

Martina Doppio Department of Computer Science, University of Verona, Verona, Italy;
Etifor | Valuing Nature, Padova, Italy

Maria-Camilla Fiazza Department of Computer Science, University of Verona, Verona, Italy

Paolo Fiorini Department of Engineering for Innovation Medicine, University of Verona, Verona, Italy

Michele Ginesi Department of Computer Science, University of Verona, Verona, Italy;
European Institute of Oncology, Milan, Italy

Bogdan Maris Department of Engineering for Innovation Medicine, University of Verona, Verona, Italy

Daniele Meli Department of Computer Science, University of Verona, Verona, Italy

Giovanni Gerardo Muscolo ECT*, Fondazione Bruno Kessler, Trento, Italy;
Department of Physics, University of Trento, Trento, Italy

Sara Patuzzo Manzati Department of Surgery, Dentistry, Paediatrics and Gynaecology, University of Verona, Verona, Italy

Andrea Roberti Department of Engineering for Innovation Medicine, University of Verona, Verona, Italy

Eleonora Tagliabue Department of Computer Science, University of Verona, Verona, Italy;
Carl Zeiss AG, Oberkochen, Germany

Chiara Zandoná Department of Computer Science, University of Verona, Verona, Italy;
ASEM Srl, Verona, Italy

Introduction

Paolo Fiorini

Abstract Robotics has been steadily growing in the attention of the public and in the number of practicing people. Professional societies include thousands of members, and media attention has changed its dystopic view of the early days. However, the dream of "A robot in every home" presented in the December 2006 issue of Scientific American is still far away. The reasons for this delay are many: cost, lack of a "killer" application, lack of suitable technologies, etc. This book addresses the technologies relevant to autonomous robots, which are the devices in the public imagination, and we consider the application of autonomy to the domain of surgery. Before starting the technical chapters, this Introduction gives a brief summary of the robotics evolution and its applications to medicine and surgery. Robotics is not the magic wand that solves difficult medical cases and simplifies complex interventions, but it provides important support to physicians to carry out their work. Robotics raises the average quality of interventions and reduces the dependence on subjective skills. Thus it should be made available everywhere to everybody, but we are still far away from this goal. In the first section of this chapter, we put robotics and medical robotics in their historical context. In the second section of this chapter, we describe the ERC-Advanced Grant project ARS (Autonomous Robotic Surgery) that funded our research from 2016 to 2023. The objective identified when the grant proposal was written, were slightly changed during the years, but we managed to maintain the overall project goals. In the third section of the chapter we give a brief summary of the experimental setup used and we describe the experiments carried out. Some of the devices and concepts described here are repeated also in the later sections, but we thought that collecting all the relevant information in a single place would have helped the readers. Finally in the last section of the chapter we describe the book outline of the chapters' structure.

P. Fiorini (✉)
Department of Engineering for Innovation Medicine, University of Verona, Verona, Italy
e-mail: paolo.fiorini@univr.it

P. Fiorini (ed.), *Towards Autonomous Robotic Surgery*, Springer Tracts in Advanced Robotics 161, https://doi.org/10.1007/978-3-032-04247-7_1

1 Brief History of Robot Development

The quest for an Artificial Life Form has been present in the human imagination since ancient times, e.g. the mythical Jewish Golems [1], the Norse legendary giants, and the bronze warrior Talos [2]. The creation of human-like devices capable of autonomous behaviors addressed first their technical aspects, and only recently designers were able to add perception and reasoning. In historical times, many cultures have developed mechanical humans, e.g. in China [3], in Europe [4] and in Japan [5]. In 18th century, life-sized automatons were built [6], and used for entertainment, such as the famous "Mechanical Turk" [7]. The first use of the word *robot* was in the 1920 play R.U.R. (Rossum's Universal Robots) [8] by the Czech author Karel Capek, referring to autonomous entities used as forced labour, *robota* in Czech, that eventually gained self-consciousness. The modern robot development started in 1949 with the design of teleoperation systems to handle radioactive materials [9], in which physical and cognitive actions were directly controlled by a human. Soon afterwards, the development focused on industrial automation, with the first Unimation robot [10] in 1960 and the commercial deployment of the The Tomorrow Tool (T3) by Cincinnati Milacron [11]. The addition of sensors, e.g. proximity, force, vision, made robots capable of some limited adaptation to their surroundings to compensate differences in the working environment. Robots carry out their tasks by executing a program stored in their memory that considers all the foreseen task options.

Industrial robotic development has accelerated since the 1980s, and current manufacturing cannot operate without robotics, which has been responsible for increased speed, accuracy, and safety of mass manufacturing. Industrial robotics enjoys wide adoption and public acceptance in spite of the early fears of impact on the workforce. Car construction is mainly robotized, and robots are used beyond the structured workplace of the automotive factory, now being deployed to deliver packages [12], drive through our neighborhoods [13], and to find and defuse mines [14]. These tasks are carried out in unstructured and dynamic environments and are fundamentally different from industrial tasks. In fact, an industrial robot executes repetitive tasks, programmed and tuned before the tasks start, and with no capability of making major changes without complete reprogramming its behavior by the robot user. On the other hand, an autonomous robot would need to make large adjustments to its program, potentially completely reprogram its task without human intervention. Current robotic capabilities are not the result of autonomous behaviors but of well designed deterministic algorithms, e.g. obstacle avoidance or handling of delicate objects, and of the software skills of the programmers. A more detailed description of robotics development can be found in [15]

In recent years, there has been also a rise in collaborative robots (cobots) [16], i.e. robots designed to operate alongside humans safely, using force-limited joints and computer vision, that allows them to interact directly with humans.

The development of autonomous robots spans already several decades, and it greatly benefited from advancements in Artificial Intelligence (AI) algorithms that use learning and big data techniques. Current autonomous technology is mostly used in mobility devices with the deployment of autonomous transportation devices, for goods and people as well. The initial development of self-driving cars started in the 1980s, but the main push was given by the DARPA Grand Challenges [17] in 2004 and 2005 that prompted many projects leading to commercial deployment. Examples of devices under commercial testing are Waymo (formerly Google Self-Driving Car Project 2009) [18] that since 2017 is operating fleets of commercial autonomous taxis in the urban areas of Los Angeles and Phoenix, and Serve Robotics [19] that has deployed autonomous delivery vehicles in some areas of Los Angeles.

1.1 Medical and Surgical Robots

Surgical and medical robotics was a niche development in parallel to mainstream of industrial robots. The original idea was to bring robotic accuracy and precision to the medical world. Surgical robots were first introduced to interact with rigid anatomical parts, i.e. guidance to neurosurgery [20] and orthopedic surgery and then extended to other anatomical districts. ROBODOC for the first commercial surgical robot used in hip surgery replacement [21]. Surgery of soft tissues started in early 1991, with transurethral resection of the prostate (TURP) [22]. In 1994, the Automated Endoscopic System for Optimal Positioning (AESOP) (Computer Motion, Inc., Goleta, CA) was developed as a laparoscopic camera holder [23]. Later on, Computer Motion introduced its Zeus surgical robot [24], soon followed by the da Vinci system manufactured by Intuitive Surgical, Inc. (Sunnyvale, CA) [25]. After Intuitive Surgical acquired Computer Motion in 2003, the da Vinci system has gained market dominance for interventions on soft tissues. Recently Medtronics and CMR Surgical introduced the surgical robots Hugo [26] and Versius [27], respectively. There are, however, more than 100 companies worldwide working on the development of competing systems for robot-assisted surgery. A more detailed description of surgical robot development can be found in [15].

Surgical automation can bring long-term benefits to all stakeholders, by enabling more consistent task execution, compensating for slow or missing human response, and by supervising the execution of surgical tasks and reducing errors. Early attempts of automation of surgical tasks were for TURP interventions [22, 28], whereas automation in Minimally Invasive Surgery has focused on the control the laparoscopic camera mounted on the AESOP robot or on the Endoassist system [29]. To better distinguish among the different automatic features, a few classifications of autonomy have been proposed. For example, the EC/TR 60601-4-1: "Medical electrical equipment" Technical Report [30], and the classifications of autonomous features presented in [31–33]. These classifications follow the standards proposed for self-driving vehicles, based on different levels of human involvement in the task. At level 0, the robot does not provide any cognitive or manual assistance to the surgeon. At level 1, the robot informs the surgeon about task options and may provide manual assistance. In the intermediate levels 2 and 3, the interaction between the robot and the operator becomes discrete, e.g. the surgeon approves a course of action at the beginning of the task. Levels 4 and 5 are different since the robot may be practicing medicine and will require a different testing and validation strategy. A more detailed description of autonomy in robotic surgery can be found in [34].

A debate is going on within the scientific community about the difference between automatic and autonomous systems. Some researchers see autonomy as an extension of automation, whereas others identify a step change between automation and autonomy, i.e. autonomy cannot be reached without a fundamental change in the paradigm of automation. In this book, we adhere to the second opinion and we will show how autonomy requires technologies that are not in the field of automation and whose integration requires a new way of approaching the problems and developing the solutions.

2 The Research Project

The ARS (Autonomous Robotic Surgery) project was conceived in 2016 with the purpose of identifying the main challenges of bringing autonomous capabilities to the surgical world. Furthermore, we aimed at developing the technologies that would eventually lead to the deployment of autonomous robots in the operating room. In addition to the obvious scientific results that such an objective would produce, there are also more practical and direct consequences of adding autonomy to a surgical robot. Currently, about 310 million major surgical operations are performed worldwide every year. The number of surgeries is steadily increasing, while economic and personnel resources for health care are decreasing. In the developed world, almost half of all harmful events (such as miscommunication, wrong medication, and technical errors) affecting patients are related to surgical care and service. These accidents are due, among others, to excessive fatigue, lack of coordination and training, lack of manual skills, and cognitive overload. Systemic and human factors are the main causes of patient harm during health care, including during surgery. Although robotic devices are used in a very small fraction of surgical interventions worldwide (approximately 2,680,000 in 2024, i.e. less than 1% of the total number of interventions), they have the potential to increase patient safety if they can be endowed with some level of autonomy. Autonomous robots can provide more assistance to surgical procedures than is currently available today. Robots can supervise the intervention progress, warn about critical situations, provide consistent and repeatable surgical actions, and compensate for time delay in future tele-surgical applications. The key to a larger diffusion and impact of surgical robots is the reduction of acquisition and operating costs. In this area, autonomy can also have an impact, allowing more cost effective design by replacing expensive hardware with low-cost "intelligent" hardware, and requiring lower operational expenses due to preventive maintenance and failure identification. Within these hypotheses, the ARS project aimed to develop technologies that would allow the introduction of an autonomous robot into the surgical scenario. We have addressed and solved specific problems that arise in surgical procedures. The project examined the steps in the diagnosis-planning-execution phases of a surgical procedure and identified the key elements that can be made autonomous. From this analysis, innovative solutions for a complete surgical workflow were developed, which were tested and validated in specific demonstrations.

The research carried out in the ARS project was expected to improve the technology of autonomous robotic surgery with the following key objectives:

- Knowledge extraction and representation: ARS aimed at analyzing and modeling real surgical interventions, integrating a priori knowledge from textbooks with the structures identified by big data analysis. Anatomical models and their properties were considered to create realistic virtual and physical phantoms.
- Intervention planning: This scientific goal aimed at developing methods to plan an intervention for a specific anatomy by instantiating the generic intervention description. On-line and reactive planning were also addressed.
- Surgical task control and execution: This objective would permit us to actuate the surgical instruments according to the developed plan and with respect of the anatomical constraints i.e. the organ positions in the surgical area and their biomechanical properties.
- Perception and situation awareness: Geometrical reasoning methods and control policies identified in the surgical data were to be used to design reactions to unexpected situations and determine when the control was to be transferred to the supervising surgeon.
- Demonstrations and validations: The algorithms and models developed in the previous objectives were to be demonstrated with the autonomous execution of representative cases using the laboratory setup and patient specific physical phantoms. The quality of the autonomous execution was to be measured by developing specific benchmarks.

One of the necessary elements to support the development outlined above was the availability of clinical data collected during robot-assisted interventions. Their analysis would have allowed one to identify the actual surgical actions performed by the operating physician and compare them to the planned actions. To this purpose, an agreement was reached with the surgical department of the City of Hope Medical Center (Duarte, CA USA) directed by Prof. Yuman Fong, with the group of prof. Joel Burdick at Caltech (California Institute of Technology, Pasadena, California USA), and with the data analysis group at Intuitive Surgical (Mountain View, California USA) directed by Dr. Simon DiMaio and Anthony Jarc. According to the agreement, data would have been collected during interventions at City of Hope and stored in an encrypted format on a support provided by Intuitive Surgical. Intuitive Surgical personnel would have decoded the data, filtered to remove sensitive information, and anonymized to remove patient information. Then, these pre-processed data would have been transferred to Caltech for the extraction of significant motion features, such as phase durations and average values of positions, speed and acceleration. These data would then have been sent to the University of Verona for task identification and analysis and for the computation of the task policy. Clearly, this was not a simple agreement to reach and it took more than one year to be signed among the participating institutions. A first data set was collected in summer 2019 and sent to

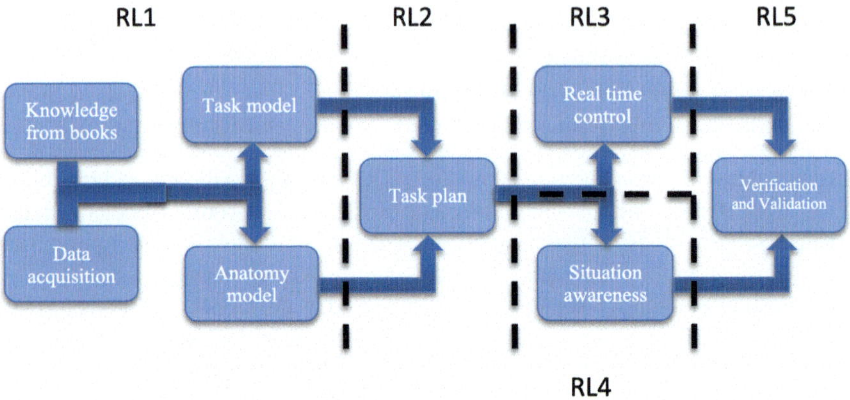

Fig. 1 The research structure of the ARS project

Intuitive Surgical for processing. Unfortunately, the COVID-19 pandemic first put the data collection on hold, and then stopped it all together. Thus, surgical task analysis was carried out using public domain data and data collected during simulations carried out in the robotics laboratory at the University of Verona.

The proposed implementation of the research objectives, as described in the ARS proposal, was coarsely divided into five research lines, addressing the main aspects of autonomous surgery, i.e.: modelling, planning, execution, monitoring, and verification, as shown in Fig. 1. Each Research Lines (RL) was further subdivided into tasks. RL1 developed models of surgical actions and anatomical environments, extracted from books and experience and learned from data. RL2 addressed surgical plans, both off-line and on-line, and their verification. RL3 addressed plan execution and the kinematic and dynamic constraints of robot-tissue interaction. RL4 addressed real time reasoning and task monitoring. Finally RL5 addressed the integration of the above elements in the da Vinci Research Kit (dVRK), our laboratory surgical robot.

Since the ERC-Advanced Grant is a single beneficiary grant, the ARS project enjoyed the freedom to select the participants and optimize its structure since all the project participants belonged to the University of Verona, the grant beneficiary. Each research line was assigned to one, or more, doctoral students of the Computer Science Department of the University of Verona. Of course each student research developed into directions that were unexpected at the beginning of the project. Furthermore, we improved our understanding of the problem complexity, allowing us to give a better perspective to the research carried out.

When we looked back at the project, we realized that our ambitious objective was to have the autonomous surgical robot to carry out an intervention by first reading and understanding a surgical manual, by interpreting the description of the intervention and planning it according to the specific patient anatomy. The robot would then carry out the intervention, react to unexpected events, and finally report about the outcome to the surgeon.

We also realized that many tools, algorithmically as well as physical, were not available and we set up to fill these gaps.

Thus, the structure of this book follows this logical, rather than temporal, structure. For example, the research lines on automatic knowledge extraction from text books, which was part of RL1 and should have started at the beginning of the project, was actually carried out at the end, because of student availability and interest. In this perspective, the main purpose of this book is not to summarize the research results achieved, which are already available in the scientific literature, but to give a coherent and logical presentation of the complete research carried out. This overall perspective and the synergies and interactions among the different research lines, are not evident in the single research publications and the purpose of this book is to give a homogeneous and complete vision of the research carried out.

3 The Experimental Setup

We demonstrated the theoretical results described in this book on the *da Vinci Research Kit* (dVRK) the research robotic platform used by many laboratories around the world to develop hardware and software for robot-assisted surgical procedures. We give here a brief description of the main hardware and software components of the dVRK system and then we present the experiments carried out to demonstrate the theoretical results. The experiments include a training task, tissue manipulation, and an anatomically relevant demonstration. Each one of them addresses a specific aspects of the theory, which is briefly summarized before describing the experimental details.

3.1 The da Vinci Research Kit

The genesis of the dVRK is described in [35]. This device consists of an out-of-market model of the da Vinci Surgical System that was donated by its manufacturer, the Intuitive Surgical Inc. (ISI), Sunnyvale, CA, USA, to laboratories proposing innovative experiments. The dVRK shown in Fig. 2 is the system used in our experiments and consists of the first version of the da Vinci system, called *classic*, augmented by hardware and software developed through a collaboration between academic institutions, Johns Hopkins University and Worcester Polytechnic Institute, and ISI in 2012 [36].

The dVRK in the Altair Robotics Laboratory of the University of Verona consists of the two standard parts, the patient side system and surgeon side control station. The patient side robot is equipped with two Patient Side Manipulators (PSM) and one Endoscopic Camera Manipulator (ECM). The surgeon side system is equipped with two Master Tool Manipulators (MTM) and the stereoscopic video console. More recent versions of the dVRK are equipped with three PSM's. Figure 3 shows the

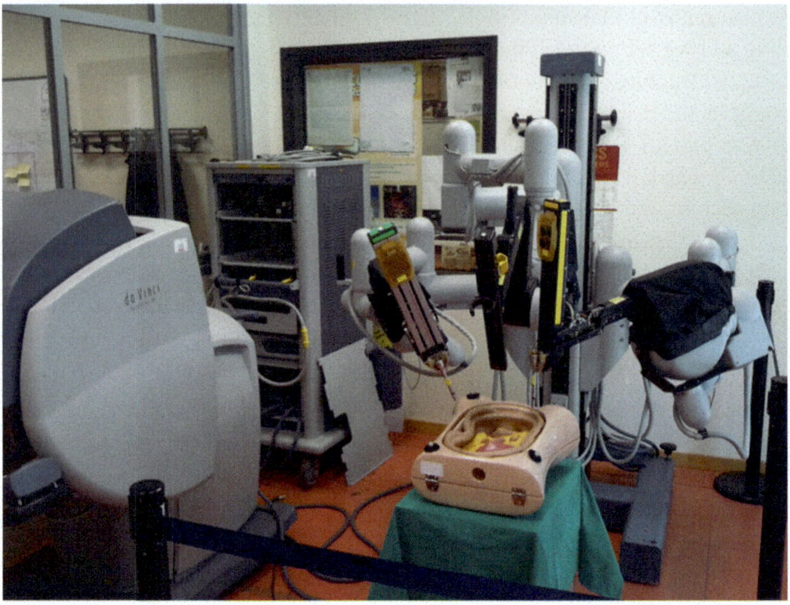

Fig. 2 The da Vinci Research Kit (dVRK) in the robotics laboratory Altair of the University of Verona

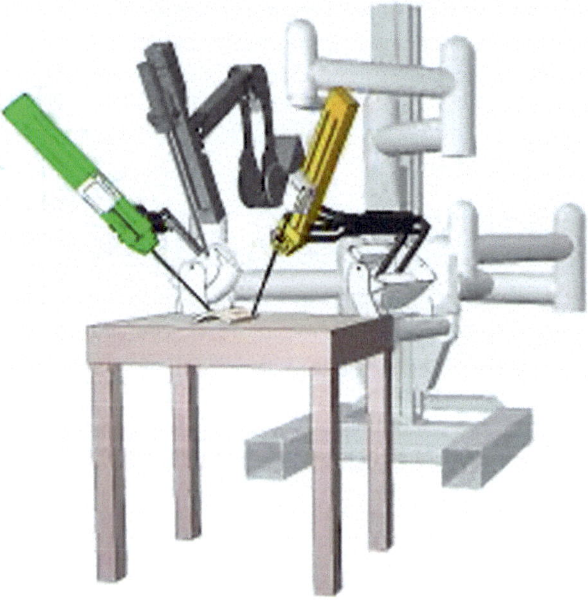

Fig. 3 Models of the patient side robot

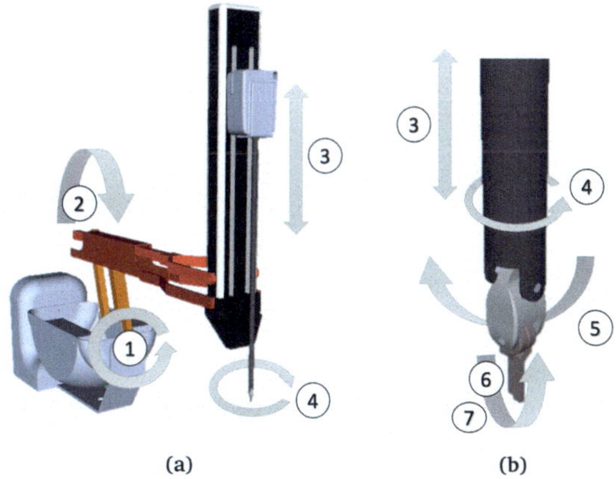

Fig. 4 Models of the PSM (**a**), the surgical instrument **b** (models are not to scale)

graphical representation of the two PSM's, in green and yellow colors, and of the ECM in gray.

The kinematic structures of each PSM is represented in Fig. 4. The instrument motion is based on the concept of Remote Center of Motion (RCM) that is fixed w.r.t. the robot body. The initial task of every intervention is to position the PSM so that the RCM position corresponds to incision position. The PSM has the following joints:

1. It is the revolute joint that moves the entire PSM with respect to its mounting base. It pivots the instrument in a yaw motion about the remote center.
2. It is a revolute joint that pivots the instrument in a pitching motion about the remote center
3. It is a prismatic joint that moves the instrument along the axis of its shaft in or out of the patient.
4. It is a revolute joint that rolls the instrument around its shaft.
5. It is a revolute joint. It is the first joint of the wrist mechanism (for standard 8mm instruments). Anthropomorphic to a human wrist knocking on a door, it controls the wrist pitch movement
6. It is a revolute joint, and it is the second joint of the wrist mechanism (for standard 8mm instruments). Anthropomorphic to a human wrist wiping a surface. It is a coordinated motion of two mechanical joints representing the two jaws of the gripper.
7. It is a revolute joint controlled in combination with Joint 6 to control wrist yaw motion and jaws opening and closing motions.

Although the command station is not used in our experiments of autonomous surgery, the MTM has to be always available to permit switching to the human operator in case of need. The MTM is shown in Fig. 5 and has the following structure:

1. Outer—Yaw This joint moves the entire MTM about the mounting base. The axis of rotation is perpendicular to the ground.

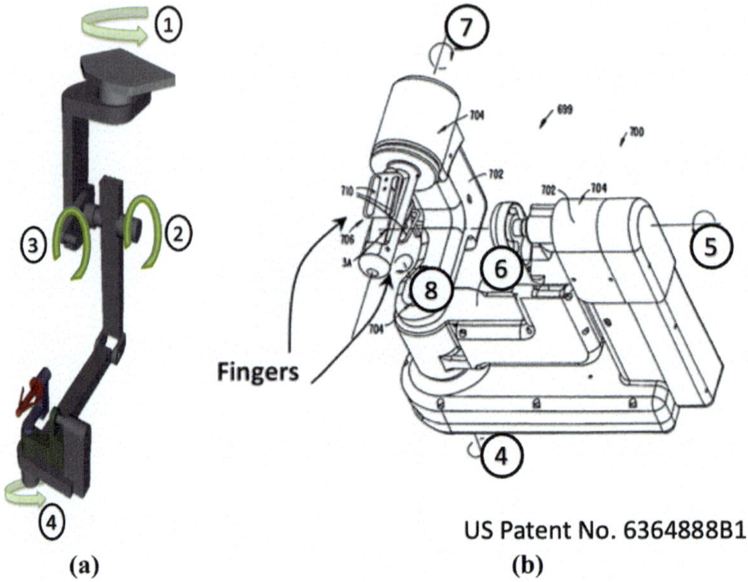

Fig. 5 Models of the MTM structure (**a**) and of its handle (**b**) (models are not to scale)

2. Outer Pitch1 (Shoulder)—This joint is one of the two joints that are responsible for the pitch and in/out translation of the MTM.
3. Outer Pitch2 (Elbow)—This joint is the second of the joint pair which together with the previous joint controls the pitch and in/out translation of the MTM.
4. Setup Joint (Platform)—This joint acts as the platform for the Gimbal arrangement for the MTM's wrist; it also provides the extra degree of freedom to enable movement in the NULL space.
5. Wrist Pitch—This joint determines the pitch of the wrist in the gimbal arrangement.
6. Wrist Yaw—This joint determines the yaw of the wrist in the gimbal arrangement.
7. Wrist Roll—This joint determines the roll of the wrist in the gimbal arrangement.
8. Finger Grips—This joint directly controls the desired motion of the jaws of the instruments.

The kinematic analysis of the PSM and MTM is available in reference [36]. An open controller developed by the John Hopkins University provides a full ROS-based control of all the dVRK robotic arms [37]. The controller allows position, velocity and current control.

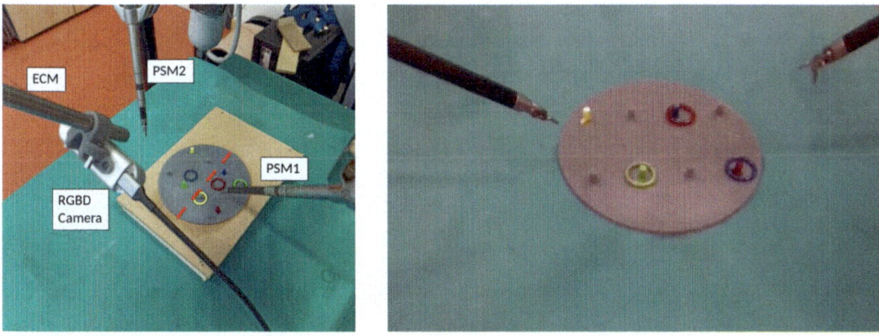

(a) (b)

Fig. 6 The ring transfer scenario used as a running example (**a**); an example scenario with occupied colored pegs for PSM1 (**b**)

3.2 The Demonstration Tasks

The experiments include a training task, tissue manipulation, and an anatomically relevant demonstration. Each one of them addresses a specific aspect of the theory, which is described in the following chapters of the book. For completeness, the Figures and the text descriptions are duplicated in this chapter and in the chapters discussing the theory.

The Ring Transfer Task

The approach taken to carry out this task is described in chapter Surgical Task Planning and Learning, and it consists of describing a task by using the Answer Set Programming (ASP) formalism. The logic program that is written in this way represents the task plan. The *ring transfer task* is a variant of the standard peg transfer task described in the fundamentals of laparoscopic surgery for novice training [38]. The goal is to place colored rings on the same-color pegs, using the Patient-Side Manipulators (PSM) of our dVRK. Our dVRK has three mechanical arms, two of which carrying a surgical instrument and indicated as PSM1 and PSM2, and the third carrying the endoscopic camera and indicated as ECM, as shown in Fig. 6–a.

Each instrument can touch the objects (rings and pegs) in the scene, depending on their reachability, which is defined by their position with respect to the red-dashed line in Fig. 6–a. For instance, the red ring can be reached by PSM1 in the picture, while the yellow peg can be reached by PSM2. Depending on the reachability, a ring may be picked and placed by the same PSM* (e.g., the red ring and peg are both reachable by PSM1), or transfer between the arms may be required (as in the case for the blue ring, whose peg is reachable only by PSM1). Moreover, if a ring is placed on a peg (e.g., the yellow ring in Fig. 6–b), it can be moved to the peg only after it has been extracted from its current position.

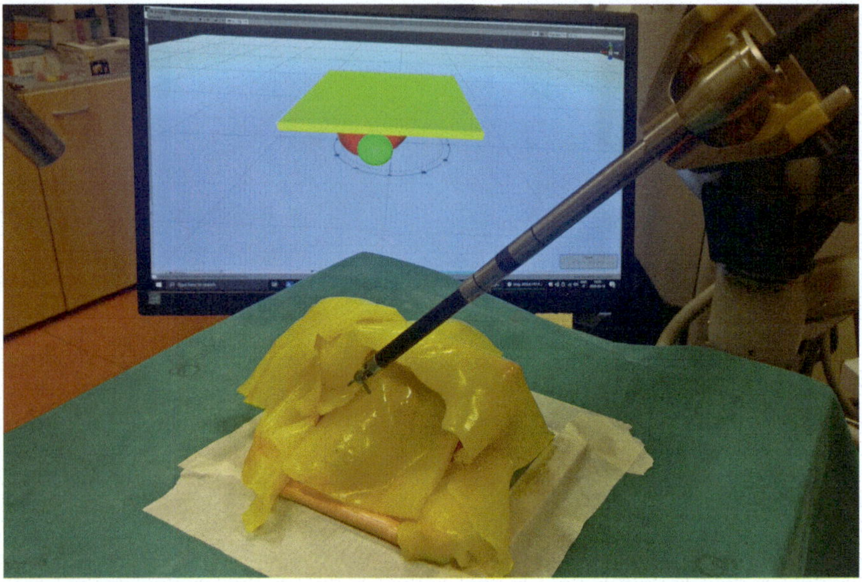

Fig. 7 A single arm of the dVRK interacts with silicone fat tissue covering a kidney phantom. The simulated scene controlling dVRK movements within *UnityFlexML* can be seen in the background

The Tissue Retraction Task

The tissue retraction demonstration is described in chapter Learning Tissue Retraction in Simulation and it consists of lifting a sheet of silicone fat tissue covering a kidney phantom, as shown in Fig. 7. We restrict the portion of fat tissue our agent interacts with to a 90×90 mm square region which is rigidly anchored to the top part of the kidney. The silicone patch representing the fat is held in place through a custom designed rigid structure, which enables to uniquely define the position of fat and kidney between the simulated and the real environment. The initial configuration of the fat tissue is obtained by letting this square region fall on the kidney phantom under gravity load. In these experiments, we consider a scenario with a single PSM arm equipped with the Large Needle Driver.

The Medical Slam Task

This task is described in chapter Situation Awareness in Autonomous Surgical Robots: Calibration and Medical SLAM' and it consists of labeling the anatomical elements that are visible in an image. This task leveraged on the availability of anatomical phantoms from the SARAS project, that was carried out at the same time in the Altair laboratory. The SARAS [39] project aimed at developing robotic bedside surgeons in robot-assisted surgical procedures. This development would have

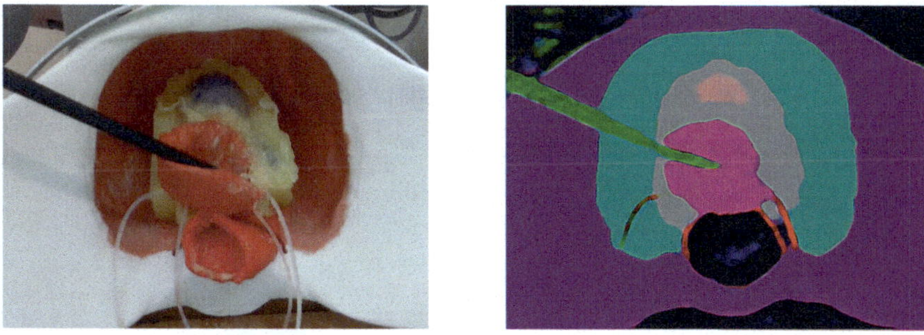

(a) RealSense® view (b) Segmented image

Fig. 8 Examples of real-time semantic segmentation computed using RealSense image

the immediate result of halving the number of surgeons needed in a procedure, potentially reducing the waiting time to access surgery. Furthermore, this application of autonomy is within reach of the technology, since the tasks required by the assistant surgeon are simpler than those of the main surgeon and usually prompted by voice commands. The results of the SARAS project are described in [40].

We could use the phantom of the pelvic area developed by the SARAS project to develop the automatic semantic segmentation of the anatomy. The task consisted of reaching the bladder and pressing the instrument on it. As illustrated in Fig. 8, the real time imagine acquired by the RealSense® camera is effetively segmented in its main components, and the target point of the instrument motion can be identified.

4 Book Outline

This book follows the structure of the Research Lines (RL) presented in Sect. 2 by organizing the book into three main parts.

Part I presents the challenges we addressed to extract, represent, and use the knowledge of robotic surgery for planning, representing RL1 and RL2. We describe the theoretical and methodological aspects of knowledge extraction from text, as described in chapter Learning Surgical Procedures from Text. In this chapter we introduce the use of LLM for surgical language interpretation, which cannot be done by the LLM trained for natural language. We then develop a knowledge representation based on the logical representation of task structures in chapter Surgical Task Planning and Learning, and we use this formalism to develop the task plan. We linked knowledge extraction from text and planning in chapter Towards Surgical Task Planning from Text to develop a method that could derive the plan directly from text. We addressed the knowledge extraction from data in chapter Learning Surgical Gestures from Data, where we learned the control policy of instrument motions and the task structure phases. We also present simulations as an alternative method to represent knowledge in the context of autonomous systems, as described in chapter Simulation and Autonomy.

Part II addresses the challenges of mapping the generic surgical plan into a specific environment, representing RL3, RL4 and RL5. We discuss how the environment is sensed and how the knowledge is mapped to a specific anatomy chapter Situation Awareness in Autonomous Surgical Robots: Calibration and Medical SLAM. Then, we give first a brief introduction to the architecture used in the demonstrations in chapter The Cognitive Architecture. Then we describe how we applied this architecture to simulate and test a plan and to forecast the expected effects of the actions, as discussed in chapter Autonomous Tissue Retraction with DEFRAS. The comparison between simulation and reality generates on-line learning, which is discussed in chapter Learning Tissue Retraction in Simulation However, not all information can be derived from existing sensors and new sensors were developed to extract data during the procedures, as described in chapter New Hardware: Design, Models and Analysis.

Part III presents the non-technical issues related to autonomy. The ethical and social issues facing an autonomous robot used in surgery are described in chapter The Ethical and Social Aspects of Autonomy. The risks and the structure of a future Human-machine relationship are briefly explored in chapter Automation on the Brink of Autonomy: Letting Go of Control. The challenges and successes achieved during the communication of the sensitive topics of robotic autonomy are described in chapter Communication Strategy of the ARS Project. Finally, the exploitation potential of autonomy in robotic surgery is addressed in chapter The Exploitation of Results.

The book is closed by chapter Conclusions that summarizes the research project and its main results.

5 Conclusions

This first chapter gives a brief introduction to the history of robotics and the development of medical and surgical robotics. Before entering the technical details of the next chapters we also summarize the features of the laboratory hardware, and of the demonstration discussed. Finally the last section gives an overview of the complete book.

References

1. Wikipedia, "The jewish golems". https://en.wikipedia.org/wiki/Golem. Accessed 15 Feb. 2025
2. Wikipedia, "The myth of talos." https://en.wikipedia.org/wiki/Talos. Accessed 15 Feb. 2025
3. Needham, J.: Science and civilisation in China: volume 2, ch. History of scientific thought. Cambridge University Press (1991)

4. Wikipedia, "Leonardo's robot". https://en.wikipedia.org/wiki/Leonardo%27s_robot. Accessed 15 Feb. 2025
5. Law, J.: Puppets of nostalgia—the life, death and rebirth of the Japanese Awaji Ningyo tradition. Princeton University Press (1997)
6. Wood, G.: Living Dolls: a Magical History of the Quest for Mechanical Life. Faber and Faber, London (2003)
7. Wikipedia, "The mechanical turk". https://en.wikipedia.org/wiki/The_Turk. Accessed 15 Feb. 2025
8. Wikipedia, "R.u.r.". https://en.wikipedia.org/wiki/R.U.R. Accessed 15 Feb. 2025
9. Goertz, R.: Fundamentals of general-purpose remote manipulators. Nucleonics **10**, 36–42 (1952)
10. Engelberger, J.: Robotics in Practice. IFS Publications, Kempston (1980)
11. Hon, R.: Application flexibility of a computer controlled industrial robot, Technical report. MR 76-603, SME Technical Paper (1976)
12. Wikipedia, Why amazon, ups and even domino's is investing in drone delivery services. https://www.insiderintelligence.com/insights/drone-delivery-services. Accessed 15 Feb. 2025
13. Metz, C.: The long road to driverless trucks. The New York Times, 28 Sept. 2022
14. Webster, G.: Mine kafon: the low-tech, high-design tumbleweed minesweeper. CNN Buis. (2013)
15. Fong, Y., Erhunmwunsee, L., Pigazzi, A., Podolsky, D., Portenier, D.D.: Robotic General Surgery. Wolters Kluwer Health (2024)
16. Villani, V., Pini, F., Leali, F. Secchi, C.: Survey on human-robot collaboration in industrial settings: safety, intuitive interfaces and applications. Mechatronics **55**, 248–266 (2018)
17. Wikipedia, "Darpa grand challenges". https://en.wikipedia.org/wiki/DARPA_Grand_Challenge. Accessed 15 Feb. 2025
18. Wikipedia, "The waymo self driving car". https://waymo.com. Accessed 15 Feb. 2025
19. Wikipedia, "Autonomous robotic delivery". https://www.serverobotics.com. Accessed 15 Feb. 2025
20. Kwoh, Y., Hou, J., Jonckheere, E., Hayati, S.: A robot with improved absolute positioning accuracy for CT guided stereotactic brain surgery. IEEE Trans. Biomed. Eng. **35**, 153–160 (1988)
21. Rassweilera, J., Binderc, J., Frede, T.: Robotic and telesurgery: will they change our future? Curr. Opin. Urol. **11**, 309–320 (2001)
22. Harris, S., Arambula-Cosio, F., Mei, Q., Hibberd, R., Davies, B.W.J. et al.: The probot—an active robot for prostate resection. Proc. Inst. Mech. Eng H. **211**, 317–325 (1997)
23. Kraft, B., Jäger, C., Kraft, K., Leibl, B., Bittner, R.: The aesop robot system in laparoscopic surgery: increased risk or advantage for surgeon and patient? Surg. Endosc. **18**, 1216–123 (2004)
24. Wikipedia, "The zeus robotic system". https://en.wikipedia.org/wiki/ZEUS_robotic_surgical_system. Accessed 15 Feb. 2025
25. Intuitive Surgical, "The da vinci robotic system". https://www.intuitive.com/en-us/products-and-services/da-vinci. Accessed 15 Feb. 2025
26. Medtronics, "The hugo robotic system". https://www.medtronic.com/covidien/en-gb/robotic-assisted-surgery/hugo-ras-system.html. Accessed 15 Feb. 2025
27. CMR Surgical, "The versius robotic system". https://us.cmrsurgical.com. Accessed 15 Feb. 2025
28. Rovetta, A., Sala, L., Tosatti, R.M.: A robotized system for the execution of a transurethral laser prostatectomy. ISIR, International Symposium on Industrial Robot (1996)
29. Kraft, B., Ger, C.J., Kraft, K., Leibl, B., Bittner, R.: The AESOP robot system in laparoscopic surgery: increased risk or advantage for surgeon and patient?. Surg. Endosc. **18**, 1216–123 (2004)
30. International Standard Organization (ISO), "The iso 60601 standard". https://www.iso.org/standard/65529.html. Accessed 15 Feb. 2025
31. Yip, M.C., Das, N.: Robot autonomy for surgery, pp. 1–33 (2017). arxiv:abs/1707.03080

32. Yang, G.-Z.E.A.: Medical robotics—regulatory, ethical, and legal considerations for increasing levels of autonomy. Sci. Robot. **2**(4) (2017)
33. Haidegger, T.: Autonomy for surgical robots: concepts and paradigms. IEEE Trans. Med. Robot. Bionics **1**(2), 65–76 (2019)
34. Fiorini, P., Goldberg, K.Y., Liu, Y., Taylor, R.H.: Concepts and trends in autonomy for robot-assisted surgery. Proc. IEEE **110**(7), 993–1011 (2022)
35. D'Ettorre, C., Mariani, A., Stilli, A., Baena, F.R.Y., Valdastri, P., Deguet, A., Kazanzides, P., Taylor, R.H., Fischer, G.S., DiMaio, S.P., Menciassi, A., Stoyanov, D.: Accelerating surgical robotics research: a review of 10 years with the da vinci research kit. IEEE Robotics Autom. Mag. **28**(4), 56–78 (2021)
36. Coils, N.B.: "da vinci research kit research wiki page". https://research.intusurg.com/index.php/Main_Page, 2012. Accessed 15 Feb. 2025
37. "John hopkins university dvrk controller git repositories". https://github.com/jhu-dvrk. Accessed 15 Feb. 2025
38. Soper, N.J., Fried, G.M.: The fundamentals of laparoscopic surgery: its time has come. Bull. Am. Coll. Surg. **93**(9), 30–32 (2008)
39. Muradore, R.: The SARAS web page. https://saras-project.eu. Accessed 15 Feb. 2025
40. Muradore, R. et al.: The Results of the SARAS Project. Springer Star Series. to be published

Knowledge Extraction, Representation and Task Planning

A truly autonomous robot should be able to find the information needed to carry out a task without human intervention, to store it in a form suitable for later use, and organize its knowledge so that it can be easily accessed. Clearly, these are difficult tasks even for a human, and we can simplify the robot task by removing some uncertainties. For example, we can provide the structure in which the knowledge should be stored, the sequence of steps necessary to convert it into a sequence of actions, and the sources from which the information should be extracted. By reducing the choices available to the robot, it can go through the different steps autonomously and eventually perform the assigned tasks.

With some hindsight, the ARS project demonstrated the validity of the above assumptions and this part of the book lays down our working hypotheses, and how we demonstrated their validity.

We use a combination of analytical models, symbolic and sub-symbolic approaches to extract and represent the surgical knowledge. Deep Learning and Large Language Models were tools used to analyze the surgical text, as discussed in Chapter "Learning Surgical Procedures from Text". To ensure execution explainability plans were formed using the Answer Set Programming (ASP) approach, a logical framework that not only represents the surgical plans, but also grounds the variables to the sensor readings, as discussed in Chapter "Surgical Task Planning and Learning". Plans can also be derived directly from the textual procedural description further simplifying the explainability of the results as discussed in Chapter "Towards Surgical Task Planning from Text".

Demonstration learning was used to define the robot control policies, so that motions could be adapted to different anatomies. This topic is presented in Chapter "Learning Surgical Gestures from Data". In the same chapter, we address the issue of tasks that are executed by the human surgeon differently than the plan described in the textbook. Therefore in the second section of the fifth chapter we present our preliminary approach on how the task structure can be extracted from data.

Chapter "Simulation and Autonomy" introduces the simulation methods available in the literature and motivates the importance of simulation as a tool for knowledge representation and task learning.

Learning Surgical Procedures from Text

Marco Bombieri

Abstract This Chapter describes the approach chosen in the research to acquire surgical knowledge "topdown", i.e. from textbooks and interviews with the physicians, so that the robot can learn autonomously how to perform surgery. The Chapter is organized into five main Sections, describing the technological instruments that were developed, how these tools work and what performance was achieved. After the Introduction, Sect. 2 describes how Large Language Models (LLM) can be used to analyze medical text and their limitations. Section 3 addresses the shortcomings of standard LLM by developing an LLM specifically tuned to recognized procedural sentences in surgical text. Section 4 develops the second stage of the pipeline able to extract relational information based on the actions and the actors involved. Section 5 uses the tools developed in an example of extraction of detailed surgical actions from the description of procedures on robot assisted surgical textbooks and papers. Finally, Sect. 6 summarizes the work described and draws some conclusions.

1 Introduction

The knowledge necessary to inform a robot on how to apply its skills to carry out a task can be acquired in different ways: we can code it directly in the robot, or we can provide the robot with the tools to acquire this knowledge autonomously. To address the goals of the ARS project, we followed the second route, and we developed the necessary tools and knowledge bases so that the robot can learn the task knowledge autonomously. These techniques are described in this Chapter. We also developed tools that allow the robot to learn the control and sensing skills necessary to carry out a task and to monitor its evolution and the environment. These techniques are described in Chaps. 5 and 7, respectively.

M. Bombieri (✉)
Department of Computer Science, University of Verona, Verona, Italy
e-mail: marco.bombieri_01@univr.it

Department of Information Engineering and Computer Science, University of Trento, Trento, Italy

P. Fiorini (ed.), *Towards Autonomous Robotic Surgery*, Springer Tracts in Advanced Robotics 161, https://doi.org/10.1007/978-3-032-04247-7_2

There are two distinct types of surgical knowledge essential for the autonomous execution of surgical interventions [1]: *procedural* and *non-procedural* knowledge.

Procedural knowledge encompasses the instructions required to carry out specific surgical interventions, whether these involve the patient's body or the positioning of the surgical robot. Generally, a procedure consists of an ordered sequence of actions that are temporally and causally linked. An action is initiated when a specific pre-condition is met and concludes upon the occurrence of a certain post-condition. An action can typically be executed if accompanied by a set of semantic details, such as the "*agent*" (the individual performing the action), the "*patient*" (the individual undergoing the action), the "*instrument*" (the tool used to perform the action), and the "*purpose*" (the reason for the action). Additional semantic information includes *temporal* and *spatial* parameters.

Conversely, *non-procedural knowledge* involves anatomical knowledge and other ontological information. It does not provide specific instructions for the surgeon's actions, but describes anatomical details, possible exceptional events during surgery, and general guidelines that are not tied to any particular step of an intervention.

To illustrate these concepts, Table 1 presents examples of procedural and non-procedural sentences.

Procedural knowledge can be expressed at various levels of granularity as described in [2] and illustrated in Fig. 1. Each level specifies the detail provided in the description.

In this framework, a procedure (e.g., partial nephrectomy) consists of a sequence of primary events, known as phases, that occur during the procedure (e.g., tumor excision or final suture). Each phase comprises a series of steps, which are sequences

Table 1 Examples of procedural and non-procedural sentences in books. In the table, "P" means *Procedural*, while "!P" is for *Non-procedural*

Type	Sentence
P	*The peritoneum is then incised*
P	*Using a combination of blunt dissection and electrocautery, the posterior aspect of the pylorus and the proximal duodenum are gently elevated off of the retroperitoneum*
P	*Allis clamps are used to tension the ileal segment against the catheter along its antimesenteric edge*
!P	*As a distinguishing feature, Gerota's fascia appears pale yellow, compared with the brighter yellow color of the mesentery*
!P	*Numerous descriptions of nerve sparing during RARP have been reported in the literature*
!P	*Longer operative times were seen with robotic procedures*

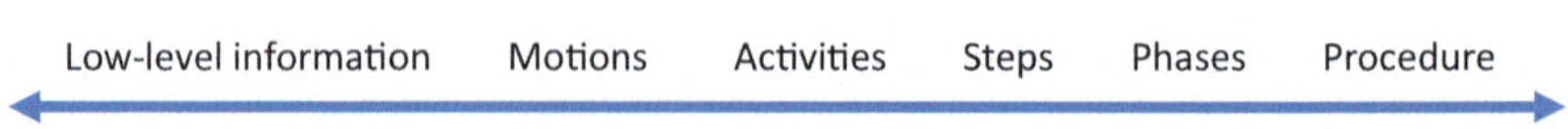

Fig. 1 Granularity axis. *Low-level information* is relative to video, image, and kinematic data

of activities aimed at achieving a surgical objective (e.g., the main steps of the final suture phase include the removal of the trocar, the extraction of the specimen, and the closure of the skin). Each activity is further broken down into a sequence of motions, which are surgical movements involving only one hand trajectory (e.g., pulling the needle to close the suture with the right arm). Finally, the low-level information consists of raw data, such as kinematic and video data captured during the surgery at a specific frequency [33].

Depending on the granularity level at which information is to be extracted, two different approaches can be followed:

- *Top-down approach*: It constructs the execution flow of a surgical procedure by exploiting the notional knowledge available in ontologies or books. Starting from these resources, the goal is to develop a plan that a robot can execute.
- *Bottom-up approach*: starting from the data captured during the execution of a surgery (kinematics and video), this approach develops methods to infer the surgical process. In this research domain, an important task is to define features useful for surgical gesture recognition: machine-learning algorithms use them to segment the intervention into phases and steps, deriving the actions in the surgical procedure.

The development of an autonomous robotic surgical system will require integrating notional knowledge extracted from textbooks to understand high-level instructions and low-granularity actions, which can only be learned from data of the actual interventions.

This Chapter deals with top-down approaches, particularly the possibility of extracting procedural surgical knowledge directly from written resources, such as textbooks, academic papers, and surgical guidelines.

Chapter 5 addresses the extraction of bottom-up knowledge from data. In the original plan of the ARS project, data would have been supplied by the City of Hope Medical Center, our clinical partner in this project. Unfortunately, the COVID-19 pandemic forced us to use public data or data from simulations, as described later.

To carry out the top-down approach, we have identified four steps, each described in one of the following sections:

1. The release of an LLM specific for the robotic-surgery language (Sect. 2)
2. the use of the above-mentioned LLM to extract from textbooks only sentences containing procedural knowledge (Sect. 3)
3. the definition of a structured template to map natural language to structured frames (Sect. 4)
4. the use of the above-mentioned LLM and template to extract the procedure using Semantic Role Labeling (SRL) [3] (Sect. 5).

Chapter 4 will expand on this by showing how it is possible to map written surgical procedures into the logical language ASP (Answer Set Programming) by using appropriate transformation rules.

2 LLM for Surgery

The literature included various language models, some of which were pre-trained on medical or clinical text, such as BioMedRoBERTa [4], trained on biomedical literature, and ClinicalBERT [5], pre-trained on clinical notes and Electronic Health Records (EHR). However, there was no pre-trained language model specifically designed for procedural surgical language—this gap was addressed by our work.

This section presents SurgicBERTa, the pre-trained language model trained on a large quantity of surgical textual material that we developed to automatically understand the semantics of written robotic-surgical procedures [18].

SurgicBERTa has been developed on top of RoBERTa, the freely available English pre-trained language model for use with the general language domain, described in [6].

We developed SurgicBERTa by training RoBERTa for the Masked Language Modeling (MLM) task on a large body of surgical-specific text. MLM is a common pretraining objective used in training transformer-based language models, such as BERT [19]. In the MLM task, a token w_t in a sentence is replaced with $\langle mask \rangle$ and predicted using all past and future tokens $\boldsymbol{W}_{\setminus t} := (\boldsymbol{w}_1, ..., \boldsymbol{w}_{t-1}, \boldsymbol{w}_{t+1}, ..., \boldsymbol{w}_{|W|})$. Figure 2 illustrates the MLM task used to obtain SurgicBERTa: consider a sentence from an operative report: "*Radical prostatectomy is the surgical removal of the prostate.*" In the example sentence, the word "*prostate*" is replaced with the special token $\langle mask \rangle$ yielding the sentence: "*Radical prostatectomy is the surgical removal of the* $\langle mask \rangle$." The language model is then trained to predict the masked

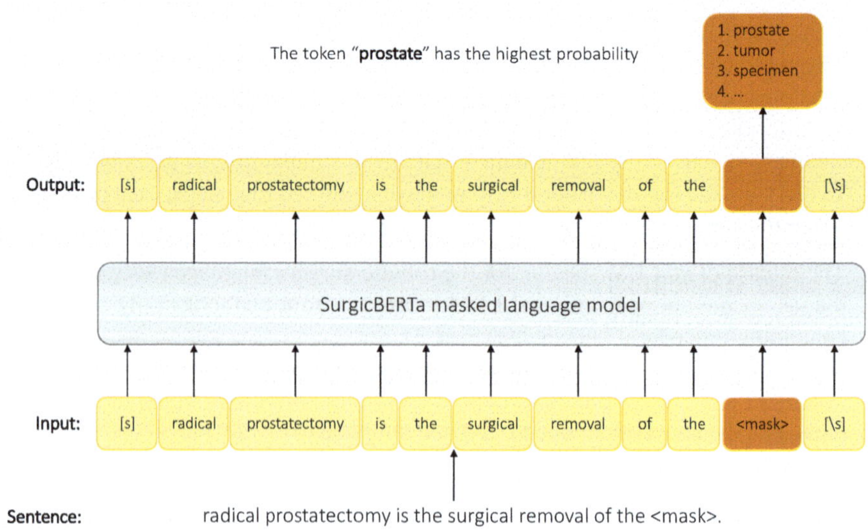

Fig. 2 MLM task used for adapting RoBERTa to the surgical domain. s and \s are special tokens denoting the sentence's beginning and end, respectively

word–"*prostate*"—based on the surrounding context. Through repeated exposure to such masked examples during pretraining, the model gradually learns to recognize and understand the specialized vocabulary of surgical procedures, anatomy, and clinical reporting. Once pretrained, the language model can be fine-tuned for specific downstream tasks such as procedure extraction, report classification, or clinical information retrieval.

In our setting, 300 K sentences from surgical textbooks (comprising 7 million words) were selected. To develop a surgical model as comprehensive as possible, the training sentences were drawn from books spanning diverse surgical fields, e.g., from abdominal surgery to orthopedics, to eye surgery. We searched for English-language surgical textbooks on the websites of various publishing houses. We used keywords such as the names of surgical macro-areas (e.g. general surgery, abdominal surgery, gynecology surgery, eye surgery). From the search results, we downloaded the digital versions of texts for which our university holds the proper legal access. Minimal pre-processing was performed on the sentences to remove URLs and bibliographic references.

In more detail, 15% of tokens were selected for possible replacement. Among the selected tokens, 80% were replaced with the special $\langle mask \rangle$ token, 10% were left unchanged, and 10% were replaced with a random token. The model was then trained to predict the initial masked tokens using cross-entropy loss. Following the RoBERTa approach, tokens were dynamically masked instead of fixing them statically for the whole dataset during pre-processing. This dynamic masking strategy increases the variability of the training data by presenting the model with different masked tokens at each epoch, rather than the same ones repeatedly. As a result, the model becomes more robust—less prone to overfitting—and better able to generalize to unseen surgical language patterns.

2.1 Evaluation

Once obtained SurgicBERTa, we evaluated it in several dimensions, comparing its performance with RoBERTa's, the starting language model we adapted to the surgical domain. Section 2.1.1 presents the intrinsic evaluation, while in Sect. 3 we show how to use SurgicBERTa for the classification of *procedural* and *non-procedural* surgical sentence. Finally, in Sect. 5, we use SurgicBERTa to extract surgical information of a specific task.

2.1.1 Intrinsic Evaluation

Evaluation metrics

Shin et al. [20] introduced the pseudo-perplexity metric to evaluate BERT-based language models. We computed the pseudo-perplexity values for both RoBERTa and SurgicBERTa on a robotic surgery test corpus to assess each model's ability

Table 2 Perplexity, accuracy and evaluation loss. Bold values mark the better scores for each metric

Pre-trained model	Perplexity	Accuracy	Evaluation loss
RoBERTa	15.410	0.546	2.735
SurgicBERTa	**4.30**	**0.699**	**1.458**

to predict unseen text from the corpus, serving as an intrinsic quality metric in the surgical domain. This comparison was valid since RoBERTa and SurgicBERTa use the same vocabulary, i.e., the same set of known words, and tokenizer, i.e., the component that breaks the input text into smaller units, like words or word pieces, so the model can understand and process it. Using the same tokenizer ensures that both models interpret the text in exactly the same way, making the evaluation consistent and comparable.

Additional intrinsic metrics used to evaluate RoBERTa and SurgicBERTa in the surgical domain included the accuracy of the MLM during the evaluation phase and the evaluation loss. Accuracy reflects how accurately the model predicts masked words by comparing predictions to actual values as a percentage. Evaluation loss represents the total errors in the model, indicating its performance; higher errors result in higher loss and poorer performance.

In general, better model performance is indicated by higher accuracy on the evaluation dataset and lower evaluation loss.

Results and discussion. Table 2 reports perplexity, accuracy, and loss values of RoBERTa and SurgicBERTa obtained during the evaluation of the MLM task. SurgicBERTa has lower perplexity (−11.11), greater accuracy (+15.30%), and lower evaluation loss (−1.277) than RoBERTa. All obtained results intrinsically confirm that SurgicBERTa deals better with surgical language than RoBERTa. For further details and other intrinsic and extrinsic evaluation metrics and tasks used, refer to [18]. Instead, Sects. 3 and 5 describe the evaluation of SurgicBERTa on the two downstream tasks needed for procedural surgical knowledge extraction from text, namely procedural sentence detection and procedural knowledge extraction. In the first, we use SurgicBERTa to identify procedural sentences within a surgical procedure description—that is, to pinpoint only those sentences that contain procedural information. In the second, we apply SurgicBERTa again to extract procedural entities from these identified sentences, such as the performed actions, the actors involved, the instruments used, as well as spatial and temporal constraints.

3 Using SurgicBERTa to Extract Knowledge of Surgical Procedures

This chapter aims to develop a model capable of automatically understanding *procedural* written text within the robotic-surgical domain, primarily targeting textbooks and academic papers. These texts are intended to describe how to perform specific surgeries by listing actions, required instruments, and spatial and temporal constraints. However, they also contain *non-procedural* information, such as the history of that surgery, annual surgery statistics, patient demographics, related anatomy, organ positions, and other ontological details. As a result, real-world documents often mix procedural descriptions with non-procedural content, which is not directly useful for deriving the procedure workflows.

This section details the method developed within the ARS project to distinguish *procedural* from *non-procedural* sentences, a crucial step towards the automatic understanding and extraction of procedural sentences. The overall research objective is divided into two main steps: first, recognizing *procedural sentences*, i.e., sentences containing procedural knowledge (this Section); and second, using the recognized sentences, extracting procedural surgical knowledge (discussed in Sect. 4).

We present our novel contribution to the first step by addressing the problem as a sentence classification task using SurgicBERTa, compared to other state-of-the-art models.

To train and evaluate these approaches, we developed a new surgical textual dataset, SPKS (Surgical Procedural Knowledge Sentences), comprising sentences from surgical texts that we manually annotated as procedural or non-procedural [1].

The following research question was investigated:

RQ1 As a continuation of the validation of Sect. 2, does SurgicBERTa perform better than RoBERTa also on the task of detecting procedural sentences of robotic-surgery?

3.1 *Proposed Methods to Detect Procedural Sentences in Robot-Assisted Surgery*

In this section, we describe the collected dataset and the proposed methods.

To train and test a supervised classification approach that would automatically identify procedural sentences, a dataset of sentences labeled as *procedural* and *non-procedural* is needed. Given the lack of such a dataset in the literature, we manually constructed and annotated a new dataset, called SPKS (Surgical Procedural Knowledge Sentences)[1] collected from surgical books and academic papers. The dataset's statistics, resources and annotation steps are reported in [1, 18].

The dataset comprises 2250 annotated sentences from 28 robotic surgery procedures, with approximately 68% procedural and about 32% non-procedural sentences. These documents, used to create SPKS, were writen by various authors, leading to significant variations in writing style. Some procedure descriptions are concise and schematic, while others are lengthier and include additional background information.

Each sentence in the selected procedure texts was manually labeled as *procedural* or *non-procedural* strictly following the guidelines provided in [1].

[1] Dataset web-page: https://gitlab.com/altairLab/spks-dataset.

3.2 Classifiers

To measure the benefit of MLM in this downstream task, we compared SURGICBERTA with ROBERTA, i.e., its base model, and ClinicalBERT [5].

To fine-tune ClinicalBERT, ROBERTA, and SURGICBERTA for procedural sentence classification in robotic-assisted surgical texts, we adapted the base model to produce a classification output (procedural or non-procedural). This adaptation involved adding a classification layer on top of the pre-trained models and training the entire model on our annotated dataset until it was well-suited for our task. Specifically, we employed a single linear layer for sentence classification, following the approach in [5]. Additionally, pre-processing of the dataset was necessary to fine-tune BERT, ClinicalBERT, ROBERTA, and SURGICBERTA, including word tokenization, index mapping to the tokenizer vocabulary, and fixed-length normalization (by truncation or padding) of all texts.

3.3 Evaluation

The results of the procedural sentence detection task are reported in Tables 3 and 4, where higher results are in bold. SURGICBERTA improves all performance metrics compared to ROBERTA and ClinicalBERT on both procedural and non-procedural classes. Overall, averaging the performances of both classes, SURGICBERTA improves the accuracy by 0.014, Macro-F1 by 0.033 and Weighted-F1 by 0.029, when compared with its base version ROBERTA, thus confirming the benefit of having a domain-specific language for surgical-related text classification. We can positively answer RQ1 because SURGICBERTA, obtained by ROBERTA with

Table 3 Aggregated classification performance of the tested methods in the second setting

Method	A	Macro			Weighted		
		P	R	F1	wP	wR	wF1
`ClinicalBERT`	0.856	0.840	0.823	0.831	0.854	0.856	0.855
`RoBERTa`	0.872	0.860	0.841	0.849	0.871	0.872	0.871
`SurgicBERTa`	**0.886**	**0.880**	**0.853**	**0.864**	**0.885**	**0.886**	**0.884**

Table 4 lassification performance of the tested methods per class in the second setting

Method	Procedural			Non-procedural		
	P	R	F1	P	R	F1
`ClinicalBERT`	0.879	0.915	0.897	0.801	0.731	0.764
`RoBERTa`	0.889	0.928	0.908	0.831	0.753	0.790
`SurgicBERTa`	**0.894**	**0.945**	**0.919**	**0.865**	**0.762**	**0.810**

the MLM domain adaptation technique, achieves higher performance. For further details, please refer to [18].

4 An Annotated Resource for Procedural Knowledge Extraction

The second stage of the pipeline aims to extract relational information based on the actions and the actors involved. Semantic Role Labeling (SRL) techniques [21] have proven to be promising and viable solutions for this task [22, 23].

These techniques rely on shallow semantic parsing to produce predicate-argument structures of sentences. In most semantic theories, predicates are verbs, verbal nouns, and other verb forms, primarily based on the PropBank [3] and FrameNet [7] lexical resources.

PropBank-based SRL methods [3] have been successfully applied to various Natural Language Processing (NLP) applications, including conversation analysis [24], video understanding [23], information extraction and ontology population [25], mining event logs written in natural language [22], and automatic image captioning [26]. However, the performance of current SRL systems on out-of-domain examples is often poor [27]. This is because PropBank annotations focus on general-purpose, newswire texts and do not fully cover specific domains, such as the surgical domain in our case.

Our goal in this section is to describe how we addressed this gap by extending PropBank to make its frames suitable to represent the semantic roles typically required in the procedures of robot-assisted surgeries.

We introduced a new linguistic resource that extends PropBank with frames describing actions and participants in the robotic-assisted surgical domain, and we released an annotated dataset to train and test automatic models. This resource, named the *Robotic Surgery Propositional Bank* (RSPB) [28, 32], is essential for adapting SRL methods from other domains to the procedural robotic-surgery domain.

4.1 Building the Robotic-Surgery Procedural Propositional Bank

The Robotic Surgery Propositional Bank (RSPB) is thus the extension of PropBank [3] to the robotic-surgical domain that is described in [28]. The standard PropBank consists of:

- a *framebank*, i.e. a collection of *frames* (a.k.a., *meaning* or *senses*) for *lemmas* denoting predicates (*verbs* or *nominalized verbs*). Frames are specific to a given lemma, and each lemma has one (*mono-sense* lemma) or more (*polysemous* lemma) associated frames. Moreover, each frame specifies its semantic *roles*, i.e.

the different labels that can be used to characterize the arguments of the corresponding predicate semantically;
- a corpus of text annotated (according to the framebank) with information about basic semantic propositions.

Following the steps described in [3], the development of RSPB is also divided into two parts, namely the creation of a lexicon of frames files (RSPF, i.e. Robotic Surgery Procedural Framebank) summarised in Sect. 4.2), and the annotated dataset with RSPF's labels, presented in 4.3.

4.2 The Robotic Surgery Procedural Framebank

Two approaches are used to identify procedural verbs and nouns in the domain of robotic surgery, utilizing the existing SPKS corpus. The first approach involves identifying actions conveyed through nominalized verbs, employing keyword extraction techniques. The second method utilizes Part-Of-Speech (POS) tagging to detect actions expressed by verbs. By combining these methods and incorporating any low-frequency or omitted candidates flagged by clinicians during validation, comprehensive coverage of robotic surgery actions within the specified domains is achieved. The full description of these steps, omitted in this section, is presented in detail in [28].

4.2.1 Adapting PropBank to the Robotic-Surgical Domain

We analyzed the semantic use of each lemma that describes an action identified in the SPKS corpus with respect to the PropBank framebank. Each candidate is then assigned to one of the four categories described in Table 5.

Table 5 Categories to which each candidate lemmas is assigned

Category	Description
PRESENT	The lemma is already present in PropBank, and there is a frame file that adequately describes the use of the predicate. For this lemma, PropBank already describes appropriate semantic roles as core entities
MISSING_ROLE	The lemma is already present in PropBank, and there is a frame file that adequately describes the use of the predicate. This frame, however, does not include domain-specific semantic roles often used in the robotic-surgical domain
MISSING_FRAME	The lemma is already present in PropBank, but a proper frame needs to be included, as the existing ones have different meanings
MISSING_LEMMA	The lemma is not present in PropBank

If a lemma is categorized under the PRESENT class, no alteration is required as PropBank adequately encompasses the robotic surgical application, providing a framework that precisely delineates the predicate usage.

However, if a lemma is categorized under the MISSING_ROLE class, certain semantic roles that are crucial to the domain of robotic surgery may be absent, and it is necessary to provide their inclusion. For instance, the action denoted by the lemma *to retract* falls into this category. PropBank offers the "*retract.01: to take back*" frame, capturing the specific nuances within the surgical context. Nonetheless, this frame only proposes two roles for it:

- **Arg0**: *taker back, agent*
- **Arg1**: *thing retracted*

The action of *to retract* finds frequent application in the realm of robotic surgery, often accompanied by additional details for precise description: the specific instrument utilized, the technique employed, and the designated endpoint or extent of retraction.

A lemma may fall into the MISSING_FRAME category for two primary reasons: i) its semantic usage significantly differs from all frames cataloged in PropBank, lacking any semantic role overlap; ii) while not entirely novel, its meaning is too specific to be covered adequately by the broad frames of PropBank, especially within the context of robotic surgery, which is focusing on a subset of existing meanings. An example of the first case is the verb *to grasp*. For it, PropBank offers a single meaning "*grasp.01: to take hold of, comprehend*" with two semantic roles:

- **Arg0**: *grasper*
- **Arg1**: *thing grasped*

The robotic-surgical domain uses this lemma with a significantly different meaning, i.e. "*to clasp or embrace especially with the fingers or arms*". For this lemma, important information is the grasper, i.e. the specific type used, the tissue grasped, the instrument used for grasping, and important spatial indications for correct grasping. An example of the second case is the verb *to approximate*. For it, PropBank has the frame "*approximate.01: to be close or similar, cause to come near to or approach again*" with only two roles:

- **Arg0**: *entity coming close*
- **Arg1**: *entity coming close to*

It offers a broader meaning than the more specific meanings used in the robotic surgery, (i.e. "*to come near in position, to bring near*"), which is typically enriched with the following information: agent, entity coming close, entity coming close to, instrument and spatial indications.

Finally, an example of a lemma of class MISSING_LEMMA is the noun "*kocherization*". In surgery, it refers to "*an operative maneuver to mobilize the duodenum before performing other procedures locally or before incising the duodenum*". For it, important information is the agent, and the anatomical entity to be kocherized.

Table 6 (Left) Example of nominalized actions extracted using the first method with the indication of the verb they refer to ("—" means missing the corresponding verb) and the modification required. (Right) Example of domain lemmas extracted using the second method with the indication of the type of modification required

Nominalized actions	Verbs
<Placement , Place , PRESENT >;	<Extraperitonealize , MISSING_LEMMA >
<Reflection , Reflect , MISSING_FRAME >;	<Resect , MISSING_ROLE >
<Retraction , Retract , MISSING_ROLE >;	<Spatulate , MISSING_LEMMA >
<Exposure , Expose , PRESENT >;	<Skeletonize , MISSING_LEMMA >
<Resection , Resect , MISSING_ROLE >;	<Kocherize , MISSING_LEMMA >
<Mobilization ,Mobilize , MISSING_FRAME >;	<Insufflate , MISSING_LEMMA >
<Traction , —, MISSING_LEMMA >;	<Redock , MISSING_LEMMA >
<Administration , Administer , PRESENT >;	<Detubularize , MISSING_LEMMA >
<Identification , Identify , MISSING_FRAME >;	<Grasp , MISSING_FRAME >
<Excision , Excise , MISSING_ROLE >	<Incise , MISSING_ROLE >

To extend PropBank to the robotic-surgery domain, those verbs (or nominalized verbs) that are typical of the surgical domain are collected using the approach described in [28]. Examples of nominalized actions and verbs, with an indication of the type of modification required, are reported in Table 6.

4.3 The Robotic Surgery Procedural Propositional Bank

The team annotated sentences from the SPKS dataset according to the frames and roles defined in RSPF.

All sentences were procedural in the sense described in [1]. Approximately 80% of the sentences were taken from robotic-surgery textbooks describing how-to of surgical procedures, while 20% were taken from academic papers or case reports dealing with academic research on surgical procedures or descriptions of real interventions of specific patients.

4.3.1 The Framebank (RSPF)

The approach described in [28] has been utilized to examine 252 lemmas. Among these, 109 instances needed at least one adjustment from those outlined in Table 5. Specifically, out of the 252 lemmas scrutinized, 24 fell under the MISSING_LEMMA category, indicating that novel lemmas (both verbs and nouns) should be included to describe precise actions within the surgical context, that are absent in the original PropBank. Additionally, 22 lemmas fell into the MISSING_FRAME category, indi-

Table 7 Semantic type of the core roles added to modified lemmas

Type	Description	Subtype	Number
Who and What	Core-role roles indicating who (or what) performs the action and who (or what) instead undergoes it. Often they respectively coincide with the robotic or the human operator and the anatomical part that is object of the action	Agent	44
		Patient	46
How	Core-role arguments indicating how the action is performed by specifying the surgical technique or the manner to follow to carry out the action or the instrument to use	Manner or technique	36
		Instrument used	30
Spatial information	Core-role arguments specifying different kind of spatial information to know during the execution the corresponding action. These core-roles reply to questions "where?" or "through which passage or port?" or "starting from where?" or "ending where?" or final other frame-specific information such as orientation or spatial constraint to follow for safety reasons	Where	22
		Through	9
		Starting point	2
		Ending point	4
		Other	32
Purpose	Core-role argument explicitly describing the purpose of the main action. It is inserted as core-role only if very frequently present in our sample sentences	—	6
Other	Core-roles very specific to a particular lemma and thus not fitting in any of the above classes	—	13

cating that new senses should be added to existing lemmas to cover meanings not previously addressed by PropBank. Furthermore, 63 lemmas exhibited the MISSING_ROLE issue, prompting the enhancement of the corresponding sense of existing predicates with the new semantic roles commonly used in robotic surgery. With the incorporation of new lemmas, frames, and core roles into the existing structures, a total of 244 core roles were introduced. Table 7 illustrates the semantic types of these core roles added to the robotic-surgery domain lemmas. While the initial row of the table shows a significant number of core roles added, most roles stem from MISSING_LEMMA and MISSING_FRAME cases, indicating frames not present in the original PropBank.

The introduction of these semantic roles underscores the crucial need in surgical procedural language to specify, for each operative action, the agent (Arg0), the affected anatomical structure (typically Arg1), the instrument employed, the surgical methodology, the objective, and various spatial descriptors aiding in the anatomical localization within the body. Overall, the inclusion of new and revised lemmas and frames underscores the substantial expansion of PropBank to encompass the robotic-surgical domain, emphasizing the distinctions between procedural surgical language and general English in terms of predicates utilized and roles required.

4.3.2 The Annotated Dataset

Following the annotation process and guidelines described in [28], the first annotated dataset specific for SRL of robotic-surgery textbooks was obtained. 28 surgical operative descriptions have been annotated for 1,559 sentences and 32,448 tokens. The obtained dataset is composed of 12,202 annotations. Of them, 3,601 are predicate-level annotations, and 8,601 are argument-level annotations, both core and modifier. Further details about the dataset are given in [28].

5 Extraction of Surgical Actions from Text

This section describes the application of RSPB to train an SRL model, presenting an initial benchmark for the extraction of detailed surgical actions from the description of procedures on robotic-surgery texts and papers. Utilizing the RoBERTa, BioMedRoBERTa, and SurgicBERTa pre-trained language models, we initially explored a zero-shot scenario, where no additional SRL-annotated domain-specific data was employed, and compared results with the fine-tuned setup, where such data were utilized. This section explains how we applied RSPB to train a surgical role labeling (SRL) model and provides an initial benchmark for extracting detailed surgical actions from robotic surgery procedure descriptions in scientific texts and papers. Using the pre-trained language models RoBERTa, BioMedRoBERTa, and SurgicBERTa, we first tested a zero-shot approach—where the model was applied without any additional domain-specific SRL annotations—and then compared these results with those obtained from a fine-tuned model trained on annotated surgical data.

We examined various dataset splits, including one in-domain and two out-of-domain splits, and we also evaluated the effectiveness of the approach in a few-shot learning scenario, where only a portion of the SRL-annotated domain-specific sentences was used for training.

The ARS project addressed the following research questions:

RQ2 How effectively can general-English and bio-medical pre-trained language models perform SRL on surgical annotated texts without resorting to supervised learning?
RQ3 Does fine-tuning of surgical annotated texts significantly enhance the performance compared to the zero-shot setting using off-the-shelf models from existing literature?
RQ4 Does further unsupervised learning of pre-trained language models (as in SurgicBERTa) contribute to a better understanding of surgical language?
RQ5 Can SRL models generalize across surgical sub-domains?

In addition to conventional evaluation measures for the SRL task, we proposed a novel method for evaluating SRL systems based on joint disambiguation of arguments and predicates. This entails correctly disambiguating semantic arguments relative to the framing of the actual predicate. Results presented in Sect. 5.6 indicate that fine-tuning SurgicBERTa on the SRL task leads to the highest performance across all splits and sub-tasks.

5.1 The Method Developed for Procedural Knowledge Extraction

We framed the operation of extracting procedural surgical knowledge from the text as an SRL problem since SRL is also applied for information extraction in various biomedical domains [8–10]. In this Section, we use the PropBank-based SRL, exploiting the Robotic-Surgery Propositional Bank described in Sect. 4 for carrying out the knowledge extraction.

The typical SRL task is composed of two sub-tasks. The first is the *predicate identification and disambiguation* task. It is aimed to identify each predicate in a sentence, assigning the appropriate meaning (i.e. sense in RSPF) to the predicate in the given context. The meaning is selected among the available ones for that predicate lemma codified in the target lexical resource. The second task is *argument identification and classification*. It aims to detect the argument spans or syntactic argument heads of a predicate. It also assigns to each predicate the appropriate semantic role label according to the target lexical resource.

As an example in the robotic-surgery domain, consider the following sentence, focusing on the verb "*grasp*":

Using the cadiere grasper (robot arm #3), grasp the soft tissues along the lesser curvature of the stomach to straighten out the lga perpendicular to the celiac axis.

In the predicate identification and disambiguation phase, "*grasp*" is recognized as a predicate, assigning it the RSPF meaning of *grasp.02*: "*to clasp or embrace especially with the fingers or arms*", rather than *grasp.01*: "*to take hold of, comprehend*". Then, in the argument identification and classification phase, SRL produces the following output:

[**Arg2**: Using the cadiere grasper (robot arm #3)], [**grasp.02** grasp] [**Arg1**: the soft tissues] [**Arg3**: along the lesser curvature of the stomach to straighten out the lga perpendicular to the celiac axis].

where, for the sense *grasp.02* in RSPF, Arg2 represents the "*instrument used for grasping*", Arg1 is the "*thing grasped*", and Arg3 identifies an "*important spatial indication for correct grasping*".

Another example related to the verb "*dissect*" is the following:

The lymphatic tissue is dissected off with meticulous hemostatic and lymphatic control, using bipolar electrocautery and hem-o-lok clips, to improve visualization.

the text is annotated as follows:

[**Arg1**: The lymphatic tissue] is [**dissect.02** dissected] off [**Arg3**: with meticulous hemostatic and lymphatic control], [**Arg2**: using bipolar electrocautery and hem-o-lok clips], [**ArgM-PRP**: to improve visualization.]

where Arg1 is the entity dissected, Arg3 is the surgical technique, Arg2 is the instrument, ArgM-PRP is the modifier role for purpose, and *dissect.02: "to cut apart (an animal body, plant, etc.) to examine the structure, relation of parts, or the like"*) is the main action.

5.2 The SRL Neural Architecture Adopted

SRL is traditionally performed with data-driven methods. Since recent approaches leverage self-attention techniques [11] and transformer-based architectures with pre-trained language models [29], we also followed this trend and adopted a neural approach, thus addressing the SRL task in an end-to-end fashion while testing different pre-trained language models. The pre-trained language models considered in this section are the state-of-the-art RoBERTa, BioMedRoBERTa [4] and SurgicBERTa, described earlier in Sect. 2. In particular, BioMedRoBERTa is obtained from RoBERTa via continuous pre-training on 2.68M full-text biomedical papers from S2ORC [12]. This amounts to 7.55B tokens and 47GB of data. With this configuration, we wanted to implicitly verify if the biomedical domain was similar to the surgical domain and if we can obtain performance improvements by adopting a more accurate pre-trained language model than the general domain RoBERTa. All pre-trained language models use the same transformer-based architecture [13] and are trained with an MLM objective. The word representations learned in the pre-trained models have then been reused for the SRL task through fine-tuning. In more detail, the SRL models used in this Section are instantiated on top of the ROBERTA encoder (the same also used by BIOMEDROBERTA and SURGICBERTA). Figure 3 illustrates the neural architecture we used. First, we encoded the input text using contextualized word embeddings for each token using the pre-trained language model; we then used linear transformations of the word embeddings to obtain a concatenated input for a two-layer ReLU, which is next input to a linear layer followed by softmax activation to produce a probability distribution over labels for each word (to avoid overfitting, a standard dropout layer [14] with probability 0.5 is used). To capture the sequential dependencies between labels, we used a standard CRF layer [30] to produce at testing the most probable label sequence using standard Viterbi decoding.

For training and validation, the CoNLL-2012 dataset [15], we used a large-scale ($\sim 318k$ annotated SRL predicates), multi-genre general-English corpus to train and validate the "*zero-shot*" models, while we used RSPB dataset in combination with CoNLL-2012 for the "*few shot*" and "*full fine-tuning*" models that will be described later. RSPB contains four different robotic surgery domains:

- *Urology*—51.51% of the sentences;
- *Gastrointestinal procedures*—24.82% of the sentences;
- *Thoracic procedures*—13.02% of the sentences;
- *Gynecology*—10.65% of the sentences.

We therefore used the CoNLL-2012 dataset to make the architecture learn the standard SRL task and RSPB to specialize the model to better understand the surgical language and to perform the SRL task in the given surgical sub-domains.

Evaluation was carried out on different test splits of the robotic-surgery annotated dataset, detailed next in Sect. 5.3. Sentences of the test sets were never seen during the training and validation phase.

5.3 *Splits of the Robotic-Surgery Annotated Dataset*

Due to the high computational costs needed for training, validating and testing the SRL models, we adopted the classical evaluation protocol of manually splitting the RSPB dataset into three components (train, validation, and test) instead of following a more computationally demanding cross-validation protocol. More in detail, we split the robotic-surgery annotated dataset into three different combinations:

- **BAL**: Data division into training, testing, and validation sets is equitable across various surgical fields. Each type of procedure, such as thoracic, gynecological, urological, and gastrointestinal, is allocated accordingly in the split. Specifically, 80% of the sentences were designated for training, with 10% reserved for validation, and the remaining 20% form the test set.

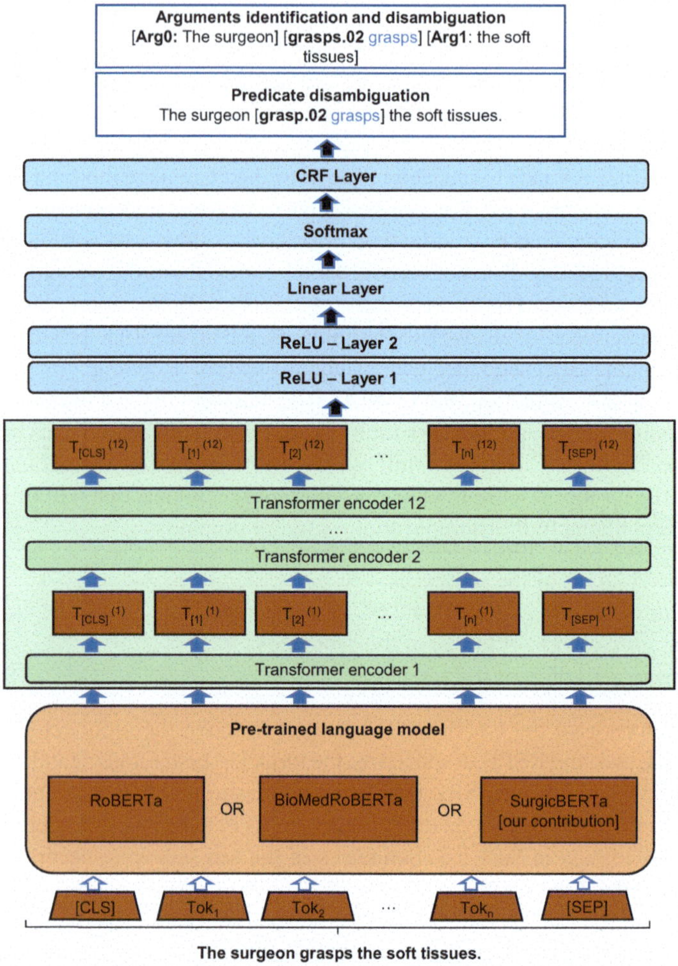

Fig. 3 The neural architecture used for SRL. Sentences are tokenized and each token is input to a pre-trained language model to produce a contextualized representation, which is then fed into ReLU layers and a linear layer. Next, a softmax layer produces a probability distribution over the labels. A CRF layer finally captures dependencies between labels by decoding the resulting representations into the most probable label sequence

- **GYN**: the training and validation datasets encompassed sentences from thoracic, gastrointestinal, and urological descriptions, while the test dataset exclusively comprised sentences from the gynecological domain. Notably, no sentence pertaining to gynecological surgeries were encountered during the training and validation phases.
- **THO**: the training and validation datasets included all sentences pertaining to gynecological, gastrointestinal, and urological descriptions. Conversely, the test

dataset exclusively comprised sentences from the thoracic domain. Notably, sentences detailing thoracic surgeries were absent during the training and validation phases.

The BAL split wants to investigate the ability of the method to learn a general surgical domain procedural language from a limited set of annotated sentences. The GYN and THO splits aim instead to verify if the annotations are general across different surgical sub-domains, i.e. if the models trained on them perform comparably with the one trained with the BAL split. The statistics and in-depth description of these splits are left to the original paper [31].

5.4 Fine-Tuning of Language Models on the SRL Downstream Task

We trained 18 different models, six for each split. In particular, for each one, we fine-tuned RoBERTa, BioMedRoBERTa, and SurgicBERTa on two different scenarios:

- **Zero-Shot**: We refined the language models solely using CoNLL-2012 annotated data, excluding any surgical data. Subsequently, we assessed these models on the surgical test set across various divisions.
- **Full Fine-Tuning**: Building upon the refined models from the Zero-Shot phase, we further refined them using the train and validation sets of the robotic-surgery annotated dataset's different divisions. Subsequently, we evaluated the resultant models on the respective surgical test set matching the division used in the Zero Shot phase.

5.5 Evaluation Methodology

Performance was evaluated according to three different dimensions:

- *argument identification and disambiguation*: the capability of assigning the correct semantic role label to the predicate arguments mentioned in the text, after identifying it. This is the traditional dimension used for benchmarking SRL tools [16, 17, 29], adopted also in the CoNLL-2012 Shared Task evaluation (and corresponding script);
- *predicate disambiguation*: the capability of assigning the correct RSPF frame (i.e. meaning) to the predicate in the text. In our domain setting, this evaluation was particularly useful to assess if the models were capable to discriminate the domain-specific usage of some verbs with respect to their general-English usage;
- *predicate-argument disambiguation*: the capability of assigning the correct semantic role label to the predicate arguments as well as to assign the correct sense (i.e. frame) to the corresponding predicate.

Table 8 Performance (overall) on the arguments-disambiguation task for BAL, THO and GYN splits. FFT means *Full Fine-Tuning* scenario, while ZS stands for *Zero-Shot* scenario. The best scores are highlighted in bold

SPLIT	BAL			THO			GYN		
MODEL	P	R	F1	P	R	F1	P	R	F1
RoBERTa$_{ZS}$	0.714	0.688	0.701	0.692	0.677	0.685	0.775	0.767	0.771
BioMedRoBERTa$_{ZS}$	0.718	**0.696**	0.707	0.708	0.684	0.696	0.788	0.777	**0.782**
SurgicBERTa$_{ZS}$	**0.724**	**0.696**	**0.710**	**0.726**	**0.700**	**0.713**	**0.827**	**0.781**	0.775
RoBERTa$_{FFT}$	0.771	0.752	0.762	0.753	0.744	0.748	0.799	0.781	0.790
BioMedRoBERTa$_{FFT}$	**0.779**	0.764	0.772	0.756	0.738	0.747	0.798	0.794	0.796
SurgicBERTa$_{FFT}$	0.778	**0.768**	**0.773**	**0.759**	**0.749**	**0.753**	**0.813**	**0.796**	**0.804**

5.6 Results

In this section, we report and discuss the results obtained using the methods described in Sect. 5.1. Each score reported in the section is the average over three distinct runs of the considered method.

5.6.1 Argument Disambiguation

We first evaluated the obtained models on the traditional argument disambiguation task. The results are summarized in Table 8.

The findings indicate that access to annotated domain-specific data is crucial for enhancing the disambiguation performance of arguments. Specifically, fine-tuning language models with such data significantly boosts the performance metrics across all subsets. Focusing on the F1 metric within the BAL subset, transitioning from zero-shot to full fine-tuning yields notable enhancements: a 0.061 improvement for RoBERTa, 0.065 for BioMedRoBERTa, and 0.063 for SurgicBERTa. Similar improvements are observed in precision (RoBERTa +0.057; BioMedRoBERTa +0.061; SurgicBERTa +0.054) and recall (RoBERTa +0.064; BioMedRoBERTa +0.065; SurgicBERTa +0.072). These outcomes confirm that utilizing annotated domain data enables models to enhance both the accuracy of positive identifications and the detection of actual positives. As expected, RSPF, an extension of PropBank for the surgical domain, contains labels not present in the CoNLL-2012 dataset utilized for zero-shot models. Consequently, the absence of annotated examples for these labels in the training material prevented some accurate predictions on the test set, where such labels may be prevalent. Moreover, domain-specific data is indispensable for comprehending surgical procedural language nuances, which often differ from those of general English [32].

The THO split's performance mirrored that of the BAL split, with full fine-tuning resulting in notable enhancements across precision (RoBERTa +0.061; BioMed-

RoBERTa +0.048; SurgicBERTa +0.033), recall (RoBERTa +0.067; BioMedRoBERTa +0.054; SurgicBERTa +0.049), and F1-score (RoBERTa +0.063; BioMedRoBERTa +0.051; SurgicBERTa +0.040) for all models considered. The GYN split also benefited from full fine-tuning, albeit to a lesser extent compared to the other splits: precision (RoBERTa +0.024; BioMedRoBERTa +0.010; SurgicBERTa −0.014), recall (RoBERTa +0.014; BioMedRoBERTa +0.017; SurgicBERTa +0.016), and F1-score (RoBERTa +0.019; BioMedRoBERTa +0.014; SurgicBERTa +0.029). The modest improvement in GYN could be attributed to fewer sentences that needed RSPF specializations, as evidenced by higher zero-shot scores compared to the other splits. This result stated that incorporating domain-specific sentences during training substantially enhanced the performance across all scenarios, even when utilizing general English and biomedical models. Furthermore, the comparable improvement from zero-shot to full fine-tuning across splits indicated the satisfactory model performance on unseen surgical sub-domains, answering RQ2, RQ3, and RQ5.

SurgicBERTa achieved superior results in both zero-shot and full fine-tuning scenarios across nearly all metrics and splits, except for the F1 metric of the GYN split in the zero-shot scenario, where BioMedRoBERTa achieves a marginally higher score. This underscored the efficacy of employing unsupervised domain adaptation techniques like MLM to enhance performance, even when dealing with limited or absent annotated data. Notably, SurgicBERTa outperformed BioMedRoBERTa, which is specifically tailored for biomedical domain texts. This suggested that the procedural robotic-surgery domain, which is a specialized subset of the biomedical domain, possessed a unique language that needed specialized training resources for comprehensive coverage by language models. Thus, we can confidently state that RQ4 was answered in an affirmative way.

The detailed results in [31] showed that full-fine tuning for the BAL split improved the disambiguation of almost all core and modifier arguments.

5.7 *Predicate and Predicate-Argument Disambiguation*

Table 9 shows the results of the other two dimensions considered in our analysis, i.e. predicate disambiguation and predicate-argument disambiguation.

Similar considerations apply to both assessments as those discussed for argument disambiguation: leveraging domain annotations enhances model performance. The enhancements were particularly significant for the BAL and THO splits, while they were less pronounced in the GYN split. Similarly, employing a domain-specific language model (SurgicBERTa) often boosted performance for both predicate disambiguation and predicate-argument disambiguation tasks. The most substantial improvements occured with full-fine tuning. This reiterated the trends observed in the data for argument disambiguation, confirming the findings for RQ2, RQ3, RQ4, and RQ5.

Additionally, it is worth noting that the scores for argument disambiguation (Table 8) were notably lower than those for predicate-argument disambiguation (Table 9). For instance, SurgicBERTa$_{FFT}$ achieved an F1 score of 0.773 for argument disambiguation in the BAL split, but only 0.732 (i.e., a decrease of 0.041) for predicate-argument disambiguation. The score disparity between argument disambiguation and predicate-argument disambiguation was even more pronounced in the Zero-Shot scenario (e.g., 0.701 vs. 0.534 for RoBERTa$_{ZS}$). This indicates that while the argument label suggested by the models might be correct independently (ignoring the predicate it refers to), it might correspond to the wrong predicate sense, resulting in an incorrect argument label overall, given that argument labels were predicate-sense specific in resources like PropBank. This underscored the importance of evaluating joint predicate-argument when assessing the disambiguation performance in SRL, alongside the traditional (and separate) evaluation of argument disambiguation and predicate disambiguation.

6 Conclusion

This chapter focused on extracting procedural knowledge from existing textbooks and academic papers that describe how to perform specific surgeries. We introduced a novel pre-trained language model, SurgicBERTa, specialized in surgical literature, and combined it with state-of-the-art approaches to identify procedural sentences in the context of robotic surgery. We approached this as a sentence classification task, addressed through supervised machine learning. To train and evaluate our models, we compiled a new dataset of sentences from the robotic surgery domain, manually annotated as either procedural or non-procedural based on their content. After filtering out the procedural sentences, we tackled the challenge of extracting structured procedural knowledge. This was achieved by fine-tuning language models for the SRL task. Due to the lack of existing training and evaluation data, we created a custom dataset. Following the PropBank methodology for annotating semantic roles, we

Table 9 Performance (overall) on the predicate disambiguation and predicate-argument disambiguation tasks for BAL, THO, and GYN splits. The best scores are highlighted in bold

SPLIT	BAL				THO				GYN			
TASK	Pred	Pred-Args			Pred	Pred-Args			Pred	Pred-Args		
MODEL	Acc	P	R	F1	Acc	P	R	F1	Acc	P	R	F1
RoBERTa$_{ZS}$	0.731	0.544	0.525	0.534	0.769	0.555	0.543	0.549	**0.835**	**0.649**	0.642	**0.645**
BioMedRoBERTa$_{ZS}$	**0.748**	0.560	0.543	0.551	**0.777**	**0.573**	**0.555**	**0.564**	0.810	0.641	0.632	0.636
SurgicBERTa$_{ZS}$	0.735	**0.565**	**0.544**	**0.555**	0.732	0.559	0.540	0.549	0.827	0.646	**0.643**	**0.645**
RoBERTa$_{FFT}$	0.907	0.706	0.689	0.697	**0.910**	0.680	0.672	0.676	0.930	0.745	0.729	0.737
BioMedRoBERTa$_{FFT}$	0.897	0.707	0.694	0.700	0.887	0.669	0.653	0.661	0.935	0.752	**0.748**	**0.750**
SurgicBERTa$_{FFT}$	**0.925**	**0.737**	**0.727**	**0.732**	**0.910**	**0.690**	**0.680**	**0.685**	**0.938**	**0.756**	0.741	0.749

structured our work in two phases: first, identifying key semantic elements relevant to robotic surgery, and second, annotating the corresponding sentences accordingly. Using this annotated dataset and a fine-tuned version of SURGICBERTA, we trained an SRL model capable of accurately identifying and categorizing surgical content within procedural sentences. Chapter 4 will build on this work by applying SRL to simple use cases, exploring the potential of translating constrained natural language descriptions into logical rules.

References

1. Bombieri, M., Rospocher, M., Dall' Alba, D., Fiorini, P.: Automatic detection of procedural knowledge in robotic-assisted surgical texts. Int. J. Comput. Assisted Radiol. Surg. **16**(8), 1287–1295 (2021)
2. Lalys, F., Jannin, P.: Surgical process modelling: a review. Int. J. Comput. Assist. Radiol. Surg. **9**(3), 495–511 (2014)
3. Palmer, M., Kingsbury, P.R., Gildea, D.: The proposition bank: an annotated corpus of semantic roles. Comput. Linguist. **31**(1), 71–106 (2005)
4. Gururangan, S., Marasović, A., Swayamdipta, S., Lo, K., Beltagy, I., Downey, D., Smith, N.A.: Don't stop pretraining: adapt language models to domains and tasks. In: Proceedings of the 58th Annual Meeting of the Association for Computational Linguistics, (Online), pp. 8342–8360. Association for Computational Linguistics, July 2020
5. Alsentzer, E., Murphy, J., Boag, W., Weng, W.-H., Jin, D., Naumann, T., McDermott, M.: Publicly available clinical BERT embeddings. In: Proceedings of the 2nd Clinical Natural Language Processing Workshop (Minneapolis, Minnesota, USA). Association for Computational Linguistics, June 2019, pp. 72–78
6. Liu, Y., Ott, M., Goyal, N., Du, J., Joshi, M., Chen, D., Levy, O., Lewis, M., Zettlemoyer, L., Stoyanov, V.: Roberta: a robustly optimized BERT pretraining approach, vol. abs/1907.11692 (2019)
7. Baker, C.F., Fillmore, C.J., Lowe, J.B.: The berkeley framenet project. In: Boitet, C., Whitelock, P. (eds.), 36th Annual Meeting of the Association for Computational Linguistics and 17th International Conference on Computational Linguistics, COLING-ACL '98, 10–14 Aug. 1998, Université de Montréal, Montréal, Quebec, Canada. Proceedings of the Conference, pp. 86–90. Morgan Kaufmann Publishers/ACL (1998)
8. Barnickel, T., Weston, J., Collobert, R., Mewes, H.-W., Stümpflen, V.: Large scale application of neural network based semantic role labeling for automated relation extraction from biomedical texts. PLOS One, vol. 4, pp. 1–6, July 2009
9. Bethard, S., Lu, Z., Martin, J.H., Hunter, L.: Semantic role labeling for protein transport predicates. BMC Bioinform. **9**(1), 1–15 (2008)
10. Eckert, F., Neves, M.: Semantic role labeling tools for biomedical question answering: a study of selected tools on the BioASQ datasets. In: Proceedings of the 6th BioASQ Workshop A challenge on large-scale biomedical semantic indexing and question answering. Brussels, Belgium, pp. 11–21. Association for Computational Linguistics, Nov. 2018
11. Strubell, E., Verga, P., Andor, D., Weiss, D., McCallum, A.: Linguistically-informed self-attention for semantic role labeling. In: Riloff, E., Chiang, D., Hockenmaier, J., Tsujii, J. (eds.), Proceedings of the 2018 Conference on Empirical Methods in Natural Language Processing, Brussels, Belgium, Oct. 31–4 Nov. 2018, pp. 5027–5038. Association for Computational Linguistics (2018)
12. Lo, K., Wang, L.L., Neumann, M., Kinney, R., Weld, D.S.: S2ORC: the semantic scholar open research corpus. In: Proceedings of the 58th Annual Meeting of the Association for Computational Linguistics, pp. 4969–4983 (2020)

13. Zhang, X., Yang, H., Young, E.F.Y.: Attentional transfer is all you need: technology-aware layout pattern generation. In: 58th ACM/IEEE Design Automation Conference, DAC 2021, San Francisco, CA, USA, 5–9 Dec. 2021, pp. 169–174. IEEE (2021)
14. Srivastava, N., Hinton, G., Krizhevsky, A., Sutskever, I., Salakhutdinov, R.: Dropout: a simple way to prevent neural networks from overfitting. J. Mach. Learn. Res. **15**(56), 1929–1958 (2014)
15. Pradhan, S., Moschitti, A., Xue, N., Ng, H.T., Björkelund, A., Uryupina, O., Zhang, Y., Zhong, Z.: Towards robust linguistic analysis using ontonotes. In: Hockenmaier, J., Riedel, S. (eds.), Proceedings of the Seventeenth Conference on Computational Natural Language Learning, CoNLL 2013, Sofia, Bulgaria, 8–9 Aug. 2013, pp. 143–152. ACL (2013)
16. Carreras, X., Màrquez, L.: Introduction to the conll-2005 shared task: semantic role labeling. In: Dagan, I., Gildea, D. (eds.), Proceedings of the Ninth Conference on Computational Natural Language Learning, CoNLL 2005, Ann Arbor, Michigan, USA, 29–30 June 2005, pp. 152–164. ACL (2005)
17. Màrquez, L., Carreras, X., Litkowski, K.C., Stevenson, S.: Semantic role labeling: an introduction to the special issue. Comput. Linguist. **34**(2), 145–159 (2008)
18. Bombieri, M., Rospocher, M., Ponzetto, S.P., Fiorini, P.: Surgicberta: a pre-trained language model for procedural surgical language. Int. J. Data Sci. Anal. **18**(1), 69–81 (2024)
19. Devlin, J., Chang, M.-W., Lee, K., Toutanova, K.: Bert: pre-training of deep bidirectional transformers for language understanding,. In: Proceedings of the 2019 Conference of the North American Chapter of the Association for Computational Linguistics: Human Language Technologies (NAACL-HLT), Oct 2018
20. Shin, J., Lee, Y., Jung, K.: Effective sentence scoring method using bert for speech recognition. In: Lee, W.S., Suzuki, T. (eds.), Proceedings of The Eleventh Asian Conference on Machine Learning, vol. 101 of Proceedings of Machine Learning Research, PMLR, pp. 1081–1093, 17–19 Nov. 2019
21. Gildea, D., Jurafsky, D.: Automatic labeling of semantic roles. Comput. Linguist. **28**(3), 245–288 (2002)
22. Rebmann, A., van der Aa, H.: Extracting semantic process information from the natural language in event logs. In: La Rosa, M., Sadiq, S., Teniente, E. (eds.), Advanced Information Systems Engineering, pp. 57–74. Springer International Publishing, Cham (2021)
23. Sadhu, A., Gupta, T., Yatskar, M., Nevatia, R., Kembhavi, A.: Visual semantic role labeling for video understanding. In: IEEE Conference on Computer Vision and Pattern Recognition, CVPR 2021, virtual, 19–25 June 2021, pp. 5589–5600. Computer Vision Foundation/IEEE (2021)
24. Xu, K., Wu, H., Song, L., Zhang, H., Song, L., Yu, D.: Conversational semantic role labeling. IEEE/ACM Trans. Audio Speech Lang. Process. **29**, 2465–2475 (2021)
25. Humphreys, L., Boella, G., van der Torre, L., Robaldo, L., Caro, L.D., Ghanavati, S., Muthuri, R.: Populating legal ontologies using semantic role labeling. Artif. Intell. Law **29**(2), 171–211 (2021)
26. Chen, L., Jiang, Z., Xiao, J., Liu, W.: Human-like controllable image captioning with verb-specific semantic roles. In: IEEE Conference on Computer Vision and Pattern Recognition, CVPR 2021, virtual, 19–25 June 2021, pp. 16846–16856. Computer Vision Foundation/IEEE (2021)
27. Do, Q.T.N., Bethard, S., Moens, M.-F.: Domain adaptation in semantic role labeling using a neural language model and linguistic resources. IEEE/ACM Trans. Audio Speech Lang. Process. **23**(11), 1812–1823 (2015)
28. Bombieri, M., Rospocher, M., Ponzetto, S.P., Fiorini, P.: The robotic-surgery propositional bank. Language Resources and Evaluation, June 2023
29. Li, T., Jawale, P.A., Palmer, M., Srikumar, V.: Structured tuning for semantic role labeling. In: Proceedings of the 58th Annual Meeting of the Association for Computational Linguistics, (Online), pp. 8402–8412. Association for Computational Linguistics, July 2020
30. Reimers, N., Gurevych, I.: Reporting score distributions makes a difference: performance study of LSTM-networks for sequence tagging. In: Proceedings of the 2017 Conference on Empirical

Methods in Natural Language Processing, (Copenhagen, Denmark), pp. 338–348. Association for Computational Linguistics, Sept. 2017
31. Bombieri, M., Rospocher, M., Ponzetto, S.P., Fiorini, P.: Machine understanding surgical actions from intervention procedure textbooks. Comput. Biol. Med. **152** (2023)
32. Bombieri, M., Rospocher, M., Ponzetto, S.P., Fiorini, P.: The robotic surgery procedural framebank. In: Proceedings of the Thirteenth International Conference on Language Resources and Evaluation (LREC 2022), (Marseille, France), pp. 3950–3959. European Language Resources Association (ELRA), 21–23 June 2022
33. Bombieri, M., Dall'Alba, D., Ramesh, S., Menegozzo, G., Schneider, C., Fiorini, P.: "Joints-Space Metrics for Automatic Robotic Surgical Gestures Classification," 2020 IEEE/RSJ International Conference on Intelligent Robots and Systems (IROS), Las Vegas, NV, USA, pp. 3061–3066 (2020). https://doi.org/10.1109/IROS45743.2020.9341094

Surgical Task Planning and Learning

Daniele Meli

Abstract This Chapter describes how "top-down" knowledge can be used to plan a robotic task. A crucial concept in modern cognitive systems is deliberation, which is the ability to make decisions that are motivated by reasoning on the available resources, i.e. the capabilities of the robot, the actual description of the environment, and the given mission. Deliberation marks a fundamental difference between automatic and autonomous robotic systems, the former merely executing pre-defined sequences of operations, with possible small adaptations to the sequence, while the latter actively reasoning on their goals and taking actions (possibly within pre-designed bounds, e.g., for safety) accordingly. To this aim, our proposed methodology is based on the use of logic programming to represent human-interpretable concepts and relations about the planning domain. In Chap. 2 we presented the process of extracting knowledge about surgical procedures from textbooks and scientific papers, and in Chap. 4 we show how the task sequence of a plan is extracted from text using techniques of Natural Language Processing (NLP). In this Chapter we present the details of how the deliberation process was carried out and demonstrated in the task shown in Fig. 12. This Chapter is organised in two main sections. First, we introduce action languages as a formal representation method for planning domains. We then show how to express an action language representation in answer set programming, a state-of-the-art logic programming formalism supporting contingent planning and knowledge revision via non-monotonic logics. Then, we consider the problem of planning knowledge extraction from task execution records, combining unsupervised action identification, semantic labeling and inductive logic programming. For clarity, the proposed approaches are exemplified in the context of a paradigmatic surgical pick-and-place training exercise, the ring transfer task, inspired from the peg transfer task described in the Fundamentals of Laparoscopic Surgery. We report preliminary results of our methodology in the end of the Chapter, finally discussing some limitations and future research directions to overcome them.

D. Meli (✉)
Department of Computer Science, University of Verona, Verona, Italy
e-mail: daniele.meli@univr.it

P. Fiorini (ed.), *Towards Autonomous Robotic Surgery*, Springer Tracts in Advanced Robotics 161, https://doi.org/10.1007/978-3-032-04247-7_3

A crucial concept in modern cognitive systems is *deliberation*, which is the ability to make decisions that are motivated by reasoning on the available resources, i.e. the capabilities of the robot, the actual description of the environment, and the given mission [1]. Deliberation marks a fundamental difference between *automatic and autonomous* robotic systems, the former merely executing pre-defined sequences of operations, with possible small adaptations to the sequence, while the latter *actively reasoning* on their goals and taking actions (possibly within pre-designed bounds, e.g., for safety) accordingly.

This Chapter explains how deliberation is implemented in the ARS project, to autonomously plan and execute surgical phases. Many different solutions to deliberative planning have been proposed [1–4]. However, ARS is strongly human-centric and safety-aware, which require the deliberation process to be explainable and trustworthy, to comply with the latest international regulations for safe autonomous systems [5]. To this aim, our proposed methodology is based on the use of logic programming [6, 7] to represent human-interpretable concepts and relations about the planning domain, which are then combined with sensor information and fed to a logic reasoner for situation-based planning and re-planning.

In Chap. 2 we presented the process of extracting knowledge about surgical procedures from textbooks and scientific papers, and in Chap. 4 we show how the task sequence of a plan is extracted from text using techniques of Natural Language Processing (NLP). In this Chapter we present the details of how the deliberation process was carried out and demonstrated in the task shown in Fig. 1a.

This Chapter is organised in two main sections. First, we introduce action languages [8] as a formal representation method for planning domains. We then show how to express an action language representation in answer set programming [9], a state-of-the-art logic programming formalism supporting contingent planning and knowledge revision via non-monotonic logics [10]. Then, we consider the problem of planning knowledge extraction from task execution records, combining unsupervised action identification [11], semantic labeling and inductive logic programming [12]. For clarity, the proposed approaches are exemplified in the context of a paradigmatic surgical pick-and-place training exercise, the ring transfer task, inspired from the peg transfer task described in the Fundamentals of Laparoscopic Surgery [13]. We report preliminary results of our methodology in the end of the Chapter, finally discussing some limitations and future research directions to overcome them.

This Chapter summarizes the results published in peer-reviewed research papers [14–21].

1 The Planning Approach Developed in ARS

Deliberative planning in ARS relies on the formal representation of the specific surgical phase to be automated, expressed in an action language. Action languages [8] encode a robotic planning domain Π (i.e., the ensemble of robotic agents and environmental description) as a tuple $\langle V, C, P, A, \mathcal{P}, \mathcal{E}, \mathcal{C}, G\rangle$, with the following meaning:

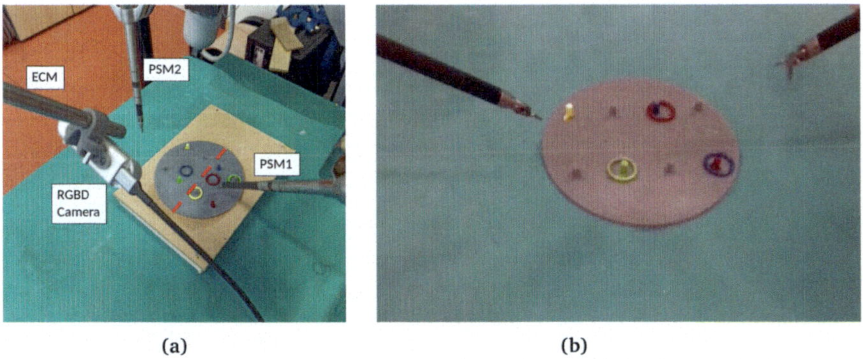

Fig. 1 The ring transfer scenario used as a running example (**a**); an example scenario with occupied colored pegs for PSM1 (**b**)

- V is the set of variables;
- C is the set of constant values, representing the range of assignment for V;
- P are properties or predicates built hierarchically on V, describing task-level concepts;
- A is the subset of predicates representing task actions;
- $\mathcal{P}$ is the set of pre-condition rules for actions, representing necessary conditions for their execution;
- $\mathcal{E}$ is the set of rules denoting effects of actions on the environment;
- $\mathcal{C}$ is the set of constraints determining the feasibility of actions, given specific environmental conditions;
- G is the set of goal conditions for the task.

To clarify the action language formalization, we consider the *ring transfer task* carried out with our da Vinci Research Kit (dVRK)[22], the laboratory version of the *da Vinci Surgical System* (donated by Intuitive Surgical, Mountain View, CA-USA) [23]. Our laboratory set-up is described in Chap. 1 and here we are focusing on its instruments used in the task, and shown in Fig. 1a . The *ring transfer task* is a variant of the standard peg transfer task described in the fundamentals of laparoscopic surgery for novice training [13]. The goal is to place colored rings on the same-color pegs, using the Patient-Side Manipulator (PSM) of our dVRK. Our PSM consists of three mechanical arms, two of which carrying a surgical instrument and indicated as PSM1 and PSM2, and the third carrying the endoscopic camera and indicated as ECM, as shown in Fig. 1a -a. Each instrument can touch the objects (rings and pegs) in the scene, depending on their reachability, which is defined by their position with respect to the red-dashed line in Fig. 1a -a. For instance, the red ring can be reached by PSM1 in the picture, while the yellow peg can be reached by PSM2. Depending on the reachability, a ring may be picked and placed by the same PSM* (e.g., the red ring and peg are both reachable by PSM1), or transfer between the arms may be required (as in the case for the blue ring, whose peg is reachable only by PSM1).

Moreover, if a ring is placed on a peg (e.g., the yellow ring in Fig. 1a)-b, it can be moved to the peg only after it has been extracted from its current position.

We start by formally representing this knowledge in the Planning Domain Definition Language (PDDL), a state-of-the-art action language [24], as follows:

```
(define(domain peg_transfer)
    %defining equality and universal quantifiers
    (:requirements :equality, :universal-precondition)
    (:types Ring, Peg, Arm, Color)                                  (1a)
    (:predicates (holding ?a, ?r, ?c - Arm, Ring, Color);
                                                                    (1b)
        (on ?r, ?c1, ?p, ?c2 - Ring, Color, Peg, Color)
                                                                    (1c)
        (reachable ?a, ?p, ?c - Arm, Peg, Color)                    (1d)
        (reachable ?a, ?r, ?c - Arm, Ring, Color)                   (1e)
    (:action move                                                   (1f)
        parameters: (?a - Arm; ?r - Ring; ?c - Color)               (1g)
        precondition: (reachable ?a, ?r, ?c)                        (1h)
        effect: (holding ?a, ?r, ?c))                               (1i)
    (:action move
        parameters: (?a - Arm; ?p - Peg; ?c1 - Color)
        precondition: (and (reachable ?a, ?p, ?c1)
            (holding ?a, ?r, ?c2)
            (not (on ?r, ?c3, ?p, ?c1))))
            (not (on ?r, ?c2, ?p, ?c4))))
        effect: (on ?r, ?c2 ?p, ?c1))

  (:action extract
    parameters: (?a - Arm; ?r - Ring; ?c1 - Color)
    precondition: (holding ?a, ?r, ?c1)
    effect: (not (on ?r, ?c1, ?p, ?c2)))
  (:action transfer                                                 (1j)
    parameters: (?a1 - Arm; ?r - Ring; ?c1 - Color)                 (1k)
    precondition: (and (holding ?a1, ?r, ?c1)                       (1l)
        (not (on ?r, ?c1, ?p, ?c2)))                                (1m)
    effect: (and (holding ?a2, ?r, ?c1)                             (1n)
        (not (holding ?a1, ?r, ?c1))                                (1o)
        (not (= (?a1, ?a2)))))                                      (1p)

        (:goal (forall (?c - Color; ?r - Ring)                      (1q)
```

```
(and (on ?r, ?c ?p, ?c)                          (1r)
(reachable ?a, ?r, ?c)))))                       (1s)
```

In the above statements, the set V of variables corresponds to `types Ring, Peg, Arm Color` (line (1a)), representing the main entities of the task. On top of them, the environmental `predicates` P are built (lines (1b) - (1e)), denoting that an arm is holding a ring, a ring is on a peg, a peg and a ring are reachable by an arm (PSM*), respectively. Similarly, the `action` predicates A are defined in the following lines, depending on variables identified as `parameters`. For instance, at lines (1f)-(1g), `move` is an action depending on the arm (agent) and ring with its color (target). For each action, preconditions $\mathcal{P}$ and effects $\mathcal{E}$ are defined. For instance, for the previous `move` action, the only precondition is that the target ring is reachable (line (1h)), while the effect is that the arm holds the ring eventually (line (1i)). Finally, the goal is defined in lines (1q)-(1s), as the requirement that all rings (line (1q)) which are reachable by any arm (line (1s)) shall be placed on the same-colored peg eventually (line (1r)).

The above planning domain definition describes the *rules of the task*, i.e., the capabilities of the robot (actions), the environment (predicates and variables), and their mutual interaction (preconditions and effects). Combining this with the definition of the goal and information coming from sensors and actuators, it is possible to derive a plan, i.e., a sequence of actions to reach the goal of the task.

The description of the sensing system and how the information about the positions and colors of the rings and pegs is described in Chap. 7. Sections 5 and 1.2 describes how this information is used to control the arms to reach the desired targets.

To this aim, it is convenient to represent the planning domain definition in a logical formalism, which preserves the interpretability of the domain description and allows to reason on its concepts and relations to derive consequences (the plan).

In the following, we show how to translate the above domain description to a logical formalism, which allows to perform autonomous planning as deductive reasoning, as we did in [15, 20]. Specifically, we opt for the Answer Set Programming (ASP) language [9], which is the state of the art of logic-based planning in artificial intelligence and robotics [25, 26].

1.1 From PDDL to Logic Programming

A planning domain Π expressed in an action language can be translated to a knowledge base in First-Order Logic (FOL) syntax [27]. Indeed, preconditions and effects of actions can be expressed as logical implications between predicates (or atoms). For instance, the rules for moving a ring (PDDL lines (1f)-(1i)) may be expressed as:

$$\texttt{move(A,ring,C)} \leftarrow \texttt{reachable(A,ring,C)}$$
$$\texttt{holding(A,ring,C)} \leftarrow \texttt{move(A,ring,C)}$$

Given a FOL knowledge base, it is possible to perform deductive reasoning on it, thus to derive feasible plans. To this aim, several logic programming paradigms exist. In the ARS project, we adopted the Answer Set Programming (ASP), an established formalism for autonomous planning and robotics [25, 26]. ASP supports high expressive power to represent planning domains, including temporal abstractions, default negation and the semantics of possible worlds [28]. Specifically, default negation (`not` in ASP syntax) implements the closed-world assumption [29], which makes the knowledge base satisfiable when certain facts are not observed in the real world (a practical assumption in partially observable robotic domains). The semantics of possible worlds allows to represent the multiple planning options available to the robotic system, hence allowing the choice among available actions in a given environmental context. For instance, when multiple rings are yet to be placed in the ring transfer domain, any order of pick-and-place operations can be executed equivalently (according to the PDDL specifications defined above). Finally, temporal relations can be expressed by assigning a specific variable for the (discrete) time step to predicates. The ASP encoding as of the standard syntax [30], corresponding to the PDDL description of the ring transfer task, is as following.

```
%Preconditions                                                                  (2a)
0{move(A,ring,C,T) : reachable(A,ring,C,T);                                     (2b)
 move(A,peg,C1,T) : reachable(A,peg,C1,T), holding(A,ring,C2,T);               (2c)
 transfer(A1,ring,C1,T) : holding(A1,ring,C1,T);                                (2d)
 extract(A,ring,C,T) : holding(A,ring,C,T)} 1 :- time(T).                       (2e)
%Constraints                                                                    (2f)
:- move(A,peg,C1,T), on(ring,C3,peg,C1,T).                                      (2g)
:- move(A,peg,C1,T), on(ring,C2,peg,C4,T), holding(A,ring,C2,T).               (2h)
:- transfer(A1,ring,C1,T), on(ring,C1,peg,C2,T), holding(A1,ring,C1,T).
                                                                                (2i)
%Effects                                                                        (2j)
holding(A,ring,C,T) :- move(A,ring,C,T-1).                                      (2k)
holding(A2,ring,C1,T) :- transfer(A1,ring,C1,T-1), arm(A2), A2!=A1.            (2l)
holding(A1,ring,C1,T) :- holding(A1,ring,C1,T-1),
  not transfer(A1,ring,C1,T-1).                                                 (2m)
on(ring,C2,peg,C1,T) :- move(A,peg,C1,T-1), holding(A,ring,C2,T-1).            (2n)
on(ring,C1,peg,C2,T) :- on(ring,C1,peg,C2,T-1),
  not extract(A,ring,C1,T-1), arm(A).                                           (2o)
```

Preconditions are represented using the aggregate construct l `{a` $_i$ `:` $\bigwedge$ `b`$_j$ `}` `u :- time(T)`, which collects preconditions for each head action `a`$_i$ (represented as the logical conjunction between body predicates `b`$_j$'s) and defines the minimum (l) and maximum (u) number of actions allowed per time step `T`. This supports the semantics of the possible worlds, when multiple actions are available but the robotic system can only execute one per time. Preconditions are extended with constraints, which forbid actions under specific environmental conditions. A constraint in the form `:-` $\bigwedge \mathtt{b}_j$ is logically equivalent to $\perp \leftarrow \bigwedge \mathtt{b}_j$, meaning that the conjunction of body atoms $\mathtt{b}_j$'s leads to logical inconsistency. For instance, the preconditions for the transfer action (PDDL lines (1l)-(1m)) state that a ring can be transferred if it is held by an arm and it is not placed on any peg. This is expressed in the constraint (2i) as the *inconsistency* of transferring the held ring when it is placed on any peg. Finally, effects of actions are expressed as normal rules, where `:-` denotes the logical implication $\leftarrow$. In particular, we assume environmental predicates to be inertial [31], i.e., they keep holding until specific conditions occur. For instance, following the effect of moving to a ring at PDDL line (1i), a ring is held after this action occurs (statement (2k)). Moreover, according to the effects of transfer action (PDDL lines (1n)-(1p)), the ring is held by an arm after another arm performed transfer (statement (2l)), or if it was held by an arm at the previous time step and the same arm did not perform transfer (statement (2m)).

1.1.1 Planning in ASP

Given the ASP formalization of Π, denoted $\Pi(AS)$, an ASP solver can be used to compute the feasible plans from a set of initial conditions and the goal definition. *Solving an ASP program* means computing its *answer sets*, i.e., the minimal sets of ground atoms, which can be inferred from the axioms. A ground atom is an atom with all variables assigned to specific constants. Given an ASP program $\Pi(AS)$, the set of ground atoms which can be inferred from it is defined as the Herbrand base of $\Pi(AS)$, denoted as $H(\Pi(AS))$. As an example, consider the ASP formalization of the ring transfer task. Assume that variables have the following ranges:

```
time(0;1).
color(red;blue).
arm(psm1;psm2).
```
(3)

and the following initial conditions hold:

```
reachable(psm1,ring,red,0).
reachable(psm1,peg,red,0).
reachable(psm1,ring,red,1).
reachable(psm1,peg,red,1).
reachable(psm1,ring,blue,0).
reachable(psm2,peg,blue,0).
reachable(psm1,ring,blue,1).
reachable(psm2,peg,blue,1).
```
(4)

An ASP solver starts grounding body atoms corresponding to the initial conditions. Then, the head of axioms can be grounded via logical deduction. In our case, at time `T=0` the following atoms can be grounded, according to aggregate preconditions (2b)-(2e): either `move(psm1,ring,red,0)` or `move(psm1,ring,blue,0)`. As a consequence, by performing a deduction at time `T=1`, the following sets of grounded atoms can be generated: either

```
holding(psm1,ring,red,1).
move(psm1,peg,red,1).
```
(5)

or

```
holding(psm1,ring,blue,1).
transfer(psm1,ring,blue,1).
```
(6)

The union of atoms (3), (4) and (5) is an answer set for $\Pi(AS)$. Similarly, another answer set consists of the union of atoms (3), (4) and (5). An answer set then encodes *a feasible plan* for the ASP task description, including the set of actions to be executed and the corresponding environmental conditions. This provides a unique advantage of ASP over other popular logic programming formalisms, e.g., Prolog [32]. The latter is based on queries, i.e., it performs deduction from a knowledge base and returns the logically consequent answer *at the given time step*. On the contrary, an ASP solver computes all possible plans and corresponding environmental contexts, enhancing workflow monitoring and verification and supporting optimal plan selection over multiple choices.

In the ARS project, we adopt the state-of-the-art ASP solver Clingo [33], which supports *incremental planning* to reason over time and compute the *shortest plan* towards the given goal. This is implemented organizing the ASP program into 3 sub-programs:

- `#program base`, containing the definition of variables and constants, as well as initial conditions and time-independent axioms;
- `#program step(t)`, containing the time-dependent axioms encoding preconditions, effects and constraints on actions;
- `#program check(t)`, containing the definition of the goal as `:- not goal (t).`

After evaluating the initial conditions in `base` sub-program, at each time step `t`, the program first evaluates the constraint in the `check(t)` sub-program. If it is violated (i.e., the goal is not satisfied at that time step), the solver evaluates `step(t)` and grounds new atoms according to task knowledge. Then, time progresses and the loop continues until `check(t)` is satisfied, i.e., the goal is achieved. In this way, it is possible to encode the temporal operator *eventually* from temporal logic into ASP. Indeed, evaluating the `check(t)` sub-program until the goal is satisfied is equivalent to asking that the goal is satisfied eventually.

Apart from the enhanced interpretability of the planning phase in ARS and the other aforementioned advantages in terms of expressiveness, the use of ASP also provides greater compactness of representation for the planning domain. For instance, consider the scenario depicted in Fig. 1b , where the right arm (PSM1) can directly pick and place the red and blue rings. However, both pegs of the corresponding colors are occupied. In this case, the task description in $\Pi(ASP)$ is able to successfully solve the problem, placing either one of the red and blue rings on a grey peg as an intermediate step. Notice that, in statements 2, this option is not explicitly represented; however, an ASP solver is able to deduce this plan from the available knowledge, thanks to goal-oriented reasoning. On the contrary, an explicit representation of the planning problem (encoded, e.g., in a finite state machine) would need an explicit branch with this option.

2 Learning to Plan in ARS

The logic-based approach to planning adopted for ARS requires the availability of task knowledge (expressed, e.g., in PDDL), as discussed earlier in this Chapter. This is unrealistic in complex robotic scenarios, especially in surgery, where only a nominal procedural description is usually available (e.g., from surgical manuals), but the workflow of task execution may vary with different patients or contingencies.

In this Section, we then address the problem of deriving a formal description Π of the surgical planning domain. In particular, we aim at automatically extracting an ASP problem representation as in $\Pi(ASP)$ presented in the previous Section, starting from available sources of information. We adopt an approach based on Inductive Logic Programming (ILP) [12], allowing to extract task knowledge as in Π from visual and kinematic recordings of the procedure, assuming a common signature (constants, variables and predicates) is available. In other words, given the sets V, C, P, A, we are interested in discovering the axioms governing the robotic task, i.e., the sets of preconditions $\mathcal{P}$, effects $\mathcal{E}$ and constraints $\mathcal{C}$. Notably, ILP has the advantage to require relatively little datasets compared to more established machine learning approaches, e.g., deep neural learning [34], thus mitigating the problem of scarcity of surgical data [35].

In the rest of this Section, we first provide theoretical details about the ILP framework, specializing it under the ASP semantics. Then, we show how to learn task knowledge via ILP, starting from labelled examples annotated by experts (*supervised ILP)* as in [16, 18], and how to relax the labelling assumption via *unsupervised ILP* from uncertain (noisy) examples as in [19, 21]. We finally present the results of our methodology in the context of the ARS project, with a focus on the paradigmatic ring transfer task.

2.1 The ILP Problem Under the ASP Semantics

We now provide relevant definitions to introduce the problem of inductive learning of ASP theories, with specific reference to the ring transfer scenario chosen as a leading example. Additional details can be found in [36].

A generic ILP problem T for ASP theories is defined as the tuple $T = \langle B, S_M, E\rangle$, where B is the *background knowledge*, i.e. a set of axioms and atoms in ASP syntax; S_M is the *search space*, i.e. the set of candidate ASP axioms that can be learned; and E is a set of *examples*. The goal of T is to find a subset $H \subseteq S_M$ such that $H \cup B \models E$. Examples are *partial interpretations* defined as follows.

Definition 1 (*Partial interpretation*) Let P be an ASP program. Any set of ground atoms that can be generated from axioms in P is an *interpretation* of P. Given an interpretation I of P, we say that a pair of subsets of grounded atoms $e = \langle e^{inc}, e^{exc}\rangle$ (respectively the included and excluded set) is a *partial interpretation (extended by interpretation I)* if $e^{inc} \subseteq I$ and $e^{exc} \cap I = \emptyset$.

In particular, we consider *context-dependent partial interpretations*, as introduced by [36].

Definition 2 (*Context-dependent partial interpretation (CDPI)*) A CDPI of an ASP program P with an interpretation I is a tuple $e_c = \langle e, C\rangle$, where e is a partial interpretation and C_e is an ASP program called *context*. I is said to extend e_c if $e^{inc} \cup C_e \subseteq I$ and $(e^{exc} \cup C_e) \cap I = \emptyset$.

We consider two different kinds of examples, namely *positive and negative examples*. Positive examples are denoted as E^+, while negative ones as E^-, such that $E = \langle E^+, E^-\rangle$. We now specialize T to CDPIs as follows:

Definition 3 (Learning ASP theories from CDPIs) An ILP task from CDPIs is a tuple $T = \langle B, S_M, E\rangle$, where $E = \langle E^+, E^-\rangle$ is a set of positive and negative CDPIs. We say that $H \subseteq S_M$ is a solution to T if the following hold:

$$\begin{aligned} &\forall e \in E^+ \ \exists AS \ s.t. \ B \cup H \cup C_e \models AS : \ e \text{ is extended by } AS \\ &\forall e \in E^- \ \nexists AS \ s.t. \ B \cup H \cup C_e \models AS : \ e \text{ is extended by } AS \end{aligned} \tag{7}$$

Positive examples then lead to *brave induction* [37], in the sense that we require the hypothesis to entail *at least one* answer set supporting them. On the contrary, negative examples lead to *cautious induction*, since *no answer set* supporting them shall be generated (thus leading to learning constraints).

In the presence of uncertainty (noise) about examples, the task in Definition 3 is extended with E as a set of N *noisy CDPIs*, i.e., CDPIs annotated with an integer weight $w_i, \forall i = 1 \dots N$ [38].

In ARS, we adopted a state-of-the-art implementation for solving ILP tasks under the ASP semantics, i.e., ILASP [36]. In the case of the task in Definition 3, ILASP seeks for a hypothesis H such that its length λ is minimal, where λ is defined as the number of atoms occuring H. For the noisy version of the task, ILASP minimizes $\lambda + \eta$, where $\eta = \sum_{i=1}^{K} w_i^u$, being $\{w_i^u\}_{i=1}^{K}$ the set of weights for $K \leq N$ uncovered examples, i.e., CDPIs not satisfying (7). In other words, [38] introduces the possibility to "ignore" some examples, if their weight is low (i.e., their uncertainty is high).

2.2 *Supervised ILP*

We now specify how the task in Definition 3 (i.e., learning ASP rules from CDPIs) is implemented in the ARS project, following the methodology published in [16, 18]. We refer to the leading example of ring transfer for clarity.

The input of our learning system was a record of synchronized visual and kinematic acquisitions $R = \langle V, K \rangle$ from our robotic system (the da Vinci Research Kit, dVRK [22]). In this Section, we assume that the records can be partitioned in segments S, such that there exist a *positive labeling function* and a *negative labeling function* $L_p : S \rightarrow H(A)$ and $L_n : S \rightarrow H(A)$, respectively, mapping each segment to a specific ground action label (or a set of ground action labels) from $A \in \Pi(ASP)$. L_p defines the action executed at each segment, while L_n defines the forbidden actions at each segment. We then rely on a prior annotation (e.g., by experts) of the visual-kinematic record, specifying the occurring action in each portion of the record itself.

Under these assumptions, we now show how to define an ILP task as in Definition 3 for learning preconditions P, constraints C and effects E separately.

2.2.1 Learning Action Preconditions and Constraints

We defined the ILP task as follows:

- we set the background knowledge $B = \langle V, C \rangle$, where $V, C \in \Pi(ASP)$ are the definitions of variables and constants in the ASP task definition;
- we set the search space S_M as the set of normal and constraint rules having predicates in P as body atoms, and predicates in A in the head;
- we build two CDPIs e_p, e_n as in Definition 2 for each segment $s_i \in S$, $i = 1, \ldots, |S|$, selecting $\langle v_{0,i}, k_{0,i} \rangle \in S$, corresponding to the first record in the segment. Specifically, e_p is a positive example with $e^{inc} = \{l_{i,p}\}$, $e^{exc} = \emptyset$, $C_e = H(P)|_{\langle v_{0,i}, k_{0,i} \rangle}$, where $l_{i,p} = L_p(s_i)$ and $H(P)|_{\langle v_{0,i}, k_{0,i} \rangle}$ represents the grounded environmental predicates holding at the beginning of s_i (recognized from sensors as, e.g., in [15]). e_n is a negative example analogous to e_p, but $e^{inc} = l_{i,n} = L_n(s_i)$ is the set of forbidden actions for that segment.

With the above task implementation, we learned the action preconditions and constraints which specified when actions should occur (thanks to e_p) and when they must not occurr (thanks to e_n).

With reference to the paradigmatic ring transfer task, let us consider for instance the scenario shown in Fig. 1b , and assume the video frame shown in Figure corresponds to the beginning of the visual-kinematic segment where the action `move(psm1,ring,red)` occured, hence $l_{i,p}$ = `move(psm1,ring,red)`. Moreover, the set of forbidden actions in this segment was $l_{i,n}$ = {`move(psm2,ring,red)`, `move(psm2,ring,blue)`} (due to reachability conditions). We then built one positive example and two negative examples as following[1]:

```
#pos(id1, {l_{i,p}}, {}, {reachable(psm1,ring,red), reachable(psm1,ring,blue), ...}).
#neg(id2, {move(psm2,ring,red)}, {}, C_e).
#neg(id3, {move(psm2,ring,blue)}, {}, C_e).
```

Given a search space S_M = { `h :-` $\bigwedge_{i=1}^{N}$ b_i | h∈{`move(A,ring,C)`, ⊥ }, $b_i \in P\ \forall i = 1, \ldots, N$ }, ILASP could discover the following rule:

```
move(A,ring,C) :- reachable(A,ring,C).
```

Note that the learned axioms come without the temporal argument `t`, since CDPIs represent an instantaneous ASP representation of the task *under specific context conditions*. Hence, the temporal argument can be added after the ILP process, by including it in the final set of rules to be used for planning.

2.2.2 Learning the Effects of Actions

Learning the set $\mathcal{E}$ of task knowledge is more challenging, since the effects occur at the following time step with respect to the actions (ref. Section 1.1). Moreover, due to the inertial property (atoms remain grounded unless specific actions are executed) learning requires the use of default negation (`not`) in the body of effect axioms. Learning default negation in the body of rules is not trivial, since it represents the non-occurrence of specific atoms, but multiple atoms may be "not grounded" in a particular context. For instance, in Fig. 1b , all the atoms representing the placement of PSMs with respect to the rings and pegs are not grounded, i.e., `at(A,ring,C)`, `at(A,peg,C)`.

In order to mitigate the issue, we redefine the effects of actions according to the equivalent formalization of *event calculus* [39]. The effect of an action can then be expressed with the following axioms:

```
effect(t) :- init(effect, effect, t).
effect(t) :- effect(t-1), not term(effect, t).
```

[1] We report examples in the syntax of ILASP tool, where the CDPI is expressed as a sequence of unique identifier, e^{inc}, e^{exc} and C_e.

where `init(effect, t)` and `term(effect, t)` are atoms defining the events which lead to the grounding and ungrounding of `effect(t)`, respectively[2]. Instead of directly defining the axioms with `effect(t)` as a head, we can define the axioms with `init(effect, t)` and `term(term, t)` in the head, and combine them with the above event calculus rules. With reference to the ring transfer task, consider for instance the effect for `on(ring,C2,peg,C1)` (axioms (2n)-(2o)). In the event calculus, it can be equivalently expressed as:

```
on(ring, C2, peg, C1, t) :- init(on(ring,C2,peg,C1), t).                      (8a)
on(ring, C2, peg, C1, t) :- on(ring, C2, peg, C1, t-1),
  not term(on(ring,C2,peg,C1), t).                                             (8b)
init(on(ring,C2,peg,C1), t) :- move(A,peg,C1,t-1), holding(A,ring,C2,t-1).
                                                                               (8c)
term(on(ring,C2,peg,C1), t) :- extract(A, ring, C1, t-1).                      (8d)
```

without default negations in the body of axioms.

Following this scheme, we can now define the ILP task for learning E as follows:

- we set the background knowledge $B = \langle V, C\rangle$, where $V, C \in \Pi(ASP)$ are the definitions of variables and constants in the ASP task definition;
- for each predicate $p \in P$, we set the search space S_M as the set of normal rules having $\texttt{init}_p\texttt{(t)}$ and $\texttt{term}_p\texttt{(t)}$ as head atoms (i.e., the starting and ending event definitions for p), and predicates in $A \cup P$ in the body;
- we build up to two CDPIs $e_{p,i}, e_{p,t}$ as in Definition 2 for each segment $s_i \in S,\ i = 1, \ldots, |S|$, selecting $\langle v_{0,i}, k_{0,i}\rangle \in S$, corresponding to the first record in the segment. For each ground atom $\bar{p} \in H(P)|_{\langle v_{0,i}, k_{0,i}\rangle}$, if $\bar{p} \notin H(P)|_{\langle v_{0,i-1}, k_{0,i-1}\rangle}$ (i.e., it is not grounded in the previous segment s_{i-1}, meaning that a starting event has occurred), we build $e_{p,i}$ as a positive example with $e^{inc} = \{\texttt{init}_{\bar{p}}\}$, $e^{exc} = \{\texttt{init}_{\bar{q}}\ \ \forall \bar{q} \in H(P)|_{\langle v_{0,i-1}, k_{0,i-1}\rangle} \setminus \{\bar{p}\}\}$, $C_e = H(P)|_{\langle v_{0,i}, k_{0,i}\rangle} \cup \{L_p(s_{i-1})\}$, where $\texttt{init}_{\bar{p}}$ is the grounding of $\texttt{init}_p$ at $\langle v_{0,i-1}, k_{0,i-1}\rangle$. Note that we add $L_p(s_{i-1})$ to C_e, in order to link the starting condition to the formerly executed action, as in axiom (8c). In this way, we do not need the explicit definition of the temporal variable in the ILP task. Similarly, if $\bar{p} \notin H(P)|_{\langle v_{0,i+1}, k_{0,i+1}\rangle}$ (i.e., it is not grounded in the sequent segment s_{i+1}, meaning that an ending event has occurred), at s_{i+1} we build a positive example $e_{p,t}$ analogous to $e_{p,n}$, where `init` is replaced by `term`.

Differently from CDPIs for learning action preconditions and constraints, for effects of actions CDPIs have $e^{exc} \neq \emptyset$, but containing the ungrounded instances of $\texttt{init}_p$, $\forall p \in P$. Indeed, in this case we could not generate negative examples, since there are no *forbidden* effects of actions, but rather *unobserved* effects of actions (hence, cautious induction required by Definition 3 would be too tight). As a consequence, we needed to define unobserved facts (either starting or ending event

---

[2] For simplicity, this formalization utilizes a shorter notation than [39], where `effect(t)` is equivalent to `holds(effect, t)` and so forth.

groundings) in e^{exc}, in order to learn more specific axioms to be included in E, relying only on brave induction.

For instance, in the ring transfer scenario depicted in Fig. 1b , the PSM1 moved to the red ring in the current segment, i.e., $L_p(s_i) =$ `move(psm1,ring,red)`. In the following segment s_{i+1}, PSM1 would be at the location of the ring red, hence `at(psm1,ring,red)` *would have started* at s_{i+1}. We then built a CDPI in the form:

```
#pos(id1,{init(at(psm1,ring,red))}, {init(at(psm1,ring,blue)), …},
        {move(psm1,ring,red), reachable(psm1,ring,red), …}).
```

In this way, ILASP could find a logical connection between being at a ring and previously moving to it:

```
init(at(A,ring,C), t) :- move(A,ring,C,t-1).
```

where the variable `t` was added after learning, accounting for the construction scheme of the CDPI with $L_p(s_{i-1})$ in the context.

2.3 *Unsupervised ILP*

The knowledge of labeling maps L_p and L_n is unrealistic in practice. Indeed, most recordings of surgical procedures come without an explicit annotation of the exact actions performed by the surgeon or her / his assistants (only high-level phases are usually available [40]). Furthermore, the map for negative (forbidden) annotations L_n cannot be easily implemented, due to the complexity and patient specificity of surgical procedures.

In this Section, we follow the published research in [21] and relax the assumption of having access to the two annotation maps. Instead, we relied on unsupervised action identification algorithms [11], which formally represented a map $\Gamma : R \rightarrow H(A)$ assigning each data point $\langle v, k \rangle \in R$ to a specific ground (executed) action in the available (ASP) action space A (hence, defining segments of R with shared annotation). In this way, unsupervised action identification took the place of L_p (to build e^{inc} of CDPIs) in the methodology described in Sect. 2.2. However, two challenges remained unsolved:

- the map Γ produced uncertain ground action assignments, due to the inherent statistical nature of the action identification algorithm;
- L_n could not be defined, hence negative CDPIs could not be exploited by ILASP, since Γ may generate false negatives, i.e., it could badly unrecognize specific action groundings.

The first problem was partly solved via the ILASP task definition from noisy CDPIs [38]. Indeed, assuming the designed action identification algorithm achieved a performance score ρ_a (e.g., F1-score or accuracy) in the assignment of data points in R to $\bar{a} \in H(a),\ a \in A$, we could set $w_{\bar{a}} = \frac{\rho_a}{\sum_{x \in A} \rho_x}$[3], being $w_{\bar{a}}$ the weight of CDPIs having $e^{inc} = \{\bar{a}\}$.

In order to compensate for missing negative CDPIs, we adopted a similar approach as for learning the effects of actions, setting $e^{exc} \neq \emptyset$. More specifically, we assumed the segment $s \in R$ was such that $\Gamma(s) = \bar{a} \in H(a),\ a \in A$. We then defined positive examples with $e^{exc} = H(x) \setminus \{\bar{a}\},\ \forall x \in A$. This was not semantically equivalent to generating negative CDPIs, since positive examples were subject to brave induction; however, ILASP could exploit e^{exc} to learn more specific preconditions for actions (inglobating constraints, e.g., as default negations).

Our approach still does not guarantee the correctness of learned axioms, since the ILASP task from noisy CDPIs identifies only *probably-correct* rules. For this reason, we also introduced an algorithm for the *online refinement* of learned knowledge, allowing a human expert to provide a feedback to the autonomous system. Specifically, whenever the robot logically deduces an action $\bar{a}$ to be executed, the human expert decides whether the action is correct or not. If it is correct, a positive noise-free CDPI is generated; otherwise, a negative noise-free CDPI is provided, together with another positive noise-free CDPI having $e^{\mathrm{inc}} = \{\mathtt{a}_e\}$, $\mathtt{a}_e$ being an action suggested by the expert. In all these CDPIs, the context is given by the current situation of the environment, as retrieved from the sensors. The ILASP task is then solved again, in order to progressively improve the task knowledge in a continual learning fashion.

3 Results of the Ring Transfer Scenario

We now present the main results attained by our ASP approach to planning, and unsupervised ILP methodology for task knowledge learning, with reference to the benchmark ring transfer task. We evaluated two performance measures:

- the *semantic validity* of learned ASP task rules ($\mathcal{P}, \mathcal{C}, \mathcal{E} \in \Pi(ASP)$), evaluating whether they can correctly ground atoms in $P \cup A$, as expert-defined rules would;
- the *semantic improvement* induced by the expert feedback for online continual learning;
- the *planning performance* with learned ASP rules, compared against expert defined task knowledge.

We denoted expert-defined task knowledge as in axioms Π^e (2), while learned task knowledge as Π^l. We used the state-of-the-art unsupervised action identification algorithm proposed by [19], and consider 3 real task executions performed

[3] We normalized the performance score to guarantee the unitary sum over A.

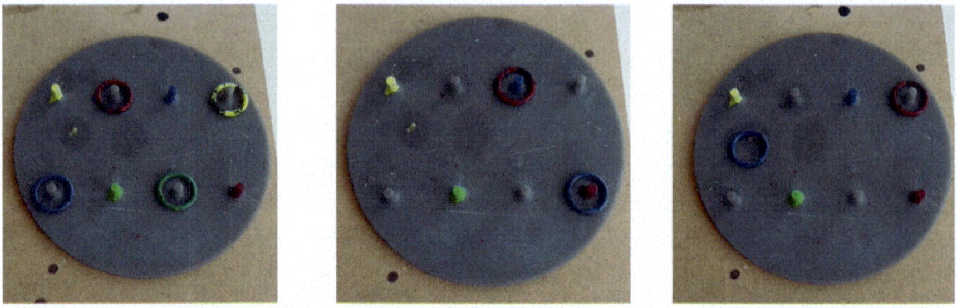

(a) (b) (c)

Fig. 2 Initial environmental conditions for the task executions used for unsupervised ILP

by humans, as shown in Fig. 2. In Fig. 2a, the task started in the nominal situation described in FLS [13], with all 4 colored rings placed on grey pegs, on the opposite side with respect to the corresponding pegs. Hence, PSMs must transfer the ring from one PSM* to the other, before placing the rings on the pegs. In Fig. 2b, a more challenging situation is depicted. The relevant rings and pegs (i.e., the blue and red ones) were on one side of the peg base, hence no transfer was needed. However, the rings occupied the pegs with mismatched color, thus one of the colored peg must be freed (by placing a ring on a grey peg temporarily), before completing the task. Figure 2c shows an unconventional scenario with the red ring on the same side as its peg, while the blue ring is on the opposite side out of any peg. Hence, not all rings required extraction in this task instance. Furthermore, before placing the blue ring on its peg (hence, after transfer), the ring fell, hence it had to be grasped again to complete the task.

We slightly reformulated axioms (2), introducing 2 gripper actions: `grasp(A,ring,C)` for gripper closure and `release(A)` for gripper opening. These actions were interleaved with others already defined in $\Pi(ASP)$, e.g., rings were moved or extracted after grasping, and they were placed to a peg (after moving) or transferred via releasing. In the following, we summarize the learned task knowledge and the results for our two performance metrics.

3.1 Learned Task Knowledge

Π^e according to this formulation is reported in [18]. Π^l is defined as following.

```
release(V1,t) :- not reachable(V1,peg,V2,t),not reachable(V1,ring,V2),
  closed_gripper(V1,t),placed(ring,V2,peg,V3,t).                          (9a)
grasp(V1,ring,V,t) :- not closed_gripper(V1,t),at(V1,ring,V2,t).          (9b)
move(V1,peg,V2,t) :- at(V1,ring,V2,t),reachable(V1,peg,V2,t).             (9c)
transfer(V1,center,V2,t) :- not closed_gripper(V3,t),at(V1,ring,V2,t),
  reachable(V3,peg,V2,t),V3!=V1.                                          (9d)
extract(V1,ring,V2,t) :- closed_gripper(V1,t),placed(ring,V2,peg,V3,t),
  at(V4,ring,V2,t).                                                       (9e)
move(V1,ring,V2,t) :- not closed_gripper(V1,t),reachable(V1,ring,V2,t),
  reachable(V1,peg,V2,t).                                                 (9f)
term(at(V1,peg,V2),t+1) :- move(V1,center,V3,t),color(V2).                (9g)
init(at(A,peg,C),t+1) :- move(A,peg,C,t).                                 (9h)
term(at(V1,ring,V2),t+1) :- move(V1,peg,V3,t),color(V2).                  (9i)
init(at(V1,ring,V2),t+1) :- move(V1,ring,V2,t).                           (9j)
term(closed_gripper(A),t+1) :- release(A,t).                              (9k)
init(closed_gripper(A),t+1) :- grasp(A,ring,C,t).                         (9l)
term(placed(ring,C1,peg,C2),t+1) :- extract(A,ring,C1,t),color(C2).       (9m)
init(placed(ring,V3,peg,V1),t+1) :- move(V2,peg,V1,t),color(V3).          (9n)
init(at(V1,center),t+1) :- move(V1,center,V2,t).                          (9o)
```

Unsupervised ILP required on average ≈ 66 s to learn the axioms for each atom in $A \cup P^{ec}$.

3.2 Semantic Validity Results

The semantic validity of learned ASP task rules was evaluated generating 1000 random contexts C_e for each atom in $P \cup A$. For atoms in A, each context was in $H(P)$, while for atoms in P, each context was in $H(P) \cup \{\bar{a}\}$, where $\bar{a} \in H(A)$ accounted for the effects of actions. We use Clingo ASP solver [33] to compute $H(\Pi^e \cup c)$, $H(\Pi^l \cup c)$, $\forall c \in C_e$. We then compared whether elements in $H(\Pi^l \cup c)$ match with elements in $H(\Pi^e \cup c)$ for each atom in $x \in A \cup P^{ec}$, where $P^{ec} = \{\text{init}(p) \vee \text{term}(p) \mid p \in P\}$. We then computed the precision Pr, recall Rec and F1-score $F1$ of rules describing preconditions or constraints for x. These metrics were computed depending on the True Positives TP, False Positives FP and False Negatives FN, respectively defined as elements occurring in $H(\Pi^l \cup c) \cap H(\Pi^e \cup c)$, in $H(\Pi^l \cup c) \setminus H(\Pi^l \cup c) \cap H(\Pi^e \cup c)$ and in $H(\Pi^e \cup c) \setminus H(\Pi^l \cup c) \cap H(\Pi^e \cup c)$. In other words, TP counts the segments *correctly identified* as the grounding of specific atoms, according to ground truth task knowledge $H(\Pi^e)$; FP counts segments *wrongly identified* as the atom grounding; FN counts segments *wrongly not identified* as an atom grounding. The following definitions then hold:

$$Pr = \frac{TP}{TP + FP}$$
$$Rec = \frac{TP}{TP + FN}$$
$$F1 = 2\frac{Pr}{Pr + Rec}$$

Hence, precision measures, for each atom in $x \in A \cup P^{ec}$, the rate of segments correctly identified as belonging to $H(x)$, across all segments *identified as belonging to* $H(x)$ by unsupervised ILP. Conversely, recall measures the rate of segments correctly identified as belonging to $H(x)$, across all segments *actually belonging to* $H(x)$. Finally, F1-score measures a geometric average between the two other metrics.

Table 1 shows the median and Inter-Quartile Range (IQR) for rules corresponding to each single atom in $A \cup P$. Our unsupervised ILP procedure achieved 100% precision over all atoms, on average. Mean recall and F1 were also high, except for `move(A,ring,C)` and atoms representing the location of the PSMs (`at(A,center)` and `at(A,peg,C)`). The imperfect performance arise from the limited and heterogeneous dataset in Fig. 2, where actions were executed with different frequency (e.g., `transfer(A,ring,C,t)` was executed only 5 times, while `release(A,t)` 21 times) and under different environmental conditions.

3.3 Semantic Improvement Results

After 13 interactions with a human expert, rules (9) were refined as follows:

Table 1 Semantic validity results (median ± IQR range). We aggregate the results for `init` and `term` conditions for effects of actions

$x \in A \cup P$	Pr	Rec	$F1$
`move(A, ring, C)`	1.00 – 0.00	0.50 – 0.50	0.67 – 0.33
`move(A, peg, C)`	1.00 – 0.00	1.00 – 0.75	0.40 – 1.00
`transfer(A, ring, C)`	1.00 – 0.00	1.00 – 1.00	1.00 – 1.00
`grasp(A, ring, C)`	1.00 – 0.00	1.00 – 0.00	1.00 – 0.00
`extract(A, ring, C)`	1.00 – 0.00	1.00 – 0.00	1.00 – 0.00
`release(A)`	1.00 – 0.00	1.00 – 1.00	1.00 – 1.00
`closed_gripper(A)`	1.00 – 0.00	1.00 – 0.00	1.00 – 0.00
`at(A, center)`	1.00 – 0.00	0.67 – 1.00	0.75 – 1.00
`at(A, ring, C)`	1.00 – 0.00	1.00 – 0.88	1.00 – 0.78
`at(A, peg, C)`	1.00 – 0.00	0.75 – 0.88	0.83 – 0.78
`on(ring, C1, peg, C2)`	1.00 – 0.00	1.00 – 0.00	1.00 – 0.00
Mean	**1.00**	**0.90**	**0.88**

```
release(V1,t) :- closed_gripper(V1,t).                                    (10a)
grasp(V1,ring,V2,t) :- not closed_gripper(V1,t),at(V1,ring,V2,t).         (10b)
move(V1,peg,V2,t) :- not at(V1,peg,V2,t),closed_gripper(V1,t),
  reachable(V1,peg,V2),not at(V3,center),arm(V3).                         (10c)
move(V1,peg,V2,t) :- not at(V1,peg,V2,t),closed_gripper(V1,t),
  reachable(V1,peg,V2),at(V3,center),not closed_gripper(V3).              (10d)
move(V1,center,V2,t) :- at(V1,ring,V2,t).                                 (10e)
extract(V1,ring,V2,t) :- closed_gripper(V1,t),placed(ring,V2,peg,V3,t),
  at(V4,ring,V2,t).                                                       (10f)
move(V1,ring,V2,t) :- reachable(V1,ring,V2).                              (10g)
term(at(V1,peg,V2),t+1) :- placed(ring,V3,peg,V3,t),
  reachable(V1,peg,V2),move(V1,ring,V4,t).                                (10h)
init(at(A,peg,C),t+1) :- move(A,peg,C,t).
term(at(V1,ring,V2),t+1) :- at(V1,center,t),move(V3,peg,V2,t).            (10i)
term(at(V1,ring,V2),t+1) :- release(V1,t),reachable(V1,ring,V2),
  at(V1,peg,V3,t).                                                        (10j)
init(at(V1,ring,V2),t+1) :- move(V1,ring,V2,t).                           (10k)
init(at(V1,ring,V2),t+1) :- reachable(V1,peg,V2),move(V3,center,V2,t).    (10l)
term(closed_gripper(A),t+1) :- release(A,t).                              (10m)
init(closed_gripper(A),t+1) :- grasp(A,ring,C,t).                         (10n)
term(placed(ring,V1,peg,V2),t+1) :- reachable(V3,peg,V2),
  extract(V3,ring,V1,t),at(V3,ring,V1,t).                                 (10o)
init(placed(ring,V1,peg,V2),t+1) :- release(V3,t),at(V3,ring,V1,t),
  at(V3,peg,V2,t).                                                        (10p)
term(at(V1,center),t+1) :- reachable(V1,peg,V2),move(V3,center,V2,t).     (10q)
init(at(V1,center),t+1) :- move(V1,center,V2,t).                          (10r)
```

Table 2 shows the semantic accuracy of the learned rules, after 13 interactions with a human expert. In general, the average F1-score increased from 88% (Table 1) to 93%, i.e., overall task knowledge was refined. This is a consequence of the increased recall (90% vs. 93%). Specifically, axioms for actions improved or maintained the same performance achieved from offline learning. About the effects of actions, `at(A, ring, C)` achieved lower performance. A closer look at finally learned axioms for the corresponding initiating conditions, in equations (10k)-(10l), the atoms start to be grounded when either `move(A, ring, C)` action is executed, or the arm which cannot reach the peg moves to the center for transfer (in this case, indeed, the other arm reaches the ring at the transfer location). These initiating conditions are complete for the atom, and extend the only partial knowledge encoded in the original axioms learned offline (9). However, the terminating conditions in equations (10i)-(10j) only specify, respectively, that `at(A, ring, C)` stops holding when, at transfer location, the other arm moves to the peg to place the ring, or the ring is released on a peg. Compared with ground-truth axioms

Table 2 Semantic validity results (median ± IQR range). We aggregate the results for `init` and `term` conditions for effects of actions. In brackets, we mark the atoms for which F1-score is invariant with "=", and the ones with better performance with "+"

$x \in A \cup P$	Pr	Rec	$F1$
`move(A, ring, C)`	0.50 – 1.00	1.00 – 0.00	0.67 – 1.00
`move(A, peg, C)`	1.00 – 1.00	1.00 – 0.00	**0.93 – 1.00**(+)
`move(A, center, C)`	1.00 – 1.00	1.00 – 0.00	1.00 – 1.00(=)
`grasp(A, ring, C)`	1.00 – 0.00	1.00 – 0.50	1.00 – 1.00
`extract(A, ring, C)`	1.00 – 0.00	1.00 – 0.00	1.00 – 0.00(=)
`release(A)`	1.00 – 0.00	1.00 – 0.00	**1.00 – 0.00**(+)
`closed_gripper(A)`	1.00 – 0.00	1.00 – 0.00	1.00 – 0.00(=)
`at(A, center)`	1.00 – 0.00	0.83 – 1.00	**0.90 – 1.00**(+)
`at(A, ring, C)`	1.00 – 0.33	0.63 – 0.89	0.29 – 1.00(=)
`at(A, peg, C)`	1.00 – 0.00	0.75 – 1.00	0.83 – 1.00
`placed(ring, C1, peg, C2)`	1.00 – 0.00	1.00 – 0.00	1.00 – 0.00(=)
Mean	**0.95**	**0.93**(+)	**0.93**(+)

(2k)-(2m), these terminating conditions are still incomplete, since `at(A, ring, C)` should stop holding *whenever* `A` *moves away*. Collecting examples for all such occurrences would require more task iterations and variants. Moreover, these considerations hold for all atoms representing the current location of arms, thus justifying the slightly worse performance achieved for `at(A, peg, C)` (higher IQR). The median improvement on `at(A, center)`, instead, rose from the scarce examples for `transfer(A, center, C)` in the dataset for offline learning (only 5 instances in scenarios depicted in Fig. 2). Thus, while the results for the action did not vary after the online ASP refinement, the results for its effect improved.

3.4 Planning Performance Results

Given Π^e, Π^l as in axioms (2) and (10), respectively, we wanted to assess whether they are actually effective and efficient for planning in ARS.

To this aim, similarly to the previous experiments, we generated 1000 random contexts consisting of atoms in $H(P \cup A)$. We then used Clingo to compute corresponding plans, and compared the planning time and plan size (i.e., the number of actions to be executed to accomplish the task). Figure 3 shows the results (mean ± standard deviation for clusters of contexts resulting in plans of the same length, when using Π^e). Null plan size was only achieved with Π^e in 6 cases. This corresponds to contexts where Clingo was not able to compute a feasible plan within a maximum allowed time of 600 s. Results show that Π^l (Learned curve) entails plans of simi-

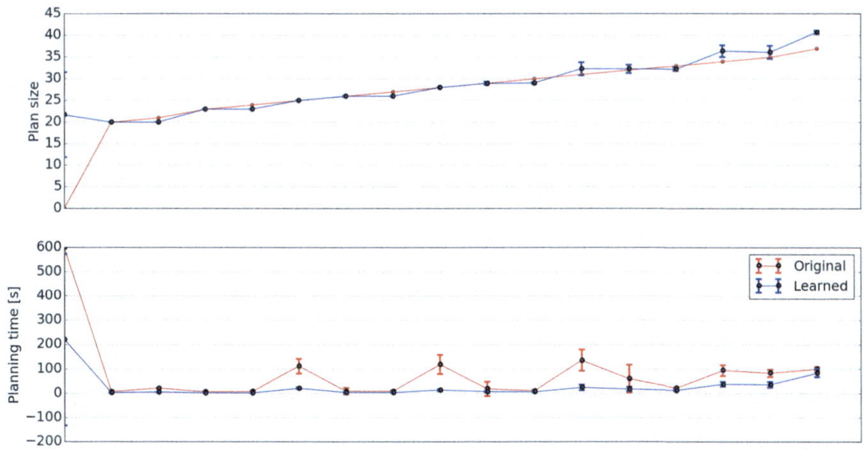

Fig. 3 Comparison between learned and original axioms in simulation for scenarios that involve sequential execution of actions

lar length as Π^e (Original curve), but Clingo required significantly less time (up to $\approx$ 100 s less for longer plans) to compute them.

4 Discussion

Preliminary experiments on the paradigmatic ring transfer task have shown the feasibility of an interpretable (hence more trustworthy and reliable) approach to planning and learning in ARS with logic programming than other machine learning approaches. Several challenges remain to be addressed.

Our methodology can be extended to account for probabilistic [41] and temporal logic [42] expressiveness, in order to represent more complex surgical knowledge. While similar solutions have been already explored for robotic deliberation [7], their applicability is still limited because of the computational inefficiency of logical reasoning.

We believe that the combination of logical learning from examples (via ILP) and from expert manuals or reports of real surgical procedures (e.g., with natural language processing [43]) has the potential to increase the accuracy and generality of learned knowledge, fostering the real application of our system in the operating room of the future.

References

1. Ingrand, F., Ghallab, M.: Deliberation for autonomous robots: a survey. Artif. Intell. **247**, 10–44 (2017)
2. Ghallab, M., Nau, D., Traverso, P.: Automated Planning and Acting. Cambridge University Press (2016)
3. K. Rajan, F. Py, J. Barreiro, Towards deliberative control in marine robotics. In: Marine Robot Autonomy, pp. 91–175. Springer (2013)
4. Matarić, M.J.: Situated robotics. Encyclopedia Cogn. Sci. (2006)
5. Proposal for a regulation of the European parliament and of the council laying down harmonised rules on artificial intelligence (artificial intelligence act) and amending certain union legislative acts (2021). https://eur-lex.europa.eu/legal-content/EN/TXT/?uri=CELEX:52021PC0206. Accessed 15 Feb. 2025
6. Lloyd, J.W.: Foundations of Logic Programming. Springer Science and Business Media (2012)
7. Meli, D., Nakawala, H., Fiorini, P.: Logic programming for deliberative robotic task planning. Artif. Intell. Rev. **56**(9), 9011–9049 (2023)
8. Erdem, E., Patoglu, V.: Applications of action languages in cognitive robotics. In: Correct Reasoning, pp. 229–246. Springer (2012)
9. Lifschitz, V.: What is answer set programming? AAAI **8**, 1594–1597 (2008)
10. McDermott, D., Doyle, J.: Non-monotonic logic i. Artif. Intell. **13**(1–2), 41–72 (1980)
11. van Amsterdam, B., Clarkson, M.J., Stoyanov, D.: Gesture recognition in robotic surgery: a review. IEEE Trans. Biomed. Eng. **68**(6) (2021)
12. Muggleton, S., De Raedt, L.: Inductive logic programming: theory and methods. J. Logic Program. **19**, 629–679 (1994)
13. Soper, N.J., Fried, G.M.: The fundamentals of laparoscopic surgery: its time has come. Bull. Am. Coll. Surg. **93**(9), 30–32 (2008)
14. Ginesi, M., Meli, D., Nakawala, H.C. Roberti, A., Fiorini, P.: A knowledge-based framework for task automation in surgery. In: 2019 19th International Conference on Advanced Robotics, pp. 37–42, Dec. 2019
15. Ginesi, M., Meli, D., Roberti, A., Sansonetto, N., Fiorini, P.: Autonomous task planning and situation awareness in robotic surgery. In: IEEE/RSJ International Conference on Intelligent Robots and Systems, pp. 3144–3150. IEEE (2020)
16. Meli, D., Fiorini, P., Sridharan, M.: Towards inductive learning of surgical task knowledge: a preliminary case study of the peg transfer task. Procedia Comput. Sci. **176**, 440–449 (2020)
17. Meli, D., Tagliabue, E., Dall'Alba, D., Fiorini, P.: Autonomous tissue retraction with a biomechanically informed logic based framework. In: International Symposium on Medical Robotics, pp. 1–7. IEEE (2021)
18. Meli, D., Sridharan, M., Fiorini, P.: Inductive learning of answer set programs for autonomous surgical task planning. Machine Learning, pp. 1–25 (2021)
19. Meli, D., Fiorini, P.: Unsupervised identification of surgical robotic actions from small non-homogeneous datasets. IEEE Robot. Autom. Lett. **6**(4), 8205–8212 (2021)
20. Tagliabue, E., Meli, D., Dall'Alba, D., Fiorini, P.: Deliberation in autonomous robotic surgery: a framework for handling anatomical uncertainty. In: 2022 International Conference on Robotics and Automation (ICRA), pp. 11080–11086. IEEE (2022)
21. Meli, D., Fiorini, P.: Inductive learning of robot task knowledge from raw data and online expert feedback. Mach. Learn. **114**(4), 91 (2025)
22. Kazanzides, P., Chen, Z., Deguet, A., Fischer, G.S., Taylor, R.H., DiMaio, S.P.: An open-source research kit for the da vinci® surgical system. In: 2014 IEEE international conference on robotics and automation (ICRA), pp. 6434–6439. IEEE (2014)
23. Da-vinci (2025). https://www.intuitive.com/en-us. Accessed 15 Feb. 2025
24. McDermott, D., Ghallab, M., Howe, A., Knoblock, C., Ram, A., Veloso, M., Weld, D., Wilkins, D.: Pddl-the Planning Domain Definition Language (1998)
25. Erdem, E., Gelfond, M., Leone, N.: Applications of answer set programming. AI Mag. **37**(3), 53–68 (2016)

26. Erdem, E., Patoglu, V.: Applications of asp in robotics. KI-Künstliche Intelligenz **32**(2–3), 143–149 (2018)
27. Barwise, J.: An introduction to first-order logic. In: Studies in Logic and the Foundations of Mathematics, vol. 90, pp. 5–46. Elsevier (1977)
28. Humberstone, I.L.: From worlds to possibilities. J. Philosoph. Logic 313–339 (1981)
29. Doherty, P., Lukaszewicz, W., Szalas, A.: Efficient reasoning using the local closed-world assumption. In: International Conference on Artificial Intelligence: Methodology, Systems, and Applications, pp. 49–58. Springer (2000)
30. Calimeri, F., Faber, W., Gebser, M., Ianni, G., Kaminski, R., Krennwallner, T., Leone, N., Maratea, M., Ricca, F., Schaub, T.: Asp-core-2 input language format. Theory Pract. Logic Program. **20**(2), 294–309 (2020)
31. Shanahan, M.: Solving the Frame Problem: a Mathematical Investigation of the Common Sense Law of Inertia. MIT Press (1997) <error l="308" c="Invalid command: paragraph not started." />
32. Wielemaker, J., Schrijvers, T., Triska, M., Lager, T.: Swi-prolog. Theory Pract. Logic Program. **12**(1–2), 67–96 (2012)
33. Gebser, M., Kaminski, R., Kaufmann, B., Schaub, T.: Multi-shot asp solving with clingo. Theory Pract. Logic Program. **19**(1), 27–82 (2019)
34. Adadi, A.: A survey on data-efficient algorithms in big data era. J. Big Data **8**(1), 24 (2021)
35. Maier-Hein, L., Vedula, S.S., Speidel, S., Navab, N., Kikinis, R., Park, A., Eisenmann, M., Feussner, H., Forestier, G., Giannarou, S., et al.: Surgical data science for next-generation interventions. Nat. Biomed. Eng. **1**(9), 691–696 (2017)
36. Law, M., Russo, A., Broda, K.: The ILASP System for Learning Answer set Programs (2015). www.ilasp.com. Accessed 15 Feb. 2025
37. Sakama, C., Inoue, K.: Brave induction: a logical framework for learning from incomplete information. Mach. Learn. **76**, 3–35 (2009)
38. Law, M.: Conflict-driven inductive logic programming. Theory Pract. Logic Program. **23**(2), 387–414 (2023)
39. Kowalski, R., Sergot, M.: A logic-based calculus of events. N. Gener. Comput. **4**, 67–95 (1986)
40. Lalys, F., Jannin, P.: Surgical process modelling: a review. Int. J. Comput. Assist. Radiol. Surg. **9**(3), 495–511 (2014)
41. De Raedt, L., Kimmig, A.: Probabilistic (logic) programming concepts. Mach. Learn. **100**, 5–47 (2015)
42. Wongpiromsarn, T., Topcu, U., Murray, R.M.: Receding horizon temporal logic planning. IEEE Trans. Autom. Control **57**(11), 2817–2830 (2012)
43. Bombieri, M., Meli, D., Dall'Alba, D., Rospocher, M., Fiorini, P.: Mapping natural language procedures descriptions to linear temporal logic templates: an application in the surgical robotic domain. In: Applied Intelligence, vol. 53, no. 22, pp. 26351–26363 (2023)

Towards Surgical Task Planning from Text

Marco Bombieri

Abstract This Chapter aims to introduce a use case and show how, after having defined some constraints on the language, the SRL method, together with other rule-based methods, can help the engineer write the logic rules needed to define the plan for the robot. In particular, we propose AUTOMATE (lAngUage To lOgic teMplATEs), a pipeline that helps the translation of natural language instructions to linear temporal logic (LTL). This chapter describes the use of a controlled language and a general English language model: state of the art in autonomous surgical robotics mainly uses two tasks as benchmarks, i.e., peg transfer and tissue retraction, presented later. Although performed with surgical robots, they are still simplified tasks whose description does not require particularly complex surgical expressions. Nonetheless, as the surgical robotics community moves to more realistic and complex benchmarks requiring more specialized surgical language, the models developed in the previous chapters will allow for more in-depth language understanding. This Chapter aims to empirically show that SRL technology is a fundamental tool for extracting logical entities from procedural natural language text and to highlight the technological deficiencies for achieving a completely automated translation.

1 Language Constraints for Surgical Texts

We proposed a set of language constraints for writing procedural descriptions that preserve much of the generality of surgical domain language while enhancing compatibility with NLP tools. The following choices are made for our benchmark texts:

- The elements of the robot are described with incremental numbering (e.g. *first arm* and *second arm*);

M. Bombieri (✉)
Department of Computer Science, University of Verona, Verona, Italy
e-mail: marco.bombieri_01@univr.it

Department of Information Engineering and Computer Science, University of Trento, Trento, Italy

P. Fiorini (ed.), *Towards Autonomous Robotic Surgery*, Springer Tracts in Advanced Robotics 161, https://doi.org/10.1007/978-3-032-04247-7_4

- The *robotic setup* is described in the first paragraph; docking of instruments to the robot can be only described by verbs such as *equip*, *place*, *install*, *use*, *mount* and *attach*;
- *verbs* are expressed in active or passive form, at present or imperative tense. Verbs such as use and synonyms are allowed to introduce the main action;
- The list of usable *instruments* is a-priori known (e.g. described in state-of-the-art ontologies such as [1]);
- *instruments* may or may not coincide with *agents*, i.e. with those who perform the action;
- *conditions* can be only expressed with *if / otherwise* and *in case / otherwise* statements;
- *temporal sequences* can only contain *then* and *once* connectors;
- *loop iterations* can only be expressed with *until / repeat* constructs; the action to be repeated must be explicitly indicated and has to coincide with a verb already mentioned before in the text;
- The use of *synonyms* is limited to those statically recognized by the state-of-the-art resources, such as WordNet [2];
- Standard logic connectors (e.g. *and, or*) are allowed in texts to specify more or alternative actions in the same sentence.

2 The AUTOMATE Pipeline

A schematic representation of the proposed pipeline is shown in Fig. 1. The first step of the pipeline is *filtering procedural knowledge* from textual resources to select only robot setup information and procedural sentences. These are processed by an SRL module and some filtering rules that highlight the *main action* of each sentence together *with procedural entities* such as agent, object, instrument and causal/temporal information. The output of this module is then automatically translated to *LTL formalism*.

2.1 Synonyms and Natural Language Variability

We used WordNet's synsets [2] to identify and cluster synonyms. WordNet is a large lexical database of English verbs, adjectives and adverbs, organized into sets of cognitive synonyms (synsets).

WordNet is designed for general English and therefore may fail to fully cover all the terms used in the surgical language: we leaved a WordNet specialization to the domain as a future work. Anyway, this section is meant to emphasize that a module of reduction of natural language variability through resolution of synonyms is fundamental to structure the natural language description of a procedure.

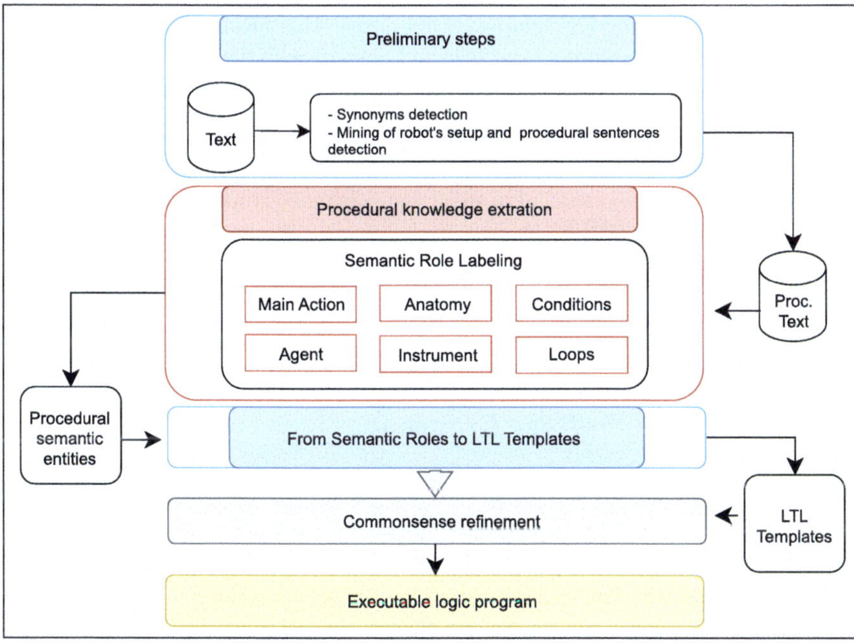

Fig. 1: Overview of the proposed AUTOMATE approach for automatic translation of procedural texts to executable ASP rules

2.2 *Identifying Robot Setup and Procedural Sentences*

Before pruning non-procedural sentences from texts, we needed to extract robotic setup information. As explained in Sect. 1, this knowledge is contained in the first paragraph of surgical text descriptions and we assumed to know in advance the list of all instrument's names: this is not a strict requirement since surgical instruments are common to most procedures, and ontologies, as the one presented in [1], already contain general surgical knowledge, in particular about surgical instruments. We then built a semantic connection between arms and instruments, searching for verbs listed in Sect. 1 (e.g. equip, place, install, use and synonyms). In this way, arms and instruments could be used interchangeably in the procedural description.

As an example, let us consider the text of the peg transfer task, in which the surgeon is the agent:

> The setup has three arms.
> The first and second arms are equipped with grippers, while the third arm mounts an endoscopic camera for vision.

Assuming *camera* and *grippers* to be known as surgical instruments, they are linked to *third arm* and *first and second arm*, respectively, after the words *equipped* and *mounted* are identified as setup-evoking terms. This means that in the descriptions, we can use, for example, *third arm* and *camera* with the same meaning.

Afterward, we exploited the methodology proposed in Sect. 3 to select only procedural sentences in surgical texts. For instance, let us consider the following sentence from the text for tissue retraction with the robot as the agent:

> A flap of adipose tissue is attached to surrounding anatomies at some points (APs), and covers a region of interest (ROI).

The sentence describes the anatomical setting and, being classified as non-procedural, it is not processed further.

2.3 *Procedural Knowledge Extraction*

For each identified procedural sentence, we extracted the actions and their relevant semantic information, which represented the procedural knowledge needed for LTL template extraction.

To this purpose, we exploited PropBank-based SRL, described in Chap. 2 and the rules defined on the language constraints presented in Sect. 1.

2.3.1 Selecting Main Action

Given a procedural sentence, we first used Part-Of-Speech (POS) algorithm [3] to identify verbs (hence potential actions). However, multiple verbs may occur in a sentence. For instance, consider the following excerpt from the text for peg transfer:

> If the ring is close to first arm, the surgeon uses first arm to reach it; [...]

Three verbs are identified in this sentence, i.e. *is*, *uses* and *reach*. However, only *reach* is the main action. In order to identify it, we proceeded as follows: first, we excluded *-ing* forms, modals and auxiliaries (e.g. *is*), as well as verbs such as *use* and its synonyms, which only introduce main task actions; we then excluded all the candidate verbs that appear in a span of text that SRL has labeled with semantic roles referred to causal and temporal relations (c.f., next section). This approach is robust with respect to different verbal forms, e.g. passive verbs.

2.3.2 Identifying Semantic Roles

Semantic roles from SRL must be matched to the relevant meanings for task procedural description, i.e.:

- the *agent* who performs the action
- the *object* (e.g. anatomical part) undergoing the action
- the *instrument* (or *robotic arm*) used to perform the action
- *causal and temporal relations* such as conditions, temporal sequences and loops

Assuming the language constraints from Sect. 1, we combined the spotting of connectors (e.g. *if, until*) and semantic roles to detect causal/temporal information. In particular, for detecting conditions, spans of text labeled by the SRL with ArgM-ADV (adverbial modifiers) or ArgM-DIS (discourse modifiers) and respecting the form presented in Sect. 1 (i.e. containing *if/otherwise* or *in case* words) were selected. A similar approach was adopted for loops and temporal sequences, by selecting spans of text labeled with ArgM-TMP (temporal markers) and containing connectors (i) *then* and *once* for temporal sequences and (ii) *repeat/until* for loops.

In order to identify agents, objects and instruments, we needed a different strategy for *robot-as-agent* and *surgeon-as-agent* scenarios. In the first scenario, the robot' arm or instrument plays the role of *agent* and thus span of texts labeled with Arg0 are selected. Instead, the *object* of the action always plays the role of proto-patient, and thus spans of text labeled as Arg1 are selected. For instance, in the tissue retraction text, the sentence *The camera selects a point on the tissue if it is far from APs.* was labeled as:

> [Arg0: The camera] [V: selects] [Arg1: a point on the tissue] [ArgM-ADV: if it is far from APs].

Thus, by looking at the arguments labeled with Arg0 (*camera*) and Arg1 (*point on the tissue*), the *agent* and the *object* of the action (*to select*) were identified respectively.

When the surgeon is the agent, the situation is more complex because the instrument/arm is not the agent (Arg0) and, if mentioned, it occurs in other roles of the corresponding action. In particular, the instrument/arm can be contained either in a core argument (Arg2 or Arg3) or a non-core argument (ArgM-MNR), depending on the specific verb. For instance, in the peg transfer scenario, the sentence *First, the surgeon identifies rings via camera* was annotated via SRL as:

> [ArgM-TMP: First], [Arg0: the surgeon] [V: identifies] [Arg1: rings] [ArgM-MNR: via camera].

The span *via camera* was labeled as an ArgM-MNR.

In this case, we relied on available resources (e.g. a knowledge base or ontology such as [1]) listing surgical instruments and we search the sentence for mentions of these instruments within arguments labeled as Arg-MNR, Arg2, or Arg3 by SRL. In the considered example, *camera* is a candidate instrument, it was labeled as ArgM-MNR, and thus was recognized as the instrument for the *identify* action.

The use of SRL also for instrument detection was necessarily performed since not all mentions of medical instruments in a sentence refer to the actual usage of an instrument to perform the main action. In particular, it was applied after identifying the candidate arguments possibly containing the instrument. For instance, the sentence *The surgeon uses the first arm to grasp scissors* mentions *scissors*, a surgical instrument, but without referring to its usage to perform the action herein described (*to grasp*). Indeed, SRL returned the following annotations:

[Arg0: The surgeon] uses the first arm to [V: grasp] [Arg1: scissors].

That is, *scissors* was correctly recognized as the *thing grasped* (Arg1 of *grasp*), and not as the instrument used to perform the grasping (i.e., Arg2, Arg3, or ArgM-MNR).

2.4 From SRL to LTL Relations

The output of SRL highlights relevant semantic information about task knowledge. This section shows how this information is automatically translated to LTL logic templates representing procedural relations for the task. Consider the following example sentences from the texts of our benchmark tasks described in [4]:

(A1) In case the point is close to first arm, point is reached by first arm; otherwise, the second arm reaches point.
(A2) Then, the gripper grasps the tissue.
(A3) The arm lifts the tissue until a maximum height is reached, or maximum force is reached, or the ROI is visible.

The output of SRL and filtering steps described before is, respectively:

(B1): [ArgM-ADV: In case the point is close to first arm,] [Arg1: the point] is [V: reached] [Arg0: by first arm;] [ArgM-ADV: otherwise] [Arg0: the second arm] [V: reaches] [Arg1: the point.]
(B2): [ArgM-TMP: Then,] [Arg0: the gripper] [V: grasps] [Arg1: the tissue.]
(B3): [Arg0: The arm] [V: lifts] [Arg1: the tissue] [ArgM-TMP: until a maximum height is reached, or maximum force is reached, or the ROI is visible.]

In order to highlight relevant semantic entities (verb, agents, objects, and temporal/causal information), these were re-written in a more convenient predicate form as follows, with the verb as the name of the predicate with ordered arguments *agent-object-additional information*:

(C 1):
reach(the first arm, the point, ADV:in case the point is close to first arm)
reach(the second arm, a point on the tissue, ADV:otherwise)

(C 2):
grasp(first arm, the tissue, TMP:then)

(C 3):
raise(first arm, the tissue, TMP:until a maximum height is reached, or maximum force is reached, or the ROI is visible.

Annotations *(C 1)* correctly split sentence *(A 1)* into two main *reach* actions, having either *first arm* or *second arm* as agent and *a point on the tissue* as object/anatomical target.

SRL correctly identified the conditions *if/otherwise* as ADV roles. Sentence *(A 2)* led to annotation *(C 2)*, where the temporal relation *then* was also marked. The agent *gripper* was automatically translated to *first arm*, following instruments recognition from the robot's setup description (see Sect. 2.2). Finally, in sentence *(A 3)*, the *until* temporal relation was recognized. Furthermore, the main action *lift* was automatically translated to the synonym *raise*, which was arbitrarily chosen as the representative lemma of the synset in WordNet (see Sect. 2.1) containing both *lift* and *raise*.

Given the SRL output, we translated logic/temporal connectors defined in the language constraints to corresponding LTL operators. This can be done automatically, assuming that such an injective map existed. We obtained the following LTL rule templates:

```
(D 1):
reach(first arm, a point on the tissue) ← the point is close to first arm
reach(second arm, a point on the tissue) ← ¬the point is close to first arm
```

```
(D 2):
○ grasp(first arm, tissue)
```

```
(D 3):

raise(first arm, tissue) 𝒰 (maximum height is reached ∨ maximum force is reached ∨ the ROI is visible)
```

where $\mathcal{U}$ denotes *until* operator, $\circ$ is the *next* operator, $\leftarrow$ is the logic *implication*, $\vee$ is logic *disjunction* and $\neg$ is logic *negation*.

2.5 From LTL Templates to Executable Logic Program

LTL templates encode task actions, agents, relevant objects/anatomical parts, and temporal/causal relations, which determine the flow of execution. However, they must be translated to the syntax of a specific logic program, in order to actually implement an autonomous task planner for robotics.

A logic program represents a domain of interest with a *signature* and *axioms*. The signature is the alphabet of the domain, defining its relevant attributes. Attributes may be *statics*, i.e. domain attributes whose values do not change over time, or *fluents*, i.e. time-dependent domain attributes. Attributes may be *terms*, *atoms*, predicates of terms (e.g. `atom(t1, ..., tn)` is an atom with terms $t_{1,\ldots,n}$ as arguments), and their classical or default negations (respectively, ¬a, meaning that a is false, or `not a`, meaning that a is not known to be true). Values of terms are *constants* (either integers, Booleans or strings). A term whose value is assigned is *ground*, and an atom is ground if its terms are grounded.

Axioms are logical relations between attributes. A causal rule h ← b_1, ..., b_n defines preconditions $b_{1,\ldots,n}$ (*body* of the rule) for the *head* h. A rule with an empty head defines a constraint, meaning that body atoms cannot be ground concurrently. Axioms can also represent temporal relations between atoms, thanks to the definition of an explicit time variable t for fluents,[1] as discussed in Chap. 3. For instance, `a(t)` ← `b(t-1)` is equivalent to the *next* operator in LTL, meaning that a occurs at the subsequent time step with respect to b; similarly, `a(t)` ← `a(t-1)`, ¬ `b(t)` encodes LTL *release* operator, meaning that a keeps holding until b does not.

In the classical representation of task knowledge, statics typically define agents and invariant environmental resources, while fluents are actions and dynamic environmental features. Axioms encode task specification, capturing the causal relations between the agents and the environment, following the pattern *precondition* → *action* → *effect* with *constraints* proposed in the Planning Domain Definition Language (PDDL) [6]. As an example, consider LTL relation *(D 1)*, defining the precondition for *reaching* action. Assuming that *the point is close to first arm* is encoded with an atom `close(first arm, tissue point)`, being `first arm` and `tissue point` constant values for domain variables `Agent` and `Object`, respectively, we can write the following axiom:

```
reach(Agent, Object, t) ← close(Agent, Object, t).
```

LTL templates can then be automatically implemented in the formalism of a logic program with the following steps:

- implementation of LTL operators in the specific logic programming syntax;
- definition of variables and atoms, with variables lifting information retrieved from SRL (e.g. *reach(Agent, Object)*, which can be lifted from *reach(first arm, tissue)*).

Representing operators is trivial since they are implemented in any logic program. The second step, however, requires yet missing information. In particular, underlined parts in LTL templates *(D 1–D 3)* represent low-level concepts and variables, which at the moment need to be encoded by a logic programming expert manually. They mostly represent commonsense knowledge (e.g. *the point is close to first*

[1] There exist logic programming frameworks, e.g. *telingo* [5], which implement LTL operators. However, we consider the explicit temporal variable definition to adhere to ASP syntax, which is more popular in the robotics and AI community.

arm, associated with the notion of *spatial distance*, or ROI visibility and maximum force measurement), which are not related to the specific procedure, but rather to the generic surgical and robotic domains. Hence, similarly to instrument knowledge (see Sect. 2.2), we can assume these concepts are stored and retrieved from the clinical domain [7] or even general-scope ontologies [8], in order to make the translation to an executable logic program possible.

2.6 Application of AUTOMATE

In [4], we empirically tested the utility of AUTOMATE. In other words, we verified that the extracted task knowledge is correct and general enough to compute suitable plans for our benchmark robotic tasks, given any possible initial environmental context. This required:

1. implementation of LTL templates into a specific logic programming language for autonomous planning;
2. implementation of low-level routines for robotic motion planning/control and perception, needed for environmental context evaluation and instantiations of LTL predicates;
3. an environment to replicate the benchmark tasks and the robot.

To address the first requirement, we implemented LTL templates in the formalism of ASP, specifically with Clingo 5 [9] software for ASP representation and solving (i.e. plan computation). For the second requirement, we adopted the framework for integrated planning and execution of surgical robotic tasks proposed in [10], including the dVRK and vision sensors. For the third requirement, we created simulation environments for the peg transfer and tissue retraction.

We empirically evaluated the quality of the extracted task specifications in terms of *planning success* and *planning computational performance*.

The planning success measured the percentage of successful generation of task plans in a set of random environmental contexts. It was important that random contexts were representative of the variability of the task, hence lead to the generation of multiple workflows of execution. Hence, we randomize relevant variables for our two benchmark tasks, for a total of 100 different contexts for each task.

The computational performance was calculated as the time required by Clingo solver to find a first plan (i.e. neglecting possible re-planning in case bad events occur), given some initial environmental context. We evaluated this metric for increasing size of each domain of interest, which affects the number of variables/atoms to be grounded by ASP. For each complexity class of context configuration, we replicated 20 executions to calculate the mean and variance of Clingo's planning time. In this way, we could analyze the evolution of computational effort as task complexity increased.

For both metrics, we compared the performance of the extracted ASP program with the ASP task description written by an expert in both of the domain and the logic syntax, following PDDL-like classical representation [11]. Standard task descriptions from PDDL do not always match LTL formulas extracted from texts with NLP. For example, consider relation *D 2*. It specifies that *grasp* shall occur after the previous action (*reach*). This can be encoded as:

```
grasp(Agent, Object, t) ← reach(Agent, Object, t-1).
```

In classical PDDL representation, a specific effect for *reach* should be defined, which then acts as a precondition to *reach*. An example is provided below:

```
at(Agent, Object, t) ← reach(Agent, Object, t-1).
grasp(Agent, Object, t) ← at(Agent, Object, t).
```

where `at(Agent, Object, t)` is a fluent representing the location of an arm with respect to an object. Detailed experiments and results are reported in [4].

3 Discussion

Bombieri et al. [4] shows that it is possible to extract procedural information with NLP techniques, in the form of LTL relations, from text written by a domain expert. The extracted knowledge can then be easily translated into any logic programming formalism for autonomous planning. A solver for the task planning problem (Clingo in our experiments) is then able to compute a suitable plan, given any random initial context, with a similar percentage of success as a logic program written by an expert both of the domain and the logic paradigm. Furthermore, [4] found that the logic program extracted from text is computationally more convenient for the solver since less time is needed for plan computation, thanks to the more efficient formalization with respect to PDDL-like specifications in the *precondition-action-effect* paradigm. Some of the issues that still remain to be addressed are indicated in the following. First, to automate the entire process without requiring human intervention, we should deal with the intrinsic incompleteness of natural language descriptions that often leave some knowledge unsaid. This is the case, for instance, of specific encoding of environmental fluents (see Sect. 2.4) that must be filled manually: at the moment, this pipeline significantly helps the programmer to write a logic program encoding effective task representation, for example, it can identify actions, agents, relevant environmental/domain entities as target objects and anatomies, and semantic roles which can be directly mapped to LTL syntax. Hence, the programmer shall only convert LTL expressions to a specific logic program syntax (e.g., ASP), with no required awareness of the specific task/surgical procedure. Second, encoding environmental information often involves commonsense knowledge –such as spatial relationships–or broad domain knowledge, like general surgical concepts, rather than details specific to the task. This makes automatic processing challenging. A detailed analysis of commonsense concepts can be found in [12] and discussed in Chap. 8. Finally, the extracted information will need to be mapped onto predefined ontologies to ensure proper knowledge grounding, as shown in [13].

References

1. Gibaud, B., Forestier, G., Feldmann, C., Ferrigno, G., Gonçalves, P., Haidegger, T., Julliard, C., Katić, D., Kenngott, H., Maier-Hein, L., et al.: Toward a standard ontology of surgical process models. Int. J. Comput. Assist. Radiol. Surg. **13**(9), 1397–1408 (2018)
2. Soergel, D.: WordNet. An Electronic Lexical Database. MIT Press, Oct. 1998
3. Bird, S.: NLTK: the natural language toolkit. In: Proceedings of the COLING/ACL 2006 Interactive Presentation Sessions (Sydney, Australia), pp. 69–72. Association for Computational Linguistics, July 2006
4. Bombieri, M., Meli, D., Dall'Alba, D., Rospocher, M., Fiorini, P.: Mapping natural language procedures descriptions to linear temporal logic templates: an application in the surgical robotic domain. Appl. Intell. **53**(22), 26351–26363 (2023)
5. Cabalar, P., Kaminski, R., Morkisch, P., Schaub, T.: telingo= asp+ time. In: International Conference on Logic Programming and Nonmonotonic Reasoning, pp. 256–269 Springer (2019)
6. McDermott, D., Ghallab, M., Howe, A., Knoblock, C., Ram, A., Veloso, M., Weld, D., Wilkins, D.: Pddl-the planning domain definition language (1998)
7. Pérez-Rey, D., Maojo, V., García-Remesal, M., Alonso-Calvo, R., Billhardt, H., Martín-Sánchez, F., Sousa, A.: Ontofusion: ontology-based integration of genomic and clinical databases. Comput. Biol. Med. **36**(7–8), 712–730 (2006)
8. Lemaignan, S., Ros, R., Mösenlechner, L., Alami, R., Beetz, M.: Oro, a knowledge management platform for cognitive architectures in robotics. In: 2010 IEEE/RSJ International Conference on Intelligent Robots and Systems, pp. 3548–3553. IEEE (2010)
9. Gebser, M., Kaminski, R., Kaufmann, B., Ostrowski, M., Schaub, T., Wanko, P.: Theory solving made easy with clingo 5. In: Technical Communications of the 32nd International Conference on Logic Programming (ICLP 2016), Schloss Dagstuhl-Leibniz-Zentrum fuer Informatik (2016)
10. Ginesi, M., Meli, D., Roberti, A., Sansonetto, N., Fiorini, P.: Autonomous task planning and situation awareness in robotic surgery. In: IEEE/RSJ International Conference on Intelligent Robots and Systems, pp. 3144–3150. IEEE (2020)
11. Kovacs, D.L.: Bnf definition of pddl 3.1. Unpublished manuscript from the IPC-2011 website (2011)
12. Tagliabue, E., Bombieri, M., Fiorini, P., Dall'Alba, D.: Autonomous robotic surgical systems: Needing common sense to achieve higher levels of autonomy [opinion]. IEEE Robot. Autom. Mag. **30**(3), 149–163 (2023)
13. Bombieri, M., Fiorini, P., Ponzetto, S.P., Rospocher, M.: Do LLMs dream of ontologies? ACM Trans. Intell. Syst. Technol. (2025)

Learning Surgical Gestures from Data

Michele Ginesi

Abstract In this chapter we develop methods to extract knowledge from data, in what we call "bottom-up" knowledge extraction. When we think about robot movements we usually think about optimized movements, that try to minimize the energy consumption, the time required for a task, or the stress (and consequent damage) on the motors. These optimizations can be achieved because the dynamical model of the robot allows to have a mathematical and physical description of these quantities to minimize. While this reasoning is true in industrial robotics, it becomes flawed when talking about surgical robotics. Indeed, in this scenario the goal is to perform a delicate procedure while maximizing the safety of the patient. The problem is that, while we are able to provide a mathematical description of the energy consumption and of the motor fatigue, there is not a way to define the 'patient safety' or the 'after-intervention patient health'. Additionally, while there is an exhaustive literature describing all the phases of an intervention, surgeons learn to move purely by practicing, building dexterity from experience. For these reasons, we decided to use a learning approach to describe the movements, called 'primitives' or 'surgemes'. In this way, we can learn the low-level movements that the robot should perform by imitating expert surgeons, trying to mimicking their movements. In particular, in Sect. 1 we present the framework we adopted to describe the kinematics, while in Sect. 2 we discuss the model used to extract these movements from data.

M. Ginesi (✉)
Department of Computer Science, University of Verona, Verona, Italy
e-mail: michele.ginesi@ieo.it

European Institute of Oncology, Milan, Italy

P. Fiorini (ed.), *Towards Autonomous Robotic Surgery*, Springer Tracts in Advanced Robotics 161, https://doi.org/10.1007/978-3-032-04247-7_5

When we think about robots movements we usually think about optimized movements, that try to minimize the energy consumption, the time required for a task, or the stress (and consequent damage) on the motors. These optimizations can be achieved because the dynamical model of the robot allows to have a mathematical and physical description of these quantities to minimize.

While this reasoning is true in industrial robotics, it becomes flawed when talking about surgical robotics. Indeed, in this scenario the goal is to perform a delicate procedure while maximizing the *safety* of the patient. The problem is that, while we are able to provide a mathematical description of the energy consumption and of the motor fatigue, there is not a way to define the 'patient safety' or the 'after-intervention patient health'.

Additionally, while there is an exhaustive literature describing all the phases of an intervention, surgeons learn to move purely by practicing, building dexterity from experience.

For these reasons, we decided to use a *learning approach* to describe the movements, called 'primitives' or 'surgemes'. In this way, we can learn the low-level movements that the robot should perform by imitating expert surgeons, trying to mimicking their movements.

In particular, in Sect. 1 we present the framework we adopted to describe the kinematics, while in Sect. 2 we discuss the model used to extract these movements from data.

1 Learning of Kinematics

Dynamic Movement Primitives (DMPs) [1–6] is a framework for trajectory learning based on a second-order Ordinary Differential Equation (ODE) of spring-mass-damper type in which a *forcing* (also called *perturbation*) term is "learned" in such a way to encode the shape of the trajectory of the solution.

During the *learning phase* a trajectory (or a set of trajectories) is recorded, and the forcing term is modeled so that the learned behavior resembles as close as possible the observation(s). Then, during the *execution phase*, the learned forcing term is used to generate new trajectories, allowing to change the initial and final positions, the speed of execution, while maintaining a trajectory of similar shape to the learned one, and guaranteeing convergence to the goal position.

We decided to use DMPs to encode surgical gestures because they are able to accurately imitate and replicate human movements, which is essential to encode the surgeon's dexterity.

The original formulation was proposed by Ijspeert et al. [1] and was later updated by Pastor et al. in 2009 [5] obtaining the following formulation

$$\begin{cases} \tau \dot{\mathbf{v}} = \mathbf{K}(\mathbf{g} - \mathbf{x}) - \mathbf{D}\mathbf{v} - \mathbf{K}(\mathbf{g} - \mathbf{x}_0)s + \mathbf{K}\mathbf{f}(s) & \text{(1a)} \\ \tau \dot{\mathbf{x}} = \mathbf{v} & \text{(1b)} \end{cases}$$

where vectors $\mathbf{x}, \mathbf{v} \in \mathbb{R}^d$ are the position and velocity of the system (in our case the robot end-effector), respectively.

Matrices $\mathbf{K} = \text{diag}(K_1, K_2, \ldots, K_d), \mathbf{D} = \text{diag}(D_1, D_2, \ldots, D_d) \in \mathbb{R}_+^{d \times d}$ are diagonal matrices satisfying $D_i = 2\sqrt{K_i}$. The matrices are diagonal in order to decouple the components x_i of the position. The condition $D_i = 2\sqrt{K_i}$ is needed to have a critically damped system in un-perturbed scenarios (i.e. $\mathbf{f}(s) = 0$). In this way, the system achieve the faster convergence to the goal position and is not subjected to oscillations.

Scalar $\tau \in \mathbb{R}^+$ is a temporal scaling factor that can be used to change the speed of execution of the system. Doubling the value of τ halves the speed of execution, thus doubling the duration.

Vectors $\mathbf{x}_0, \mathbf{g} \in \mathbb{R}^d$ are, respectively, the starting and goal positions. Changing this value allows to slow down or speed up the evolution of the system.

Scalar $s \in [0, 1)$ is a phase variable governed by the so-called *canonical system*

$$\tau \dot{s} = -\alpha s \tag{2}$$

where $\alpha \in \mathbb{R}_+$ is a parameter controlling the speed of decay of s. The canonical system's initial condition is $s(0) = 1$. The importance of the canonical system (2) relies in making the dynamical system (1a) with (2) an autonomous system, i.e. non directly dependent on time t. This allows to speed up or slow down the evolution of the system without any difficulty by simply changing the value of temporal scaling factor τ.

Function $\mathbf{f} : \mathbb{R}^d \rightarrow \mathbb{R}$ is a real-valued, non-linear *forcing* (also called *perturbation) term*. It is defined in terms of basis functions as

$$\mathbf{f}(s) = \frac{\sum_{i=0}^{N} \omega_i \psi_i(s)}{\sum_{i=0}^{N} \psi_i(s)} s, \tag{3}$$

where functions

$$\psi_i(s) = \exp\left(-h_i(s - c_i)^2\right), \quad i = 0, 1, \ldots, N \tag{4}$$

are *Gaussian Radial Basis Functions* (GRBFs) with centers c_i and widths h_i. Centers c_i are defined as

$$c_i = \exp\left(-\alpha\, i\, \frac{T}{N}\right), \quad i = 0, 1, \ldots, N, \tag{5}$$

while widths h_i are defined as [7]:

$$\begin{aligned} h_i &= \frac{\tilde{h}}{(c_{i+1} - c_i)^2}, \quad i = 0, 1, \ldots, N-1, \\ h_N &= h_{N-1}, \end{aligned} \tag{6}$$

where the value of $\tilde{h} \in \mathbb{R}_+$ determines the overlap between basis functions. This value is usually set to one [8, 9]: $\tilde{h} = 1$. Vectors $\boldsymbol{\omega}_i \in \mathbb{R}^d$, for $i = 0, 1, \dots, N$ are called *weights*.

During the *learning phase* a trajectory $\hat{\mathbf{y}}(t)$, $t \in [0, T]$ is shown and the weigths ω_i that best approximate it are computed via least squares optimization. In particular, for each component $\hat{y}(t)$, we define the matrix $\hat{\mathbf{Y}} = [\hat{\mathbf{y}}_t]_{t=0,1,\dots,M} \in \mathbb{R}$ whose components are the value of $\hat{y}(t)$ in $M + 1$ points of the discretized domain $[0, T]$. From this, we can use (1a) to compute the desired forcing term $\mathbf{f}(s)$ in each point of the discretization. In particular, we obtain the matrix $\mathbf{F} = [f_t^j]$ whose components are

$$f_t^j = f_j(s_t)$$

Let us also define the matrix $\boldsymbol{\Phi} = [\phi_{t,j}]_{t=0,1,\dots,M}^{j=0,1,\dots,N}$ whose components are

$$\phi_{t,j} = \frac{\psi_j(s(t))\, s(t)}{\sum_{k=0}^{N} \psi_k(s(t))}.$$

Then, the weights $\boldsymbol{\omega}_i$ are the rows of the matrix $\boldsymbol{\Omega}$ defined as

$$\boldsymbol{\Omega} = \boldsymbol{\Phi}^{\dagger}\mathbf{F},$$

where the dagger † denotes the pseudo-inverse operator.

During the *execution phase*, we simply solve numerically the dynamical system (1a), using the weights learned previously to compute the forcing term. Since the goal position can change during time, the system may need "more time" to reach convergence than the learned one. Thus, instead of solving the problem up to a final time, one may decide to let the system evolve until convergence to the goal is achieved within a given tolerance. In such case, the final part of the trajectory may not have an impactful forcing term, since $f(s(t)) \approx 0$ when $t \gg T$.

In Fig. 1 an example is shown. A desired behavior is used to compute the forcing term and the set of weights. Then, the resulting DMP is executed with the same starting position $\mathbf{x}_0$ as in the observed trajectory but different goal position. In particular, we run the DMP in two scenarios. In the first one, the new goal postion $\mathbf{g}'$ is set from the beginning of the DMP execution and it is maintained fixed. In the second one, the goal start in the same position $\mathbf{g}$ as in the observed behavior and starts moving linearly towards $\mathbf{g}'$. In both cases, the DMP converges towards the goal while retaining a trajectory of similar shape as the learned one.

1.1 Invariance Under Affine Transformations

A limit of DMPs is that the generaliziation to new starting and goal positions works properly only *locally*. Indeed, as it can be seen from Fig. 2, when the 'learned' goal

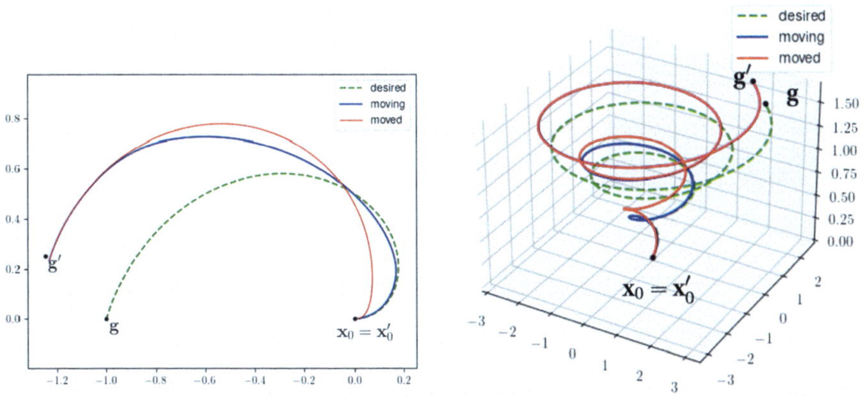

Fig. 1 Example of execution of a DMP in 2 (left) and 3 (right) dimensions. In both plots the green dashed line shows the desired trajectory. The solid lines show the trajectory of the learned DMP when the goal position $\mathbf{g}$ is changed. In particular, the red line is the trajectory obtained by fixing the goal in a new position at the start of the execution. The blue line, instead, has been obtained by moving the goal position. It starts in the same point as the learned behavior and moves linearly towards the new position. As it can been observed, in both cases the shape of the trajectory is retained

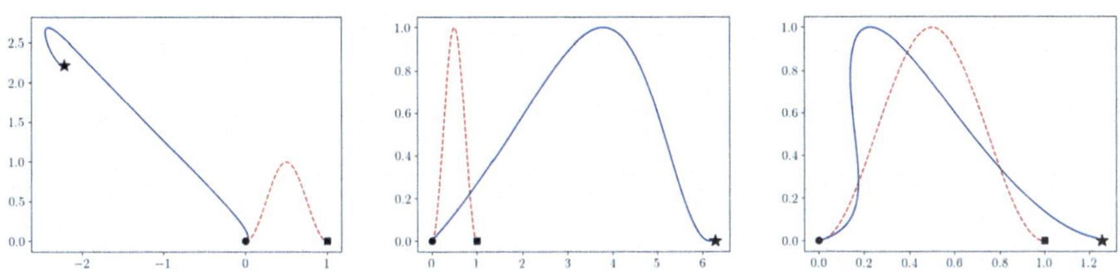

Fig. 2 Examples in which DMPs do not generalize properly to new goal positions. In all plots, the dashed red line shows the desired behavior, while the blue solid line shows the DMP execution with new goal position. The black dot denotes the starting position $\mathbf{x}_0$, the black square denotes the "learned" goal position $\mathbf{g}$, and the black star denotes the new goal position $\mathbf{g}'$

position and the new goal position differ by a large quantity, the resulting DMP is not able to retain the shape of the desired behavior.

Luckily, an important property of DMP formulation (1a) is the invariance under general invertible affine transformations.

Theorem 1.1 (Hoffmann et al. [10]) *DMP formulation (1a) is invariant under invertible affine transformations of the coordinate system.*

This property allows us to extend the generalization properties of DMPs *globally*. Indeed, following this idea, we present the *extended DMPs* [11] as

$$\tau \begin{cases} \dot{\mathbf{v}} = \mathbf{K}^{\mathbf{g}-\mathbf{x}_0}_{\mathbf{g}^\star-\mathbf{x}_0^\star}(\mathbf{g}-\mathbf{x}) - \mathbf{D}^{\mathbf{g}-\mathbf{x}_0}_{\mathbf{g}^\star-\mathbf{x}_0^\star}\mathbf{v} - \mathbf{K}^{\mathbf{g}-\mathbf{x}_0}_{\mathbf{g}^\star-\mathbf{x}_0^\star}(\mathbf{g}-\mathbf{x}_0)s + \mathbf{K}^{\mathbf{g}-\mathbf{x}_0}_{\mathbf{g}^\star-\mathbf{x}_0^\star}\mathbf{S}^{\mathbf{g}-\mathbf{x}_0}_{\mathbf{g}^\star-\mathbf{x}_0^\star}\mathbf{f}(s) & \text{(7a)} \\ \tau\dot{\mathbf{x}} = \mathbf{v} & \text{(7b)} \end{cases}$$

where we define

$$\mathbf{K}_{\mathbf{g}^\star-\mathbf{x}_0^\star}^{\mathbf{g}-\mathbf{x}_0} = \mathbf{S}_{\mathbf{g}^\star-\mathbf{x}_0^\star}^{\mathbf{g}-\mathbf{x}_0}\,\mathbf{K}\left(\mathbf{S}_{\mathbf{g}^\star-\mathbf{x}_0^\star}^{\mathbf{g}-\mathbf{x}_0}\right)^{-1}, \qquad \mathbf{D}_{\mathbf{g}^\star-\mathbf{x}_0^\star}^{\mathbf{g}-\mathbf{x}_0} = \mathbf{S}_{\mathbf{g}^\star-\mathbf{x}_0^\star}^{\mathbf{g}-\mathbf{x}_0}\,\mathbf{D}\left(\mathbf{S}_{\mathbf{g}^\star-\mathbf{x}_0^\star}^{\mathbf{g}-\mathbf{x}_0}\right)^{-1}.$$

Matrix $\mathbf{S}_{\mathbf{g}^\star-\mathbf{x}_0^\star}^{\mathbf{g}-\mathbf{x}_0}$ can be any invertible matrix such that

$$\mathbf{g}^\star - \mathbf{x}_0^\star = \mathbf{S}_{\mathbf{g}^\star-\mathbf{x}_0^\star}^{\mathbf{g}-\mathbf{x}_0}(\mathbf{g} - \mathbf{x}_0).$$

For instance, in [11] we proposed to use a roto-dilatation matrix. During the learning phase, $\mathbf{S}_{\mathbf{g}^\star-\mathbf{x}_0^\star}^{\mathbf{g}-\mathbf{x}_0}$ is fixed to be the identity matrix.

We remark that extended DMPs can be used even if the goal position changes with time during the execution of the trajectory simply by updating the matrix $\mathbf{S}_{\mathbf{g}^\star-\mathbf{x}_0^\star}^{\mathbf{g}-\mathbf{x}_0}$. We also remark that, when matrices $\mathbf{K}$ and $\mathbf{D}$ are multiple of the identity matrix, $\mathbf{K} = K\,\mathbf{I}$ and $\mathbf{D} = D\,\mathbf{I}$, we have

$$\mathbf{K}_{\mathbf{g}^\star-\mathbf{x}_0^\star}^{\mathbf{g}-\mathbf{x}_0} = \mathbf{K}, \qquad \mathbf{D}_{\mathbf{g}^\star-\mathbf{x}_0^\star}^{\mathbf{g}-\mathbf{x}_0} = \mathbf{D}.$$

In this case, extended DMPs (7) reads

$$\begin{cases} \tau\dot{\mathbf{v}} = \mathbf{K}(\mathbf{g} - \mathbf{x}) - \mathbf{D}\mathbf{v} - \mathbf{K}(\mathbf{g} - \mathbf{x}_0)s + \mathbf{K}\mathbf{S}_{\mathbf{g}^\star-\mathbf{x}_0^\star}^{\mathbf{g}-\mathbf{x}_0}\mathbf{f}(s) \\ \tau\dot{\mathbf{x}} = \mathbf{v} \end{cases}.$$

In Fig. 3 we present the same example in which the classical DMPs failed in generalizing to new goal positions, showing that, instead, the extended DMPs manage to properly adapt to the new goal position.

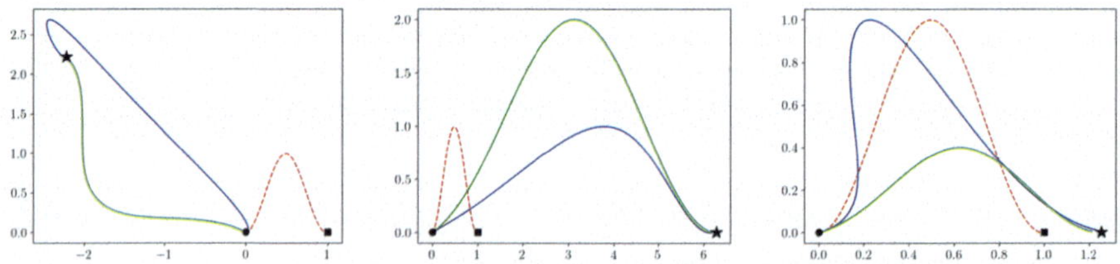

Fig. 3 Examples showing the differences between classical and extended DMPs. In all plots, the dashed red line shows the desired behavior, the blue solid line shows the classical DMP execution with new goal position, and the green solid line shows the extended DMP execution with new goal position. The black dot denotes the starting position $\mathbf{x}_0$, the black square denotes the "learned" goal position $\mathbf{g}$, and the black star denotes the new goal position $\mathbf{g}'$

1.2 Learning from Multiple Observations

Traditionally in the literature, DMPs are used as a framework for "one-shot learning", i.e. a Learning from Demonstration approach that requires only one demonstration to learn a behavior.

So-called *Stylistic DMPs* [12, 13] were developed to learn from multiple demonstrations by introducing an additional variable, called *style parameter* ζ, and by making the weights probabilistically dependent on this new variable: $p(\boldsymbol{\omega}|\zeta)$. This approach is useful when the "style" is needed to describe a trajectory, for example, if it is necessary to learn the dependency of the trajectory from the height of an obstacle. However, when the style is not an issue, this approach introduces additional and undesired variables that increase the complexity of the problem.

Other probabilistic approaches for trajectory learning can deal with learning from multiple demonstrations. These approaches include, for instance, *Probabilistic Movement Primitives* [14], *Kernelized Movement Primitives* [15], and *Gaussian Mixture Models* [16]. However, these methods necessarily require multiple trajectories to extract a common behavior, and, differently from DMPs, cannot be used as one-shot learning frameworks. Moreover, the goodness of the obtained behavior is heavily limited by the quality of the dataset. Finally, these methods have not only a probabilistic learning phase but also a stochastic execution. This aspect makes them not completely suitable in some critical scenarios, such as Robotic Minimally Invasive Surgery.

In this Section, we show how to extract a unique set of weights $\boldsymbol{\omega}_i \in \mathbb{R}^d$, $i = 0, 1, \ldots, N$, from a set of multiple observations as a single linear regression problem in the context of DMPs.

Let us consider a set of M *demonstrated trajectories*

$$\left\{\mathbf{x}^{(j)}(t), t \in \left[t_0^{(j)}, t_f^{(j)}\right]\right\}_{j=1,2,\ldots,M}.$$

Next, we transform each trajectory in such a way that all the starting and ending points are the same (we choose $\mathbf{x}_0 = \mathbf{0}$ and $\mathbf{g} = \mathbf{1}$). To do so, we compute the roto-dilatation matrices, for $j = 1, 2, \ldots, M$,

$$\mathbf{S}^{(j)} = \frac{\|\mathbf{1} - \mathbf{0}\|}{\left\|\mathbf{x}^{(j)}(t_f) - \mathbf{x}^{(j)}(t_0)\right\|} \mathbf{R}^{\widehat{\mathbf{1}-\mathbf{0}}}_{\widehat{\mathbf{x}^{(j)}(t_f)-\mathbf{x}^{(j)}(t_0)}}. \tag{8}$$

We remark that any linear invertible transformation mapping the starting point $\mathbf{x}_0$ to the origin $\mathbf{0}$ and the goal $\mathbf{g}$ to vector $\mathbf{1}$ can be used. We then use the matrices $\mathbf{S}^{(j)}$ to create the new set of transformed trajectories

$$\left\{\check{\mathbf{x}}^{(j)}(t) = \mathbf{S}^{(j)}\left(\mathbf{x}^{(j)}(t) - \mathbf{x}^{(j)}(t_0)\right)\right\}_{j=1,2,\ldots,M}.$$

In this way, all trajectories $\check{\mathbf{x}}^{(j)}$ start in $\mathbf{0}$ and ends in $\mathbf{1}$:

$$\check{\mathbf{x}}^{(j)}\left(t_0^{(j)}\right) = \mathbf{0}, \qquad \check{\mathbf{x}}^{(j)}\left(t_f^{(j)}\right) = \mathbf{1}.$$

Next, we perform a *time scaling* step, so that the time domain of each trajectory is $[0, T]$ for a fixed $T > 0$. To do so, let us define the curves $\tilde{\mathbf{x}}^{(j)}(t)$ for $j = 1, 2, \ldots, M$ as

$$\tilde{\mathbf{x}}^{(j)}(t) = \check{\mathbf{x}}^{(j)}\left(\frac{t_f^{(j)} - t_0^{(j)}}{T} t + t_0^{(j)}\right). \tag{9}$$

It's easy to verify that

$$\tilde{\mathbf{x}}^{(j)}(0) = \check{\mathbf{x}}^{(j)}\left(t_0^{(j)}\right), \qquad \tilde{\mathbf{x}}^{(j)}(T) = \check{\mathbf{x}}^{(j)}\left(t_f^{(j)}\right).$$

From these two steps, we obtain a new set of 'transformed' curves $\{\tilde{\mathbf{x}}^{(j)}(t)\}_{j=1}^M$, each with time domain $[0, T]$, and $\mathbf{0}$ and $\mathbf{1}$ as starting and ending points respectively:

$$\tilde{\mathbf{x}}^{(j)}(0) = \mathbf{0}, \qquad \tilde{\mathbf{x}}^{(j)}(T) = \mathbf{1}.$$

From (1a) we compute the set of forcing terms $\{\mathbf{f}^{(j)}\}_{j=1,2,\ldots,M}$, and we are now able to compute the set of weights $\{\boldsymbol{\omega}\}_{i=0,1,\ldots,N}$ that minimizes the sum of the squared errors (w.r.t. the L_2-norm) between the function generated using (3) and the forcing terms $\mathbf{f}^{(j)}$, $j = 1, 2, \ldots, M$.

For this purpose, we decompose the problem in each independent component. For each component $p = 1, 2, \ldots, d$, we look for the *weight vector* $\boldsymbol{\omega}^\star = [\omega_0^\star, \omega_1^\star, \ldots, \omega_N^\star]^\mathsf{T} \in \mathbb{R}^{N+1}$ satisfying

$$\boldsymbol{\omega}^\star = \arg \min_{\boldsymbol{\omega} \in \mathbb{R}^{N+1}} \underbrace{\sum_{j=1}^{M} \left\| \frac{\sum_{i=0}^N \omega_i \varphi_i(s)}{\sum_{i=0}^N \varphi_i(s)} s - f^{(j)}(s) \right\|_2^2}_{F(\boldsymbol{\omega})}.$$

The existence and uniqueness of a minimum for F is guaranteed by its continuity and strict convexity. Moreover, since F is smooth, $\boldsymbol{\omega}^\star$ is the vector that nullify its gradient: $\nabla_{\boldsymbol{\omega}} F(\cdot)|_{\boldsymbol{\omega}^\star} = \mathbf{0}$. Let us denote with G the gradient of F: $G(\cdot) \doteq \nabla_{\boldsymbol{\omega}} F(\cdot) : \mathbb{R}^{N+1} \to \mathbb{R}^{N+1}$. Its h-th component is (recalling that $\|\zeta(s)\|_2^2 = \int_{s_0}^{s_1} (\zeta(s))^2 \, ds$)

$$\begin{aligned} G_h(\boldsymbol{\omega}) &= \frac{\partial F}{\partial \omega_h}(\boldsymbol{\omega}) \\ &= \sum_{j=1}^{M} \int_{s_0}^{s_1} 2 \left(\frac{\sum_{i=0}^N \omega_i \varphi_i(s)}{\sum_{i=0}^N \varphi_i(s)} s - f^{(j)}(s) \right) \left(\frac{\varphi_h(s)}{\sum_{i=0}^N \varphi_i(s)} s \right) ds \end{aligned}$$

Function G is linear in $\boldsymbol{\omega}$, thus the minimization problem can be written as a linear system: $\mathbf{A}\,\boldsymbol{\omega} = \mathbf{b}$. The component in row h and column k of $\mathbf{A}$, $a_{h\,k}$, is, for $h, k \in \{0, 1, \ldots, N\}$,

$$
\begin{aligned}
a_{hk} &= \frac{\partial G_h}{\partial \omega_k}(\omega) \\
&= \sum_{j=1}^{M} \int_{s_0}^{s_1} 2 \frac{\varphi_h(s)\varphi_k(s)}{\left(\sum_{i=0}^{N} \varphi_i(s)\right)^2} s^2 \, ds \\
&= 2M \int_{s_0}^{s_1} \frac{\varphi_h(s)\varphi_k(s)}{\left(\sum_{i=0}^{N} \varphi_i(s)\right)^2} s^2 \, ds,
\end{aligned}
\tag{10}
$$

while the h-th component of the vector $\mathbf{b}$, b_h, is, for $h = 0, 1, \ldots, N$,

$$
b_h = \sum_{j=1}^{M} \int_{s_0}^{s_1} 2 \left(\frac{\varphi_h(s)}{\sum_{i=0}^{N} \varphi_i(s)} f^{(j)}(s) \, s \, ds \right). \tag{11}
$$

Using any quadrature formula (e.g. Simpson's rule), the integrals in equations (10) and (11) can be computed. Thus, we can solve the linear problem and obtain ω^*. We remark that this procedure has to be repeated for each direction $p = 1, 2, \ldots, d$.

Example 1.1 In this example, we generate the trajectories computing the solution of the dynamical system

$$
\begin{cases}
\dot{x}_1 = x_1^3 + x_2^2 x_1 - x_1 - x_2 \\
\dot{x}_2 = x_2^3 + x_1^2 x_2 + x_1 - x_2
\end{cases}, \tag{12}
$$

which is known to have a *alpha-limit* on the circumference of radius 1 and an attractive equilibrium at the origin. The set of (fifty) trajectories is generated by choosing a random angle $\theta_0 \in [0, 2\pi)$ and a random radius $\rho_0 \in (0.8, 1)$, and then setting as initial position $\mathbf{x}(0) = [x_1(0), x_2(0)]^\intercal = [\rho_0 \cos(\theta_0), \rho_0 \sin(\theta_0)]^\intercal$. Then, the dynamical system is integrated using the *classic fourth-order Runge-Kutta method* [17, 18] up to a random final time $T \in (5, 10)$. Choosing a final time greater than 5 allows the system to reach the origin with an error smaller than 2%: $\|\mathbf{x} - \mathbf{0}\| < 0.02$. The maximum possible value for T, $T = 10$ has been chosen so that the demonstrated trajectories have different time domains, to show the capability of the regression algorithm to extract a common behavior even when the demonstrated trajectories have different time scales. After generating the set of observations, we learn a DMP. The DMP's hyper-parameters are $\mathbf{K} = K\,\mathbf{I}_2$, $\mathbf{D} = D\,\mathbf{I}_2$, with $K = 150$ and $D = 2\sqrt{K} \approx 24.49$, and $\alpha = 4$. Finally, we randomly select an initial point $\mathbf{x}_0 : \|\mathbf{x}_0\| \in (0.8, 1)$ and execute the obtained DMP by setting as goal the attractive equilibrium of the system: $\mathbf{g} = (0, 0)$.

Figure 4 shows the results of these tests. In particular, Fig. 4a shows the set of trajectories obtained by integrating the ODE (12), together with an execution of the obtained DMP. Figure 4b shows the same trajectories when spatially rescaled to have $\mathbf{0}$ and $\mathbf{1}$ as starting and ending points respectively.

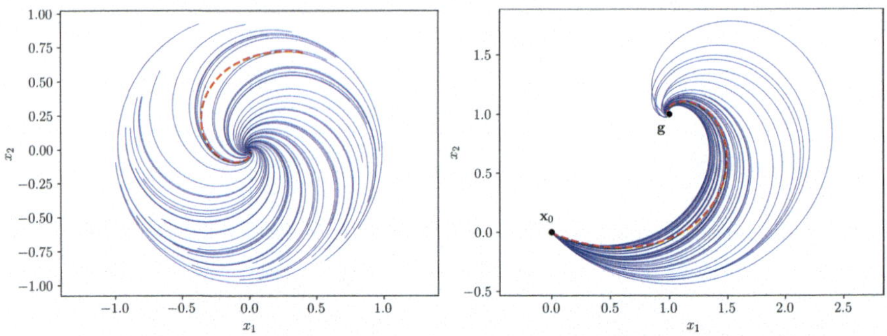

(a) Synthetic test before rescaling. **(b)** Synthetic test after rescaling.

Fig. 4 Tests for our proposed approach to perform DMPs learning from multiple trajectories. The trajectories are obtained by integrating (12) with different initial conditions. In both plots, the solid blue lines represent the demonstrated trajectories, while the dashed red one is an execution of the learned DMP. The tests are plotted both before (**a**) and after (**b**) the spatial scaling step

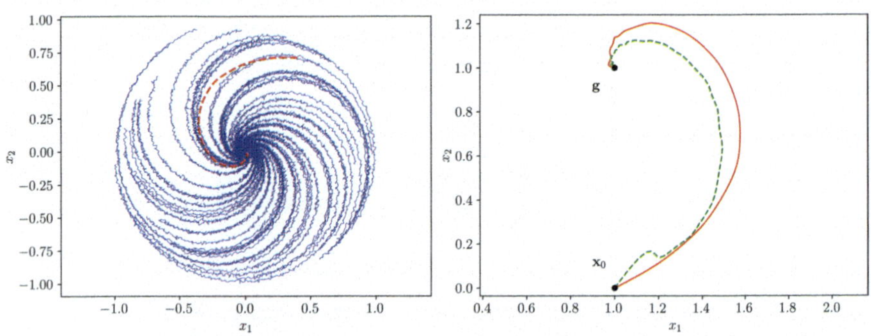

(a) Noisy data-set. **(b)** Comparison of two DMPs obtained by the noisy data-set.

Fig. 5 Tests performed added Gaussian noise to the dataset. On the left, the blue solid lines show the trajectories of the data-set, while the red dashed line shows the execution of the obtained DMP. On the right, the solid red line shows the trajectory obtained using the proposed method for regression over multiple observations. The dashed green line shows the execution of a DMP learned from one sample of the dataset

To show the importance of performing regression, we add Gaussian noise to the set of observations. The obtained, noisy, data-set is shown in Fig. 5a. In Fig. 5 it can be seen that learning from a single sample of the dataset results in a DMP with undesired oscillation. On the other hand, performing regression heavily reduces these oscillations.

1.3 Obstacle Avoidance

A crucial aspect in surgical robotics is the safety of the patient. At movement levels, this means that the autonomous system should be able to avoid collisions with blood vessels and organs. For this reason, being able to implement obstacle avoidance in the DMP system is crucial for their usage in minimally invasive surgery.

Due to the second-order ODE formulation of DMPs, the most natural way to implement obstacle avoidance is to add a repulsive term $\mathbf{p} : \mathbb{R}^d \times \mathbb{R}^d \to \mathbb{R}^d$, $(\mathbf{x}, \mathbf{v}) \mapsto \mathbf{p}(\mathbf{x}, \mathbf{v})$ to the differential equation (1a), that now reads [19]

$$\tau\dot{\mathbf{v}} = \mathbf{K}(\mathbf{g} - \mathbf{x}) - \mathbf{D}\mathbf{v} - \mathbf{K}(\mathbf{g} - \mathbf{x}_0) + \mathbf{K}\,\mathbf{f}(s) + \mathbf{p}(\mathbf{x}, \mathbf{v}). \tag{13}$$

The term $\mathbf{p}(\mathbf{x}, \mathbf{v})$ is a perturbation term that is used to "push" the trajectory away from the obstacle and is often written as the negative gradient of a *potential field* $U : \mathbb{R}^d \to \mathbb{R}$: $\mathbf{p}(\mathbf{x}, \mathbf{v}) = -\nabla_{\mathbf{x}} U(\mathbf{x}, \mathbf{v})$. The usage of potential fields in path planning and obstacle avoidance is not new in robotics [20–23] and it has been proven effective also in the DMP framework. For instance, in [24] the following potential is defined:

$$U_s(\mathbf{x}) = \begin{cases} \dfrac{\eta}{2}\left(\dfrac{1}{\rho(\mathbf{x})} - \dfrac{1}{\rho_0}\right)^2 & \text{if } \rho(\mathbf{x}) \le \rho_0 \\ 0 & \text{if } \rho(\mathbf{x}) > \rho_0 \end{cases}, \tag{14}$$

where $\eta \in \mathbb{R}_+$ is a constant gain, $\rho_0 \in \mathbb{R}_+$ is the influence radius of the obstacle, and $\rho(\mathbf{x}) \in \mathbb{R}_+$ is the distance between the obstacle and the system's position,

$$\rho(\mathbf{x}) = \|\mathbf{x} - \mathbf{o}\|,$$

where $\mathbf{o} \in \mathbb{R}^d$ denotes the position of the obstacle.

In [19] it was pointed out that a potential depending also on the velocity $\mathbf{v}$ of the system, and not only on its position $\mathbf{x}$, would result in smoother obstacle avoidance behaviors. Thus, the following 'dynamic' (i.e. velocity-dependent) potential is proposed [19]

$$U_d(\mathbf{x}, \mathbf{v}) = \begin{cases} \lambda(-\cos\theta)^{\beta}\dfrac{\|\mathbf{v}\|}{\rho(\mathbf{x})} & \text{if } \theta \in \left(\frac{\pi}{2}, \pi\right] \\ 0 & \text{if } \theta \in \left[0, \frac{\pi}{2}\right] \end{cases}, \tag{15}$$

where $\lambda, \beta \in \mathbb{R}_+$ are constant gains, and θ is the angle taken between the current velocity $\mathbf{v}$ and the system's position $\mathbf{x}$ relative to the position $\mathbf{o}$ of the obstacle,

$$\cos\theta = \frac{\langle \mathbf{v}, \mathbf{x} - \mathbf{o} \rangle}{\|\mathbf{v}\|\,\rho(\mathbf{x})}, \tag{16}$$

where $\rho(\mathbf{x})$ still denotes the distance between the system's position $\mathbf{x}$ and the obstacle $\mathbf{o}$, $\rho(\mathbf{x}) = \|\mathbf{x} - \mathbf{o}\|$. The potential U_d in (15) is set to zero when $\theta \in [0, \frac{\pi}{2}]$ so that the DMP's evolution is not influenced by the presence of the obstacle if the system is already 'going away' from the obstacle.

A shortcoming of these two potentials is the fact that they are defined for point obstacles. Thus, in order to use these approaches in surgical scenarios, the obstacles should be covered in a point cloud and each point should define its own potential field. However, this approach has two major problems. First, it is hard to decide a priori how many and where to place the point obstacles. Second, in order to properly cover the obstacle and ensure avoidance, a huge number of point obstacle may be needed, making these approach computationally demanding.

For these reasons, we defined two potential functions that allow to describe solid (or volumetric) obstacles [25, 26]. To do so, we start by defining the concept of *isopotential* for an obstacle.

Definition 1.1 (*Isopotential*) Let $\mathscr{A} \subset \mathbb{R}^d$ be a non-empty closed, simply connected subset of $\mathbb{R}^n$. An *isopotential* is a function $C : \mathbb{R}^d \to \mathbb{R}$ that satisfies the following properties:

I1 The boundary of the set $\mathscr{A}$, $\partial\mathscr{A}$, is the zero-level set of the isopotential:

$$\mathbf{x} \in \partial\mathscr{A} \Rightarrow C(\mathbf{x}) = 0;$$

I2 The value of C increases when the distance from the set $\mathscr{A}$ increases:

$$\text{dist}(\mathscr{A}, \mathbf{y}) > \text{dist}(\mathscr{A}, \mathbf{x}) \Rightarrow C(\mathbf{y}) > C(\mathbf{x}), \qquad \forall \mathbf{x}, \mathbf{y} \in \mathbb{R}^d.$$

An example of isopotential in $\mathbb{R}^3$ is the following [27]:

$$C(\mathbf{x}) = \left(\left(\frac{x_1 - \hat{x}_1}{f_1(\mathbf{x})} \right)^{2n} + \left(\frac{x_2 - \hat{x}_2}{f_2(\mathbf{x})} \right)^{2n} \right)^{\frac{2m}{2n}} + \left(\frac{x_3 - \hat{x}_3}{f_3(\mathbf{x})} \right)^{2m} - 1, \tag{17}$$

which vanishes on a *generalized ellipsoid* centered in $\hat{\mathbf{x}} = [\hat{x}_1, \hat{x}_2, \hat{x}_3]^\intercal$. By tuning parameters m, n and functions f_1, f_2, f_3 it is possible to model obstacles of any shape (their boundary will be the zero-level set of (17)). For instance, if we set $m = n = 1$, and $f_i = \texttt{const}$, we obtain the isopotential

$$C(\mathbf{x}) = \left(\frac{x_1 - \hat{x}_1}{\ell_1} \right)^2 + \left(\frac{x_2 - \hat{x}_2}{\ell_2} \right)^2 + \left(\frac{x_3 - \hat{x}_3}{\ell_3} \right)^2 - 1,$$

that vanishes on an ellipsoid of center $[\hat{x}_1, \hat{x}_2, \hat{x}_3]$ and semi-axes given by ℓ_i.
This isopotential can be generalized by using different exponents, obtaining the isopotential

$$C(\mathbf{x}) = \left(\frac{x_1 - \hat{x}_1}{\ell_1} l\right)^{2n_1} + \left(\frac{x_2 - \hat{x}_2}{\ell_2} l\right)^{2n_2} + \left(\frac{x_3 - \hat{x}_3}{\ell_3} l\right)^{2n_3} - 1, \tag{18}$$

that vanishes on a *pseudo-ellipsoid*. The main advantage of using pseudo-ellipsoids (18) is that they are both easy and computationally fast to compute. Moreover, by increasing the exponent value n_i it is possible to 'flatten' the edges, making the shape resemble a rectangle (in 2D) or a parallelepiped (in 3D). Figure 6 shows an example in 2D.

In [25] we proposed a method to implement volumetric obstacle avoidance, based on the theory of *superquadric potential functions* [27]. In this approach, the following static potential function is defined

$$U_S(\mathbf{x}) = \frac{A \exp\big(-\eta\, C(\mathbf{x})\big)}{C(\mathbf{x})}, \tag{19}$$

where $A, \eta \in \mathbb{R}_+$ are gain parameters, and $C(\mathbf{x})$ is an isopotential. Figure 7 shows an example of potential $U_S(\mathbf{x})$.

The perturbation term is defined as the negative gradient, w.r.t. the system's position $\mathbf{x}$, of the potential and can be computed as follows:

$$\begin{aligned}
\mathbf{p}(\mathbf{x}, \mathbf{v}) = \mathbf{p}_S(\mathbf{x}) &= -\nabla_{\mathbf{x}} U_S(\mathbf{x}) \\
&= -\nabla_{\mathbf{x}} \left(\frac{A \exp\big(-\eta\, C(\mathbf{x})\big)}{C(\mathbf{x})} \right) \\
&= -\frac{A}{C^2(\mathbf{x})} \Big(C(\mathbf{x}) \nabla_{\mathbf{x}} \big(\exp\big(-\eta\, C(\mathbf{x})\big)\big) - \exp\big(-\eta\, C(\mathbf{x})\big)\, \nabla_{\mathbf{x}} C(\mathbf{x}) \Big) \\
&= -\frac{A}{C^2(\mathbf{x})} \Big(-\eta\, C(\mathbf{x}) \exp\big(-\eta\, C(\mathbf{x})\big)\, \nabla_{\mathbf{x}} C(\mathbf{x}) - \exp\big(-\eta\, C(\mathbf{x})\big) \nabla_{\mathbf{x}} C(\mathbf{x}) \Big) \\
&= \frac{A}{C^2(\mathbf{x})} \exp\big(-\eta\, C(\mathbf{x})\big)\, \big(1 + \eta\, C(\mathbf{x})\big)\, \nabla_{\mathbf{x}} C(\mathbf{x}).
\end{aligned}$$

In [26] we defined the potential function

$$U_D(\mathbf{x}, \mathbf{v}) = \begin{cases} \lambda(-\cos\theta)^{\beta} \dfrac{\|\mathbf{v}\|}{C^{\eta}(\mathbf{x})} & \text{if } \theta \in \left(\frac{\pi}{2}, \pi\right] \\ 0 & \text{if } \theta \in \left[0, \frac{\pi}{2}\right] \end{cases}, \tag{20}$$

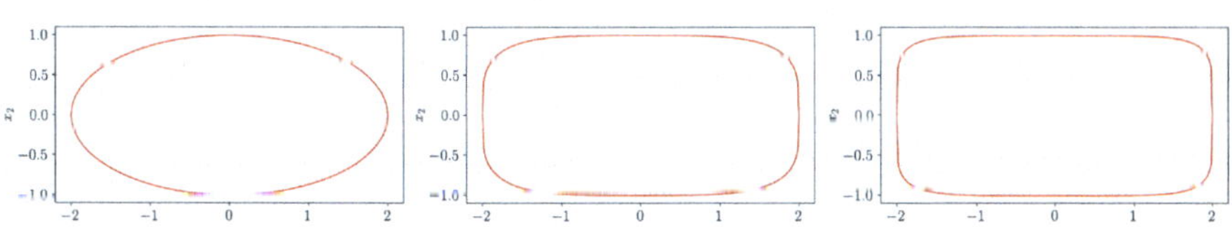

(a) $n_1 = n_2 = 1$. (b) $n_1 = n_2 = 2$. (c) $n_1 = n_2 = 3$.

Fig. 6 Example on how increasing the exponent value in the pseudo-ellipsoid definition results in a flattening of the edges

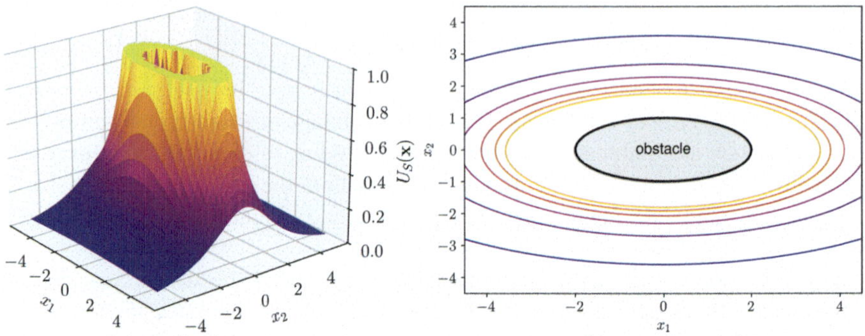

(a) Mesh plot. **(b)** Isocontour plot.

Fig. 7 Example of the static potential $U_S(\mathbf{x})$ given in (19) for an ellipse in $\mathbb{R}^2$. The gains are set to $A = 2$, and $\eta = 0.01$. The ellipse has center in $[0, 0, 0]^\mathsf{T}$, horizontal semi-axis 2, and vertical semi-axis 1

where λ, β, and $\eta \in \mathbb{R}_+$ are constant gains, and function $C(\mathbf{x})$ is any ispotential. The angle θ is taken between the system's velocity $\mathbf{v}$ and the direction between the system's position $\mathbf{x}$ and the closest point of the obstacle. Thanks to the second Property in Definition 1.1, we have that the gradient of the isopotential $C(\mathbf{x})$, $\nabla_\mathbf{x} C(\mathbf{x})$, is always perpendicular to the obstacle surface. Thus, the angle θ can be computed, for convex obstacles, using

$$\cos\theta = \frac{\langle \nabla_\mathbf{x} C(\mathbf{x}), \mathbf{v} \rangle}{\|\nabla_\mathbf{x} C(\mathbf{x})\| \, \|\mathbf{v}\|},$$

while it is not in general well defined for non-convex obstacles. An intuition for these two observations are given in Fig. 8.

Remark 1.1 For non-convex obstacles, some workarounds can be employed. First, if neither the starting position nor the goal is in the 'holes' of the obstacle, i.e. they are not in the convex hull of the obstacle, then the convex hull itself can be used as an obstacle. Second, one can think of relaxing the concept of the gradient to allow sub-differentials. In such a case, the sub-gradient exists but it is not unique. Thirdly, a non-convex obstacle can be split into multiple convex components, and each component would generate its own potential.

As an example, we show in Fig. 9 the potential (20) for an elliptic obstacle in $\mathbb{R}^2$, whose isopotential is

$$C(\mathbf{x}) = \left(\frac{x_1 - \hat{x}_1}{\ell_1} \right)^2 + \left(\frac{x_2 - \hat{x}_2}{\ell_2} \right)^2 - 1,$$

where the center of the ellipse is $\hat{\mathbf{x}} = [\hat{x}_1, \hat{x}_2]^\mathsf{T}$ and the horizontal and vertical axes are, respectively, ℓ_1 and ℓ_2.

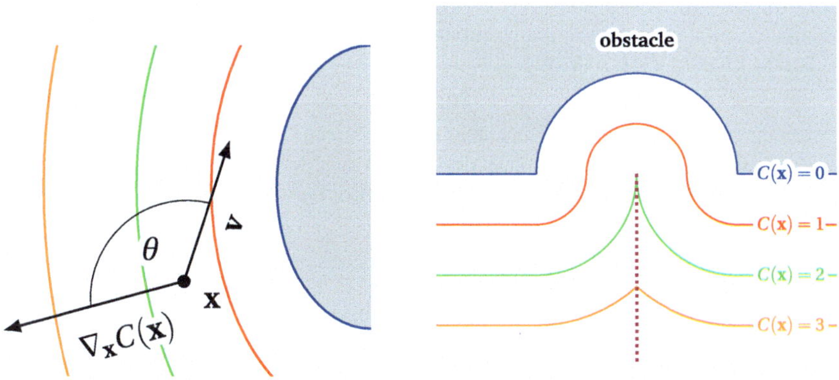

(a) Example of convex obstacle in which θ is well defined.

(b) Example of non-convex obstacle in which θ is not well defined: the purple dotted line shows the points in which $\nabla_{\mathbf{x}} C(\mathbf{x})$ is not well defined.

Fig. 8 Figure 8a shows how the angle θ is defined when the gradient $\nabla_{\mathbf{x}} C(\mathbf{x})$ of the isopotential exists. Figure 8b, instead, shows an example on how non-convex obstacles result in non differentiable isopotentials, and thus it is not possible to define the angle θ

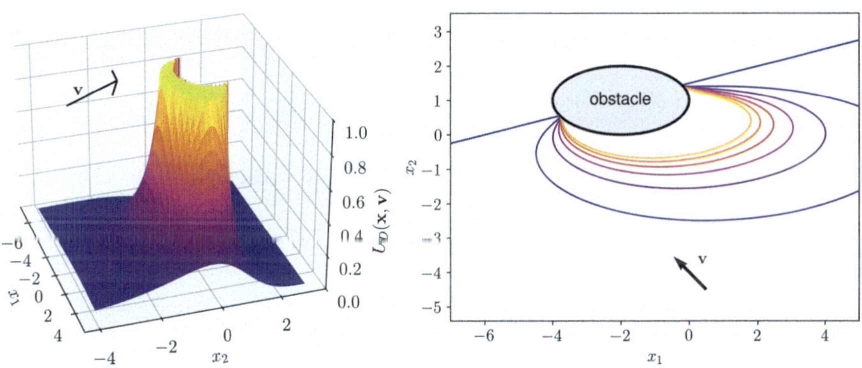

(a) Mesh plot.

(b) Isocontour plot.

Fig. 9 Example of the dynamic potential $U_D(\mathbf{x}, \mathbf{v})$ given in (20) for an ellipse in $\mathbb{R}^2$. The velocity vector $\mathbf{v}$ is set to $\mathbf{v} = [-1, 1]^\intercal$. The gains are set to $\lambda = 2$, $\beta = 2$, and $\eta = 1$. The ellipse has center in $[-2, 1]^\intercal$, horizontal semi-axis 2, and vertical semi-axis 1. In both figures, the potential has been cropped at the value of 1 for display purposes: it goes to infinity on half of the boundary of the obstacle (on the other half, the system goes away from the obstacle, so the potential is zero)

The perturbation term is defined again as the negative gradient, w.r.t. the system's position $\mathbf{x}$, of the potential, $\mathbf{p}(\mathbf{x}, \mathbf{v}) = \mathbf{p}_D(\mathbf{x}, \mathbf{v}) = -\nabla_{\mathbf{x}} U_D(\mathbf{x}, \mathbf{v})$. We can compute it as follows:

$$
\begin{aligned}
\mathbf{p}_D(\mathbf{x}, \mathbf{v}) &= -\nabla_{\mathbf{x}}\big(U_D(\mathbf{x}, \mathbf{v})\big) \\
&= -\nabla_{\mathbf{x}} \left(\lambda(-\cos\theta)^{\beta} \, \frac{\|\mathbf{v}\|}{C^{\eta}(\mathbf{x})} \right) \\
&= -\frac{\lambda \, \|\mathbf{v}\| \, (-\cos\theta)^{\beta-1}}{C^{\eta}(\mathbf{x})} \left(-\beta \, \nabla_{\mathbf{x}}(\cos\theta) + \frac{\eta\cos\theta}{C(\mathbf{x})} \, \nabla_{\mathbf{x}}\big(C(\mathbf{x})\big) \right). \qquad (21)
\end{aligned}
$$

The term $\nabla_{\mathbf{x}}(\cos\theta)$ can be computed as

$$
\begin{aligned}
\nabla_{\mathbf{x}}(\cos\theta) &= \nabla_{\mathbf{x}} \left(\frac{\langle \nabla_{\mathbf{x}} C(\mathbf{x}), \mathbf{v} \rangle}{\|\nabla_{\mathbf{x}} C(\mathbf{x})\| \, \|\mathbf{v}\|} \right) \\
&= \frac{1}{\|\mathbf{v}\| \, \|\nabla_{\mathbf{x}} C(\mathbf{x})\|^2} \Big(\|\nabla_{\mathbf{x}} C(\mathbf{x})\| \, \nabla_{\mathbf{x}}\big(\langle \nabla_{\mathbf{x}} C(\mathbf{x}), \mathbf{v} \rangle \big) - \langle \nabla_{\mathbf{x}} C(\mathbf{x}), \mathbf{v} \rangle \, \nabla_{\mathbf{x}}\big(\|\nabla_{\mathbf{x}} C(\mathbf{x})\| \big) \Big).
\end{aligned} \qquad (22)
$$

For an isopotential as (18) with $n_i = 2$, quantities $\nabla_{\mathbf{x}}\big(\langle \nabla_{\mathbf{x}} C(\mathbf{x}), \mathbf{v} \rangle \big)$ and $\nabla_{\mathbf{x}}\big(\|\nabla_{\mathbf{x}} C(\mathbf{x})\| \big)$ in (22) read, respectively,

$$
\nabla_{\mathbf{x}}\big(\langle \nabla_{\mathbf{x}} C(\mathbf{x}), \mathbf{v} \rangle \big) = 2 \begin{bmatrix} \frac{v_1}{\ell_1^2} & \frac{v_2}{\ell_2^2} & \frac{v_3}{\ell_3^2} \end{bmatrix}^{\mathsf{T}},
$$

and

$$
\nabla_{\mathbf{x}}\big(\|\nabla_{\mathbf{x}} C(\mathbf{x})\| \big) = \frac{4}{\|\nabla_{\mathbf{x}} C(\mathbf{x})\|} \begin{bmatrix} \frac{x_1 - \hat{x}_1}{\ell_1^4} & \frac{x_2 - \hat{x}_2}{\ell_2^4} & \frac{x_3 - \hat{x}_3}{\ell_3^4} \end{bmatrix}^{\mathsf{T}}.
$$

We now present a comparison between the methods presented in this chapter. In particular, for all the proposed methods, we present a 2 - dimensional test both with one and two obstacles. For point obstacle methods, the outline of the obstacle will be covered by a uniform mesh of point obstacles.

Example 1.2 In the first example, we learn the desired behavior

$$
\mathbf{x}(t) = \begin{bmatrix} x_1(t) \\ x_2(t) \end{bmatrix} = \begin{bmatrix} t \, \cos(\pi \, t) \\ t \, \sin(\pi \, t) \end{bmatrix}, \qquad t \in [0, 1].
$$

the obstacle is an ellipse centered in $[-0.5, 0.7]^{\mathsf{T}}$ with horizontal and vertical semi-axis 0.3 and 0.2 respectively. For the tests done with point obstacle methods, the outline of the ellipse is covered with fifty uniformly distributed points. The parameter of the obstacles are:

- for the static point obstacle method (14), $\rho_0 = 0.1$ and $\eta = 1$;
- for the dynamic point obstacle method (15), $\lambda = 0.2$ and $\beta = 2$;
- for the static volume obstacle method (19), $A = 10$ and $\eta = 1$;
- for the dynamic volume obstacle method (20), $\lambda = 10$, $\beta = 2$, and $\eta = 0.5$.

In Fig. 10 the behaviors of all the obstacle avoidance methods are presented.

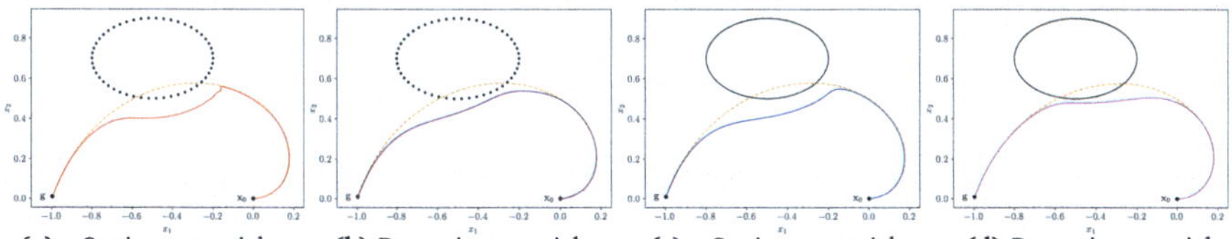

(a) Static potential (24). (b) Dynamic potential (25). (c) Static potential (29). (d) Dynamic potential (30).

Fig. 10 Obstacle avoidance behaviors from Example 1.2. In all plots, the dashed orange line shows the desired trajectory, while the solid colored line shows the adaptation of the DMP to the presence of the obstacle. In the three top figures, the black dots mark the point obstacles used as mesh. In the two bottom figures, the boundary of the obstacle is plotted using the solid black line

Example 1.3 In the second example, we maintain the same desired trajectory and obstacle as in Example 1.2; and we add a second circular obstacle. This second obstacle has center in $[0.15, 0.4]^\mathsf{T}$ and radius 0.1. For the tests done with point obstacle methods, the outline of the circle is covered with fifty uniformly distributed points. The parameter of the obstacles are the same as in Example 1.2. In Fig. 11 the behaviors of all the obstacle avoidance methods are presented.

While all four methods are able to successfully avoid the obstacle(s), we remark that the point-wise methods (14) and (15) require more computational time since more obstacles have to be modeled (one for each point of the point cloud). Moreover, tests with different parameters and/or fewer points in the cloud resulted in the trajectory colliding with the obstacle.

On the other hand, change in parameters of volumetric methods (19) and (20) results in different behaviors while always being able to properly avoid the obstacles.

Moreover, in general, we observed that dynamic methods (15) and (20) results in smoother behaviors since they take into consideration also the system velocity.

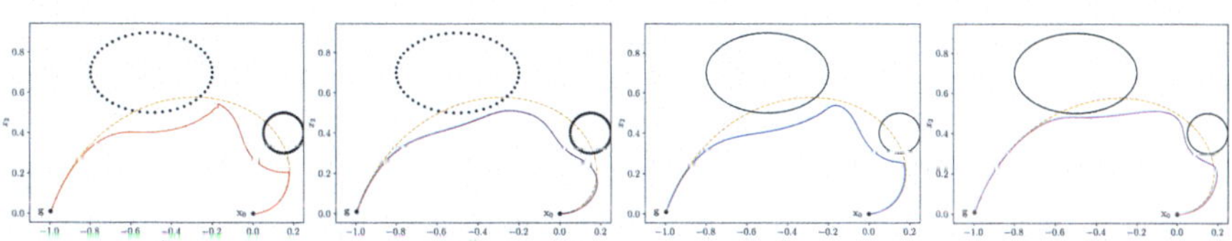

(a) Static potential (24). (b) Dynamic potential (25). (c) Static potential (29). (d) Dynamic potential (30).

Fig. 11 Obstacle avoidance behaviors from Example 1.3. In all plots, the dashed orange line shows the desired trajectory, while the solid colored line shows the adaptation of the DMP to the presence of the obstacle. In the three top figures, the black dots mark the point obstacles used as mesh. In the two bottom figures, the boundary of the obstacle is plotted using the solid black line

1.4 Application to Minimally Invasive Surgery

To prove that DMPs are a valid movement trajectory framework in surgical scenarios, in [28] we developed a framework consisting of three components: a *task reasoner*, a *situation-awareness module*, and a *low-level controller*. The goal of this framework was to perform a *Peg & Ring* task on a da Vinci surgical robot. The setup is shown in Fig. 12. It consists of a RGBD camera and two manipulators. The goal of the task is to place each colored ring on the same-colored peg. However, we add the constraint that any manipulator can act only on half of the setup. In this way, if the ring and the peg are in opposite halves of the setup, the ring should be transferred between manipulators.

Three users of different experience on the robot performed five trials, each requiring to place four rings. The initial configuration was kept the same across all trials and all users, and it was set in such a way to require to transfer all rings between manipulators before placing. We then segmented by hand all the executions. We decided to split the task in two gestures: `move` was the gesture used to both reach and place the ring, and `transfer` was the gesture used to transfer the ring between pegs. In the end, we acquired 120 `move` samples and 60 `transfer` samples (Fig. 13).

We used our proposed approach presented in Sect. 1.2 to learn a single DMP for each of the gestures. In particular, since the `transfer` gesture require cooperation between the end effectors, while `move` does not, we modeled the first as a three-dimensional DMP which is executed by any of the manipulators, while the second is modeled as a six-dimensional DMP encoding the movements of both manipulators simultaneously.

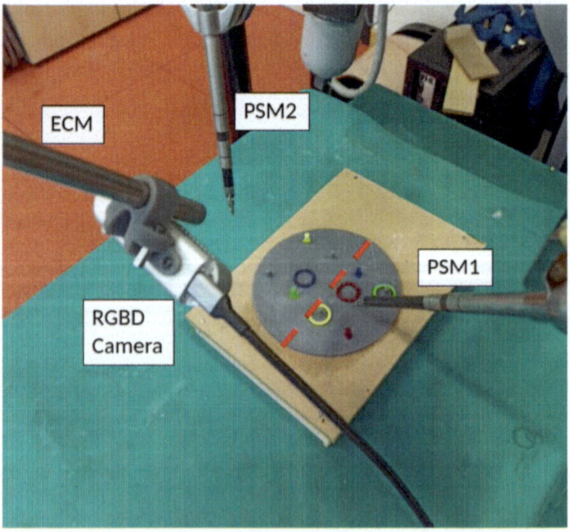

Fig. 12 Setup for the Peg and Ring task on the da Vinci surgical robot. The RGBD camera is attached to the endoscopic arm (ECM) of the robot. Each manipulator (PSM1 and PSM2) has its own reachability region, on the two sides of the red line

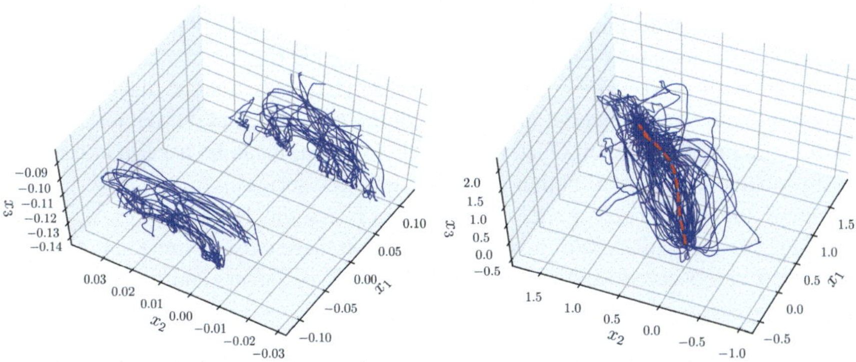

Fig. 13 On the left, the set of all trajectories for the `move` gestures. On the right, the same set of trajectories aligned to have start and end in **0** and **1** respectively. In dashed red it is plotted the obtained DMP

Each of the peg is treated as an obstacle using the avoidance behavior given by the potential field in (20) using as isosurface an ellipsoid. Moreover, to account also for the manipulators, each ellipsoid is enlarged by the size of the end-effector.

This is necessary since the DMP describes the movement of the center of the end-effector and, even if the center point avoid the obstacles, it may happen that the end-effector collides with it. By enlarging the obstacle, we are capable to maintain the end-effector center to a distance greater or equal to the end-effector size, avoiding collisions.

2 Unsupervised Trajectory Segmentation

We proved that DMPs can be effectively used as the low-level controller when automating surgical-related tasks.

However, the problem of how to extract the gestures to learn the DMPs from surgical trials remains. Manual segmentation of complete surgical tasks into subtasks is a long and tedious process. Moreover, since gestures are executed using muscular memory and are of short duration, small errors in the manual segmentation are practically unavoidable.

For this reason, unsupervised segmentation is a well-studied topic in surgical robotics. Some approaches start with an over-segmentation of the data stream, and proceed by removing false positive cuts (thus merging two segments) relying on geometrical or statistical properties of the segments [29–34]. Using the opposite strategy, some approaches start with a unique segment and perform further partitions, still based on geometric or statistical properties [35]. Other approaches look for movement repetitions within the time series to use as the basis for the segmentation [36]. Finally, semi-unsupervised approaches assume that a library of primitives is available, and uses it to perform the segmentation [37].

Instead, we proposed a model-based approach. That is, we assume that there exists a common mathematical model underlying all the time series in our dataset, and we aim at extracting this model. Once the model is known, it can be used to extract the 'most probable' segmentation that generated the time series.

One of the most used models in this context is the Hidden Markov Model (HMMs) [38–40]. This type of model assumes that there exists a finite set of *modes* that cannot be observed (and are thus called *hidden* or *latent*) and that each mode emits an *observation*.

An extension of HMMs is the *Auto-Regressive HMM* (AR-HMMs) [41–44]. In this case, each latent mode encodes a linear model which is used to evolve the observed state. Roughly speaking, the hidden mode describes which action is being executed, while the observed variables constitute the executed trajectories.

2.1 Auto-regressive Hidden Markov Models

Auto-Regressive Hidden Markov Model (AR-HMM) is an extension of the classical Hidden Markov Models (HMM) in which the observations are related by an Auto-Regressive (AR) dynamic. In this model, the latent mode encodes the (linear) vector field governing the evolution of the observed state.

Definition 2.1 An *Auto-Regressive Hidden Markov Model* (AR-HMM) is a model $\mathscr{H} = \left\{\mathscr{S}, \mathscr{Y}, \Theta = \{\boldsymbol{\varpi}, \mathbf{T}, \{\mathbf{A}_s, \mathbf{b}_s\}_{s\in\mathscr{S}}\}\right\}$ where:

- $\mathscr{S} = \{1, 2, \ldots, S\}$ is the set of (hidden) *modes*. The mode at time $t \in \{1, 2, \ldots, T\}$ is denoted by z_t.
- Vector $\boldsymbol{\varpi} = [\varpi_i]_{i=1,2\ldots,S} \in \Theta$ define the *initial probability* of hidden mode:

$$\Pr(z_1 = i) = \boldsymbol{\varpi}_i, \quad i \in \mathscr{S}.$$

  Vector $\boldsymbol{\varpi}$ satisfies $\varpi_i \in [0, 1], \forall i = 1, 2, \ldots, S$ and $\sum_{i=1}^{S} \boldsymbol{\varpi}_i = 1$.
- Matrix $\mathbf{T} = [\mathbf{T}|_{i\,j}]_{i=1,2,\ldots,S}^{j=1,2,\ldots,S} \in \Theta$ defines the *transition probabilities* between hidden modes:

$$\Pr(z_{t+1} = j | z_t = i) = \mathbf{T}|_{i\,j}, \quad i, j \in \mathscr{S}.$$

  Matrix $\mathbf{T}$ satisfies $\mathbf{T}|_{i\,j} \in [0, 1], \forall i, j = 1, 2, \ldots, S$ and $\sum_{j=1}^{S} \mathbf{T}_{i\,j} = 1, \forall i = 1, 2, \ldots, S$.
- $\mathscr{Y} = \mathbb{R}^d$ is the set of observations. The observation at time $t \in \{0, 1, \ldots, T\}$ is denoted by $\mathbf{y}_t \in \mathbb{R}^d$. The emissions are modeled by the following AR affine dynamics with Gaussian white noise:

$$\mathbf{y}_{t+1} | z_{t+1}, \mathbf{y}_t \sim \mathscr{N}\left(\mathbf{A}_{z_{t+1}} \mathbf{y}_t + \mathbf{b}_{z_{t+1}}, \boldsymbol{\Sigma}_{z_{t+1}}\right). \tag{23}$$

The set Θ contains all the parameters of the model:

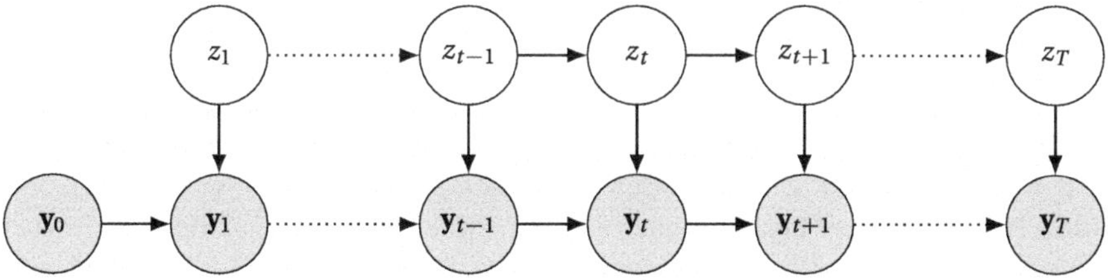

Fig. 14 Graphical representation of an AR-HMM

$$\Theta = \left\{\boldsymbol{\varpi}, \mathbf{T}, \boldsymbol{\Sigma}_s, \{\mathbf{A}_s, \mathbf{b}_s\}_{s\in\mathscr{S}}\right\}.$$

The graphical model representation is given in Fig. 14.

Two main algorithms characterize the AR-HMM (and the latent-variable models in general): the *Expectation Maximization* (EM) algorithm and the *Viterbi* algorithm. The former is used to infer the set of parameters Θ by maximizing the likelihood $p(\mathbf{Y}|\Theta)$ of the observed data. The latter, instead, allows extracting the sequence of latent mode $\hat{\mathbf{z}}$ that maximize the joint probability distribution $p(\mathbf{Y}, \mathbf{z}|\Theta)$ for a given observed sequence $\mathbf{Y} = (\mathbf{y}_0, \mathbf{y}_1, \ldots, \mathbf{y}_T)$. With the EM algorithm we 'learn' the model parameters from the data. On the other hand, the Viterbi algorithm allows to segment an observed sequence once the model parameters are known.

In brief, the EM algorithm consists of an iterative procedure that, at each iteration, maximizes, w.r.t. the set of parameters Θ, the auxiliary function

$$Q(\Theta, \Theta^{\text{old}}) \doteq Q_{\text{init}}(\Theta, \Theta^{\text{old}}) + Q_{\text{trans}}(\Theta, \Theta^{\text{old}}) + Q_{\text{out}}(\Theta, \Theta^{\text{old}}) \tag{24}$$

In the above equation,Θ^{old} denotes the current guess of the set of parameters. The three terms of the sum are defined as follows:

$$Q_{\text{init}}(\Theta, \Theta^{\text{old}}) \doteq \sum_{z_1\in\mathscr{S}} \log p(z_1|\Theta) p(z_1|\mathbf{Y}, \Theta^{\text{old}}), \tag{25a}$$

$$Q_{\text{trans}}(\Theta, \Theta^{\text{old}}) \doteq \sum_{t=1}^{T-1} \sum_{z_t, z_{t+1}\in\mathscr{S}} \log p(z_{t+1}|z_t, \Theta) p(z_t, z_{t+1}|\mathbf{Y}, \Theta^{\text{old}}), \tag{25b}$$

$$Q_{\text{out}}(\Theta, \Theta^{\text{old}}) \doteq \sum_{t=0}^{T-1} \sum_{z_{t+1}\in\mathscr{S}} \log p(\mathbf{y}_{t+1}|z_{t+1}, \mathbf{y}_t, \Theta) p(z_{t+1}|\mathbf{Y}, \Theta^{\text{old}}). \tag{25c}$$

They represent the three components of the AR-HMM: the initial condition, the transition probabilities between nodes, and the dynamic probability.

During the *Expectation Step*, the quantities that depend on θ^{old}, that is $p(z_t, z_{t+1}|\mathbf{Y}, \Theta^{\text{old}})$ and $p(z_{t+1}|\mathbf{Y}, \Theta^{\text{old}})$, are computed using the *forward-backward algorithm* [45]. During the *Maximization Step*, the set of parameters Θ that maximizes Q_{init}, Q_{trans} and Q_{out} is computed. These two steps are repeated until convergence.

Convergence is reached when the changes in the log-likelihood $\log p(\mathbf{Y}, \mathbf{z})$ is below a given tolerance.

The *Viterbi algorithm* [46] is a procedure to find the most probable sequence of hidden modes given the sequence of observations. The algorithm takes as input a hidden-variable model $\mathscr{M}$ and a stream of observations $\mathbf{Y} = (\mathbf{y}_0, \mathbf{y}_1, \dots, \mathbf{y}_T)$, and returns the sequence of hidden modes $\mathbf{z} = (z_0, z_1, \dots, z_T) \in \mathscr{S}^{T+1}$ that maximizes $p(\mathbf{Y}|\mathbf{z}, \mathscr{M})$. In its most general formulation, the Viterbi algorithm [47] works with any latent-mode model with Markov dynamics, independently of the dynamics of the observed state.

The algorithm generates two 2-dimensional tables $\mathtt{T}_1, \mathtt{T}_2$ of size $(T+1) \times S$. Element $\mathtt{T}_1|_{i\,j}$ of $\mathtt{T}_1$ contains the probability of the most likely path so far $\hat{\mathbf{z}} = (\hat{z}_1, \hat{z}_2, \dots, \hat{z}_i)$ with $\hat{z}_i = s_j$ that generates $\mathbf{Y} = (\mathbf{y}_0, \mathbf{y}_2, \dots, \mathbf{y}_i)$. Element $\mathtt{T}_2|_{i\,j}$ of $\mathtt{T}_2$ contains the mode $\hat{z}_{i-1}$ of the most likely path so far $\hat{\mathbf{z}} = (\hat{z}_1, \hat{z}_2, \dots, \hat{z}_{i-1}, \hat{z}_i = j)$. The components of $\mathtt{T}_1, \mathtt{T}_2$ are recursively computed as

$$
\begin{aligned}
\mathtt{T}_1|_{i\,j} &= \max_k \left(\mathtt{T}_{i-1,k} \Pr(z_{t+1} = j|z_t = k) \Pr(\mathbf{y}_t|z_t = s)\right), \\
\mathtt{T}_2|_{i\,j} &= \arg\max_k \left(\mathtt{T}_{i-1,k} \Pr(z_{t+1} = j|z_t = k) \Pr(\mathbf{y}_t|z_t = s)\right) \\
&= \arg\max_k \left(\mathtt{T}_{i-1,k} \Pr(z_{t+1} = j|z_t = k)\right).
\end{aligned}
$$

We remark that the last identity follows from the fact that $\Pr(\mathbf{y}_j|z_j = i)$ is positive and independent of the index k. The basis of recursion is

$$
\begin{aligned}
\mathtt{T}_1|_{1\,s} &= \Pr(z_0 = s) \Pr(\mathbf{y}_0|z_0 = s), \\
\mathtt{T}_2|_{1\,s} &= 0.
\end{aligned}
$$

For a complete overview of these algorithms in the context of Hidden Markov Models and Auto Regressive HMM, see [48].

2.2 Generalizations to AR-HMM

In [49] we proposed two generalizations to the AR-HMM model. First, we proposed a *Cartesian non-linear ARHMM* in which the Auto-Regressive dynamics in (23) is generalized to a more general dynamic $\mathbf{f}_s \to \mathbb{R}^d \to \mathbb{R}^d$ for each hidden mode $s \in \mathscr{S}$. Second, we proposed a *unit-quaternion linear ARHMM* in which the AR dynamic is a linear dynamics in the space of unit quaternions $\mathbb{S}^3$.

2.2.1 Cartesian Non-Linear ARHMM

When generalizing the AR dynamics in Cartesian space, we aim at modifying the linear AR dynamics shown in (23) with a more general dynamic $\mathbf{f}_s : \mathbb{R}^d \to \mathbb{R}^d$ for each hidden mode $s \in \mathscr{S}$. Inspired by the theory of DMPs, we will use a *basis functions*-based formulation so that the non-linear function $\mathbf{f}_s$ is written as a linear combination of non-linear basis functions $\left\{\varphi_n : \mathbb{R}^d \to \mathbb{R}\right\}_{n=0,1,\ldots,N}$:

$$\mathbf{f}_s(\mathbf{y}_t)|_i = f_i^{(s)}(\mathbf{y}_t) = \sum_{j=0}^{N} \omega_{i\,j}^{(s)} \varphi_j(\mathbf{y}_t), \tag{26}$$

where $\omega_{i\,j}^{(s)}$ is the set of *weights* that describes the vector field. By defining the *weight matrix* $\mathbf{\Omega}_s \doteq [\omega_{i\,j}^{(s)}]_{i=1,2,\ldots,d}^{j=0,1,\ldots,N}$ and the *non-linear map* $\boldsymbol{\varphi}(\mathbf{y}) \doteq [\varphi_j(\mathbf{y})]_{j=0,1,\ldots,N}$, we have that formulation (26) can be written in matrix-vector notation as

$$\mathbf{f}_s(\mathbf{y}_t) = \mathbf{\Omega}_s \boldsymbol{\varphi}(\mathbf{y}_t). \tag{27}$$

Thus, (23) now reads

$$\mathbf{y}_t | z_t = s,\ \mathbf{y}_{t-1} \sim \mathcal{N}\left(\mathbf{y}_t | \mathbf{\Omega}_s \boldsymbol{\varphi}\left(\mathbf{y}_{t-1}\right), \mathbf{\Sigma}_s\right). \tag{28}$$

We remark that, since only the formulation of the AR dynamics changes from the classical ARHMM to the non-linear case, the graphical model representation is the same as in Fig. 14.

During the *Expectation* step, the quantities that depend on the current guess of the set Θ^{old} of parameters have to be computed. Since the conditional independence properties of the model depend exclusively on its graphical representation [45], we have that the E-step for the *Non-Linear ARHMM* (NL-ARHMM) is identical to the linear case. The only difference is that the emission probability $p(\mathbf{y}_t | z_t, \mathbf{y}_{t-1})$ is given by formula (28) instead of (23).

Similarly, in the *Maximization* step, maximization of (25a) and (25b) is achieved in the same way as the linear ARHMM case, since there is no dependence on the emission probability. Thus, the only difference in the EM algorithm between a linear ARHMM and the NL-ARHMM lies in the maximization of quantity Q_{out}.

Proposition 2.1 *Denote by* $\gamma(t)$ *the quantity* $p(z_t | \mathbf{Y}, \Theta)$ *so that* $\gamma_s(t) \doteq \Pr(z_t = s | \mathbf{Y}, \Theta^{\text{old}})$. *Then, maximization of* $Q_{out}(\Theta, \Theta^{\text{old}})$ *in (25c) is achieved by setting*

$$\mathbf{\Omega}_s = \left(\sum_{t=0}^{T-1} \gamma_s(t+1) \mathbf{y}_{t+1} \boldsymbol{\varphi}(\mathbf{y}_t)^\mathsf{T}\right)\left(\sum_{t=0}^{T-1} \gamma_s(t+1) \boldsymbol{\varphi}(\mathbf{y}_t) \boldsymbol{\varphi}(\mathbf{y}_t)^\mathsf{T}\right)^{-1} \tag{29a}$$

and

$$\mathbf{\Sigma}_s = \frac{\sum_{t=0}^{T-1} \gamma_s(t+1) \mathbf{e}_t^{(s)} \mathbf{e}_t^{(s)\,\mathsf{T}}}{\sum_{t=0}^{T} \gamma_s(t+1)}; \tag{29b}$$

where the vector $\mathbf{e}_t^{(s)} \in \mathbb{R}^d$ *is defined as*

$$\mathbf{e}_t^{(s)} = \mathbf{y}_{t+1} - \mathbf{\Omega}_s \boldsymbol{\varphi}(\mathbf{y}_t).$$

Proof We aim at maximizing (by dropping Θ for notation simplicity) the quantity

$$\widetilde{Q}(\Theta, \Theta^{\text{old}}) = \sum_{t=0}^{T-1} \sum_{s=1}^{S} \gamma_s(t+1) \log p(\mathbf{y}_{t+1} | z_{t+1} = s, \mathbf{y}_t).$$

To maximize this quantity, we can maximize over each hidden mode $s \in \mathscr{S}$ independently:

$$\boldsymbol{\Omega}_s^\star, \boldsymbol{\Sigma}_s^\star = \arg\max_{\boldsymbol{\Omega}_s, \boldsymbol{\Sigma}_s} \sum_{t=0}^{T-1} \gamma_s(t+1) \log p(\mathbf{y}_{t+1} | z_{t+1} = s, \mathbf{y}_t).$$

Since the emission probability is given by (28), the function to maximize reads

$$\widehat{Q}_{\text{out}} = -\frac{1}{2} \sum_{t=0}^{T-1} \gamma_s(t+1) \log |\boldsymbol{\Sigma}_s| - \frac{1}{2} \sum_{t=0}^{T-1} \gamma_s(t+1) \left(\mathbf{y}_{t+1} - \boldsymbol{\Omega}_s \varphi(\mathbf{y}_t)\right)^\mathsf{T} \boldsymbol{\Sigma}_s^{-1} \left(\mathbf{y}_{t+1} - \boldsymbol{\Omega}_s \varphi(\mathbf{y}_t)\right). \tag{30}$$

We start by discussing the maximization over the weight matrix $\boldsymbol{\Omega}_s$. The gradient of $\widehat{Q}_{\text{out}}$ w.r.t. $\boldsymbol{\Omega}_s$ is

$$\nabla_{\boldsymbol{\Omega}_s} \widehat{Q} = \boldsymbol{\Sigma}_s^{-1} \left(\sum_{t=0}^{T-1} \gamma_s(t+1) \mathbf{y}_{t+1} \boldsymbol{\varphi}(\mathbf{y})^\mathsf{T} - \boldsymbol{\Omega}_s \sum_{t=0}^{T-1} \gamma_s(t+1) \boldsymbol{\varphi}(\mathbf{y}_t) \boldsymbol{\varphi}(\mathbf{y}_t)^\mathsf{T} \right).$$

By setting it to zero, we get formula (29a).

We now discuss the maximization over the weight matrix $\boldsymbol{\Sigma}_s$. The gradient of $\widehat{Q}_{\text{out}}$ w.r.t. $\boldsymbol{\Sigma}_s$ is

$$\nabla_{\boldsymbol{\Sigma}_s^{-1}} \widehat{Q} = \frac{1}{2} \boldsymbol{\Sigma}_s \sum_{t=0}^{T-1} \gamma_s(t+1) - \frac{1}{2} \sum_{t=0}^{T-1} \gamma_s(t+1) \left(\mathbf{y}_{t+1} - \boldsymbol{\Omega}_s \boldsymbol{\varphi}(\mathbf{y}_t)\right) \left(\mathbf{y}_{t+1} - \boldsymbol{\Omega}_s \boldsymbol{\varphi}(\mathbf{y}_t)\right)^\mathsf{T},$$

which, by setting it to zero, gives formula (29b).

We remark that the matrix $\boldsymbol{\Omega}_s$ in (29b) is the "old" guess, and not that given by the update formula (29a). Thus, when implementing the EM-algorithm, the update of the covariance matrices $\boldsymbol{\Sigma}_s$ should be performed before the update of the weight matrices $\boldsymbol{\Omega}_s$.

2.2.2 Example of Basis Functions

In this section, we present some examples of basis functions.

The first set shows how to interpret the classical, linear ARHMM as a particular case of NL-ARHMM. Indeed, by defining $\boldsymbol{\varphi}^{(\text{lin})}(\mathbf{y}) \doteq [1, y_1, y_2, \ldots, y_d]^\mathsf{T}$, we have that the resulting weight matrix is a block matrix with the offset $\mathbf{b}$ and the linear map $\mathbf{A}$ in (23) as $\boldsymbol{\Omega} = [\mathbf{b}, \mathbf{A}]$.

The second well-known set of basis functions is the family of *Gaussian Radial Basis Functions* (GRBFs) we defined in $\mathbb{R}^1$ in (5). Given a set $\{\boldsymbol{\mu}_i\}_{i=1,2,\ldots,N}$ of centers and a set $\{\boldsymbol{\Sigma}_i\}_{i=1,2,\ldots,N}$ of covariance matrices, we define the basis functions as

$$\varphi_0^{(\text{grbf})}(\mathbf{y}) \doteq 1,$$
$$\varphi_i^{(\text{grbf})}(\mathbf{y}) \doteq \exp\left(-(\mathbf{y}-\boldsymbol{\mu})\boldsymbol{\Sigma}_i^{-1}(\mathbf{y}-\boldsymbol{\mu}_i)\right), \qquad i = 1, \ldots, N.$$

Usually, the covariance matrices are set to be a multiple of the identity matrix $\boldsymbol{\Sigma}_i = \varsigma_i \mathbf{I}_d$. The main drawback of this family of basis functions lies in the fact that, even for small values of the dimension d of the observed space, a high number of basis functions is needed to 'cover' the space. Indeed, this family of basis functions is usually adopted when learning functions in bounded domains. This is why they are the standard for *Dynamic Movement Primitives*. For this reason, we suggest using this set of basis functions when dealing with bounded observation spaces, such as $d-$dimensional cubes $[0, 1]^d$.

Finally, a third family of basis functions is the set of polynomial functions up to a degree k:

$$\boldsymbol{\varphi}^{(\mathscr{P}_k)}(\mathbf{y}) \doteq \text{col}\left(\left\{\prod_{i=1}^{d} y_i^{c_i} : c_i \in \mathbb{N},\ \sum_{i=1}^{d} c_i \leq k\right\}\right). \tag{31}$$

For instance, assume that $d = 2$ ($\mathbf{y} \in \mathscr{Y} = \mathbb{R}^2$) and $k = 3$. Then the basis functions are

$$\boldsymbol{\varphi}^{(\mathscr{P}_3)}(\mathbf{y}) = \left[1, y_1, y_2, y_1^2, y_1 y_2, y_2^2, y_1^3, y_1^2 y_2, y_1 y_2^2, y_2^3\right]^\mathsf{T}.$$

As we will show in Sect. 2.5, this type of basis functions is particularly useful in low-dimensional spaces, where linear dynamics are not able to describe complex evolutions of the observed state. On the other hand, they are less useful in higher-dimensional spaces for two main reasons: firstly, linear dynamics are able to describe more complex evolutions; secondly, non-linearity in higher dimensional spaces requires a huge amount of parameters (i.e. the number of columns of $\boldsymbol{\Omega}$ increases), risking over-fitting and numerical inefficiency.

2.3 Unit-Quaternion Linear ARHMM

Orientations can be modeled in different ways. There are two preferred spaces to describe orientations: the space $SO(3)$ of *orthogonal* 3×3 *matrices*, and the space $\mathbb{S}^3$ of unit quaternions. Both representations are singularity-free. However, unit quaternions are preferred since they require only four variables to be described, instead of the nine parameters of 3×3 matrices.

The main difficulty when dealing with dynamics in $\mathbb{S}^3$ lies in the fact that the resulting quaternion must still be of unitary norm. To solve this problem, we take advantage of two properties of quaternions. The first is the fact that the exponential of a quaternion with null real part always results in a quaternion of unit norm: $\|\mathrm{Exp}(0 + a\mathtt{i} + b\mathtt{j} + c\mathtt{k})\| = 1, \quad \forall a, b, c, \in \mathbb{R}$. The second is the fact that the norm of the product between two quaternions p and q is the product of the norms: $\|p * q\| = \|p\| \; \|q\|$. Thus, we propose to describe a dynamics in $\mathbb{S}^3$ by 3 parameters $a, b, c \in \mathbb{R}$ such that

$$q_{t+1} = \mathrm{Exp}(a\mathtt{i} + b\mathtt{j} + c\mathtt{k}) * q_t .$$

From here, we will denote as 'vec' the function that maps a quaternion to its vector formulation:

$$\mathrm{vec} : \mathbb{S}^3 \to \mathbb{R}^4, \qquad q = q_r + q_i\mathtt{i} + q_j\mathtt{j} + q_k\mathtt{k} \mapsto \mathbf{q} = [q_r, q_i, q_j, q_k]^{\mathsf{T}} .$$

With this notation, we have that in this model the probability of the next observation reads

$$q_t | z_t = s, q_{t-1} \sim \mathcal{N}\big(\mathrm{vec}(q_t) | \mathrm{vec}\left(\mathrm{Exp}(a_s\mathtt{i} + b_s\mathtt{j} + c_s\mathtt{k}) * q_{t-1}\right), \mathbf{\Sigma}_s\big) \tag{32}$$

As in the case of Cartesian Non-Linear ARHMM, we need only to explain how to maximize the *emission probability*. Therefore, in the *Maximization step* we have to maximize the quantity Q_{out} in (25c) where the next-state probability is given by (32). Different from what we showed in Proposition 2.1, there is no closed-form solution to the maximization problem. Indeed, by defining $\gamma_s(t) \doteq \Pr(z_t = s | \mathbf{Y}, \Theta^{\mathrm{old}})$ we have that the function to maximize reads, similarly to (30):

$$\widehat{Q}_{\mathrm{out}} = -\frac{1}{2} \sum_{t=0}^{T-1} \gamma_s(t+1) \log |\mathbf{\Sigma}_s| - \frac{1}{2} \sum_{t=0}^{T-1} \gamma_s(t+1) \mathrm{vec}(q_{t+1} - \mu_{t+1}^{(s)})^{\mathsf{T}} \mathbf{\Sigma}^{-1} \mathrm{vec}(q_{t+1} - \mu_{t+1}^{(s)}) \tag{33}$$

where $\mu_{t+1}^{(s)}$ is the *expected orientation* at time $t + 1$ for hidden mode s:

$$\mu_{t+1}^{(s)} \doteq \mathrm{Exp}(a_s\mathtt{i} + b_s\mathtt{j} + c_s\mathtt{k}) * q_t .$$

Similarly to Proposition 2.1, maximization of (33) is achieved by setting

$$\mathbf{\Sigma}_s = \frac{\sum_{t=0}^{T-1} \gamma_s(t+1) \mathbf{e}_{t+1}^{(s)} \cdot \mathbf{e}_{t+1}^{(s)\,\mathsf{T}}}{\sum_{t=0}^{T-1} \gamma_s(t+1)}$$

where $\mathbf{e}_{t+1}^{(s)}$ is the difference between the actual orientation and the predicted one at time $t + 1$, assuming that the hidden mode s is active:

$$\mathbf{e}_{t+1}^{(s)} \doteq \mathrm{vec}(q_{t+1} - \mu_{t+1}^{(s)}).$$

On the other hand, maximization over the dynamics parameters can be formulated as

$$(a_s^\star, b_s^\star, c_s^\star) = \underset{(a_s,b_s,c_s)}{\arg\max}\left(-\sum_{t=0}^{T-1}\gamma_s(t+1)\,\|\mathrm{vec}\,(q_{t+1} - \mathrm{Exp}\,(a_s\mathtt{i} + b_s\mathtt{j} + c_s\mathtt{k}) * q_t)\|^2_{\mathbf{\Sigma}^{-1}}\right)$$

where $\|\cdot\|_{\mathbf{A}}$ is the semi-norm induced by a Symmetric Semi-Positive Definite (SPD) matrix $\mathbf{A}$: $\|\mathbf{x}\|_{\mathbf{A}} \doteq \sqrt{\mathbf{x}^\intercal\mathbf{A}\mathbf{x}}$. Unlike the Cartesian formulation, this problem cannot be solved in closed form. Therefore, to solve the Maximization step, we rewrite the maximization problem as an equivalent minimization problem

$$(a_s^\star, b_s^\star, c_s^\star) = \underset{(a_s,b_s,c_s)}{\arg\min}\left(\sum_{t=0}^{T-1}\gamma_s(t+1)\,\left\|\mathrm{vec}\left(q_{t+1} - \mathrm{Exp}\,(a_s\mathtt{i} + b_s\mathtt{j} + c_s\mathtt{k}) * q_t\right)\right\|^2_{\mathbf{\Sigma}^{-1}}\right)$$

and solve it via any minimization algorithm (e.g. *gradient descent*).

Remark 2.1 The use of our proposed generalizations can be combined with other extensions to the ARHMM model. For instance, in the EM algorithm of *Auto-Regressive Hidden semi-Markov Models*, the maximization formula for the emission probabilities can be easily extended in a similar fashion to what we proposed here.

2.4 Experiments

In this section, we will compare the results obtained with the NL-ARHMM against the linear ARHMM, showing that this novel approach results in higher segmentation scores.

2.4.1 Validation Test

At first, we show that the EM algorithm for the NL-ARHMM allows learning the parameters of the model. To do so, we define a NL-ARHMM with fixed parameters and use it to generate data samples. In our test, we set both the number of hidden modes and the dimension of the continuous state to 2: $S = 2, d = 2$. The initial mode distribution is set to $\varpi = [0.5, 0.5]^\intercal$ and the transition probability matrix is

$$\mathbf{T} = \begin{bmatrix} 0.95 & 0.05 \\ 0.05 & 0.95 \end{bmatrix}.$$

The non-linear dynamics is written as follows. We start by defining the vector field

$$\mathbf{f}\left(\begin{bmatrix} y_1 \\ y_2 \end{bmatrix}\right) = \begin{bmatrix} {y_1}^3 + {y_2}^2 y_1 - y_1 - y_2 \\ {y_2}^3 + {y_1}^2 y_2 + y_1 - y_2 \end{bmatrix}.$$

Then the dynamics of the two hidden modes are obtained using the Euler method with time step $\delta_t = 0.05$ for the dynamics $\mathbf{f}$ and its opposite $-\mathbf{f}$, with Gaussian noise with standard deviation $\varsigma = 5\mathrm{e}-03$:

$$\mathbf{y}_{t+1}|z_{t+1} = 1, \mathbf{y}_t \sim \mathcal{N}(\mathbf{y}_{t+1}|\mathbf{y}_t + \delta_t \mathbf{f}(\mathbf{y}_t), \varsigma \mathbf{I}_2),$$
$$\mathbf{y}_{t+1}|z_{t+1} = 2, \mathbf{y}_t \sim \mathcal{N}(\mathbf{y}_{t+1}|\mathbf{y}_t - \delta_t \mathbf{f}(\mathbf{y}_t), \varsigma \mathbf{I}_2).$$

We use this NL-ARHMM to generate fifty samples with $T = 100$ steps each. Next, we initialize both a NL-ARHMM (with polynomial basis functions of degree $k = 2$) and a linear ARHMM, and apply the EM algorithm to learn the model parameters. Finally, we use the Viterbi algorithm to segment a new trajectory generated from the "true" NL-ARHMM. Before applying the EM algorithm we standardize the dataset. That is, we translate it and multiply by a constant to have null mean and unit variance.

Figure 15 shows one result for these tests. As can be observed, the NL-ARHMM is able to properly segment the trajectory, being able to capture more complex dynamics. On the other hand, the linear ARHMM results in a poorer segmentation. More tests with this setup confirm that the Non-Linear ARHMM typically gives a more accurate segmentation than the linear ARHMM.

2.5 Comparison of Different Degrees Polynomial Functions

In this Section, we propose some tests to show that Non-Linear basis functions are more effective when the observation space $\mathcal{Y}$ is low-dimensional. On the other hand, for high-dimensional observation space, the difference between the two is less noticeable.

To show this aspect, we simulate three different ARHMM with nonlinear dynamics. Each of them has two hidden modes but differs in the dimension d of the observation space; $d = 1, 2, 3$. To present a fair comparison, all six dynamics (two for each value of d) are non-polynomial: in this way, none of the models we will compare (linear, quadratic, and cubic) is able to perfectly describe the dynamics.

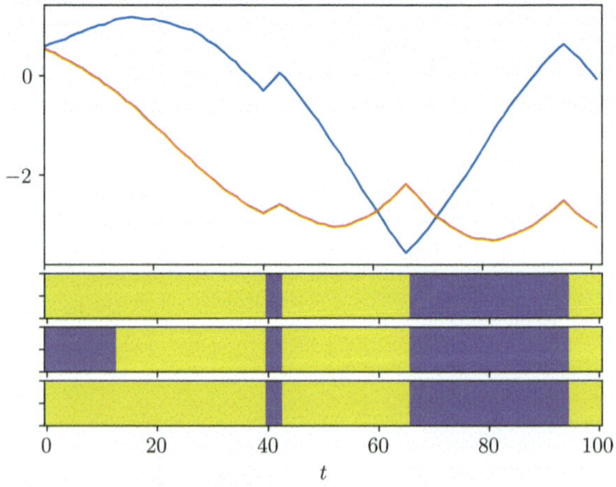

Fig. 15 Results for the validation test presented in Sect. 2.4.1. The top figure shows the components of the trajectory, the second plot shows the "true" segmentation (the first mode is represented in purple, while the second mode is represented in yellow), the third plot shows the segmentation obtained with the learned ARHMM, and the fourth plot shows the segmentation obtained with the learned NL-ARHMM

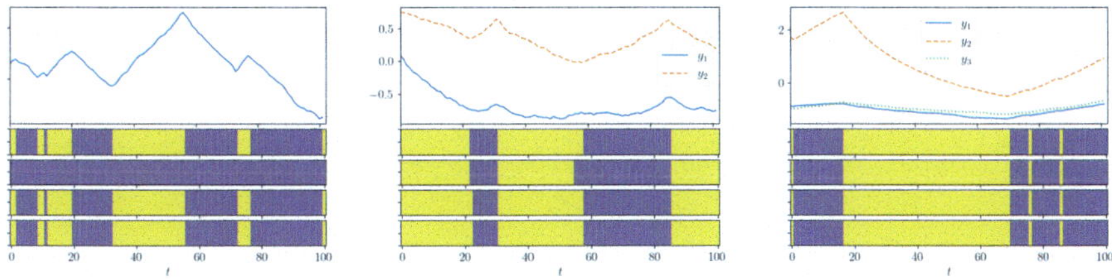

(a) $d = 1$, (b) $d = 2$ (c) $d = 3$

Fig. 16 Comparison between linear and polynomial ARHMM. In all three figures, the first plot shows the components y_i of the observed dynamics, the second plot shows the true segmentation, the third, fourth, and fifth plots shows the segmentations obtained by, respectively, the linear, quadratic, and cubic formulations of the ARHMM (i.e. $k = 1, 2, 3$ in (31))

Similarly to the previous test, for each value of d we generate a total of fifty trajectories of 100 steps. Figure 16 shows the results of these tests.

As it can be observed, with $d = 1$ (Fig. 16a) the linear model is not able to properly describe the nonlinear dynamics, failing in the segmentation of the obtained trajectory. On the other hand, for $d = 2$ and 3 (Fig. 16b and 16c respectively), the differences between the three dynamical models (linear, quadratic, and cubic) significantly reduce.

These tests show that for lower-dimensional observation spaces, the improvements in using the Non-Linear formulation for the ARHMM dynamics are more significant. We argue that the motivation lies in the fact that for high-dimensional data, linear vector fields can describe a wider range of dynamics, since the number of parameters in the dynamics grows quadratically with the space dimension. To be precise, the number of parameters for each dynamics is $d^2 + d$: d^2 elements for the matrix $\mathbf{A}_s$ and d for the vector $\mathbf{b}_s$ in (23). Oh the other hand, for smaller observation spaces, linear dynamics are too limited and the usage of polynomial functions in the definition of the dynamics provides a broader set of possible behaviors.

For this reason, in Sect. 2.6 we will propose a model in which the Cartesian position of the robot end-effector is modeled by a linear dynamics, while the gripper angle (a 1-dimensional variable) will be modeled using a polynomial dynamics.

2.6 *Experiments on Real Setups*

To prove the effectiveness of our generalizations, we propose a model combining both Non-Linear Cartesian and Linear Unit-Quaternion dynamics. In particular, we propose a pose+gripper model in which, for each hand of the robot, we model the position with a linear Cartesian model, the end-effector orientation with a linear Unit-Quaternion model, and the gripper angle with a quadratic model. The decision to use a linear model for the position and a quadratic model for the gripper angle are motivated by the tests presented in Sect. 2.5: for 3-dimensional spaces, linear,

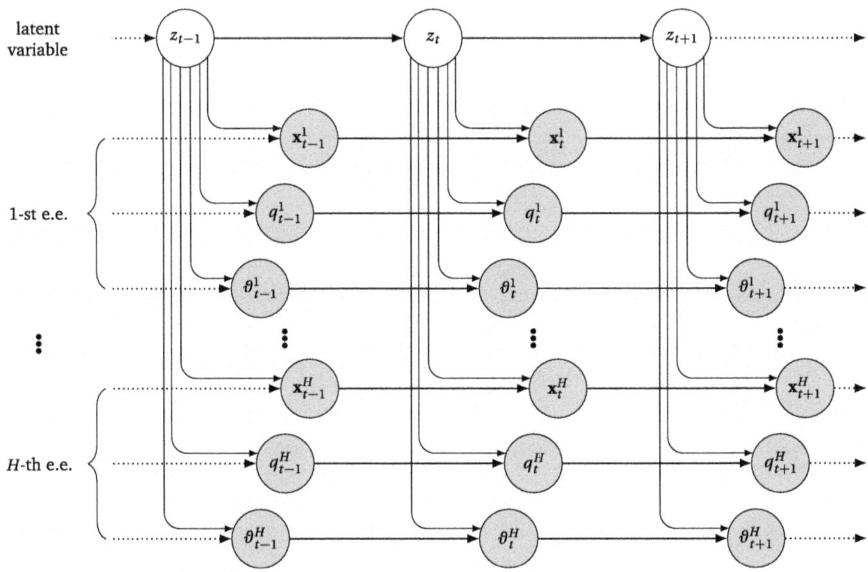

Fig. 17 Graphical representation of a Pose+Gripper ARHMM

quadratic, and cubic models are almost indistinguishable (Fig. 16c) and we thus choose the simplest one. On the other hand, for 1-dimensional trajectories, linear models fail to describe the complexity of the behavior, while a quadratic and a cubic one give similar results (Fig. 16c).

Additionally, we assume that position $\mathbf{x}_t^h$, orientation q_t^h, and gripper angle ϑ_t^h of each arm h are independent of each others when the hidden mode is given:

$$p\left(\begin{matrix}\mathbf{x}_{t+1}^1, q_{t+1}^1, \vartheta_{t+1}^1, \\ \dots, \\ \mathbf{x}_{t+1}^H, q_{t+1}^H, \vartheta_{t+1}^H\end{matrix}\,\middle|\,\begin{matrix}\mathbf{x}_t^1, q_t^1, \vartheta_t^1, \\ \dots, \\ \mathbf{x}_t^H, q_t^H, \vartheta_t^H, z_{t+1}\end{matrix}\right) = \prod_{h=1}^{H} p(\mathbf{x}_{t+1}^h | z_{t+1}, \mathbf{x}_t^h)\, p(q_{t+1}^h | z_{t+1}, q_t^h)\, p(\vartheta_{t+1}^h | z_{t+1}, \vartheta_t^h). \tag{34}$$

A graphical model representation of the model is given in Fig. 17.

To demonstrate the improvement in the segmentation quality given by the different dynamics, we compare our model against a Linear ARHMM with the same topology, so that the only difference lies in the definition of the Auto Regressive dynamics itself. This means that position, orientation, and gripper angle for each end effector is independent of each other, and the conditional probability of the next observed state follows the same law as in (34). The only difference is that the Linear ARHMM uses linear dynamics for the evolution of each observed state. Since the conditional independence (and, thus, the topology) are identical, the graphical representation of the model does not change.

To test our method, we use the *JIGSAW* dataset [50]. It consists of three different surgical tasks ('SUTuring', 'Knot Tying', and 'Needle Passing') executed by eight surgeons of different skill levels. Data consists of positions, velocities, orientations (in the form of rotation matrices), angular velocities, and gripper angle. Each variable is given for both left and right arms, and for both the patient-side and surgeon-side controllers. Moreover, JIGSAW provides a segmentation of all the tasks in gestures. We use only positions, orientations (converting from rotation matrices to unit quaternions) and gripper angle for the patient-side end-effectors. Thus, in our case, $H = 2$.

To evaluate the quality of the algorithm, we proceed as follows. For a given batch of data, we use the Expectation Maximization algorithm to infer the set of parameters Θ for both models. Then, we apply the Viterbi algorithm to segment one of the executions that were not in the training set, and we compute different scores for segmentation. This test is repeated a given number of times randomizing each time both the training and testing sets.

The scores we decide to adopt are the following: *Seg-score* and *Silhouette Index* (SI). Seg-score (also known as *Jaccard index*) [51, 52] is a *supervised score*, that is, it compares the obtained segmentation to the ground-truth; it is the size of similarity between segmentation result and ground-truth. SI [53], instead, is an *unsupervised score* and it evaluates the goodness of the segmentation by treating it as a clustering problem; it evaluates the clusters by comparing the average distance within a cluster with the average distance to the points in the nearest clusters. We decided to use these scores since they are already used for the evaluation of segmentation algorithms in the context of robotic surgery [31, 54]. The main challenge in using this dataset is that it is not consistent: the same task may contain different gestures in each trial (that is, a particular gesture is present in one trial but not in the others). This makes the segmentation a particularly hard problem: if the model has many hidden modes, but some are rare, over-fitting and over-segmentation (i.e. a segment is wrongly split in multiple smaller parts) will likely happen. On the other hand, if we use fewer hidden modes, some different gestures will be described by the same hidden mode, resulting in a lower Seg-score.

In Fig. 18, we show the results of this test. In particular, for each of the 100 trials with a given task and a given number of hidden modes, we show the histograms counting the number of occurrences of the scores in a given interval. As can be seen, the NL model is able to achieve, on average, a higher score in both the supervised and unsupervised metrics, and it is also able to achieve higher scores (see, for instance, Fig. 18d).

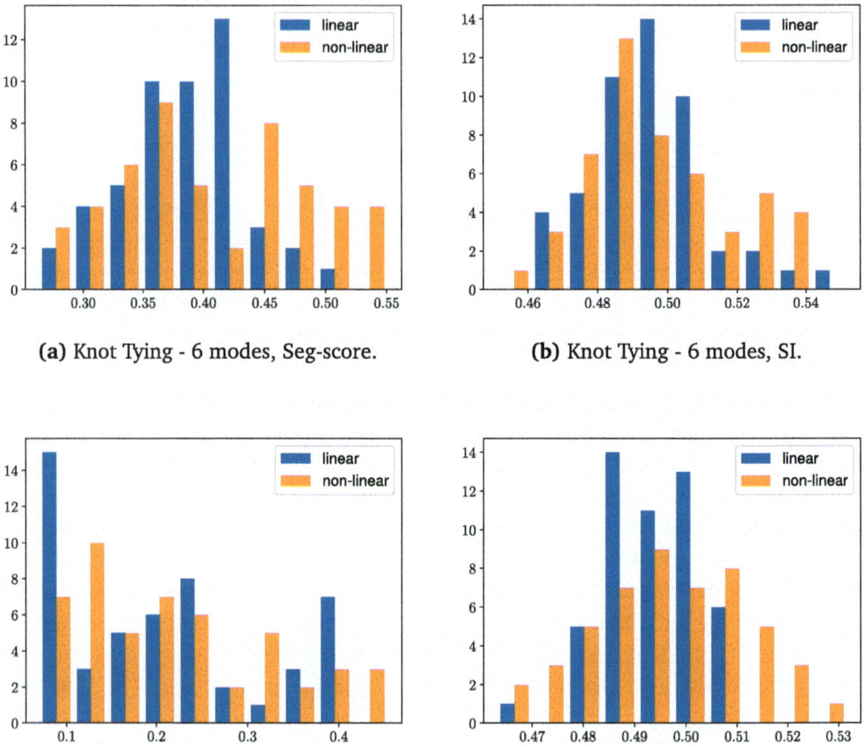

(a) Knot Tying - 6 modes, Seg-score.

(b) Knot Tying - 6 modes, SI.

(c) Suturing - 5 modes, Seg-score.

(d) Suturing - 5 modes, SI.

Fig. 18 Histograms showing the number of occurrences for different scores. Color blue marks the 'state of the art' linear ARHMM, while orange marks our proposed generalization

3 Conclusions

In this chapter, we discussed the bottom-up approach for trajectory learning in the context of Autonomous Robotic Surgery. As we discussed, this bottom-up approach is needed due to the nature of the surgical gestures: they are performed with the goal of performing the surgical task while reducing as much as possible the damage that can be inflicted on the patient. This goal cannot be described by any metric, and it is thus impossible to define a cost function to have the 'optimal' surgery. For this reason, we decided to develop a framework that allows us to learn the movements from expert surgeons.

In Sect. 1, we presented the 'Dynamic Movement Primitives' framework. It consists of a dynamical system of spring-mass-damper type that presents multiple advantages:

- it allows to learn the shape of a movement thanks to a *forcing term* that can be easily obtained from demonstrations
- there are both a Cartesian and a unit-quaternion formulation, allowing to modeling of both the movements and the orientation of the end-effector of the robot
- it can generalize to unseen scenarios thanks to the spatial-scaling properties of the system and the possibility of adding obstacles.

We tested this framework in multiple scenarios, showing that it is able to perform surgical-related tasks on the daVinci surgical robot.

Despite its effectiveness, our usage of the DMP system has a drawback: since we use DMPs to learn small movements, the definition of the dataset from which we learn the dynamics is complicated: we need to segment hours of surgical data into movements that are usually a few seconds long. For this reason, in Sect. 2, we presented our approach to perform unsupervised segmentation of time series. Our approach is based on the theory of *Auto-Regressive Hidden Markov Models*. The idea is that there is a hidden mode that, at each time, describes which action (defined as an Auto-Regressive dynamics) is being performed. This type of model is able to learn both the relation between subsequent hidden modes and the dynamics associated with each mode by observing only the time series. Moreover, once learned the parameters, it is possible to extract the most likely sequence of hidden modes that produced an observation, thus segmenting the time series. We generalized the classical AR-HMM to describe also non-linear dynamics and to work in Unit-Quaternion space, in order to have a proper segmentation also of the gestures that require mostly wrist movements.

We showed that our generalized AR-HMM is able to obtain, on average, higher scores than the classical AR-HMM on the JIGSAW surgical dataset, proving that it is a valid tool to segment surgical-related procedures in movements.

As future work, we aim at developing a joint DMP-HMM model, in which the DMP system is natively integrated in the AR-HMM model. This would allow us to simultaneously segment the time series and learn the DMP that describes the kinetics of each movement.

References

1. Ijspeert, A.J., Nakanishi, J., Schaal, S.: Movement imitation with nonlinear dynamical systems in humanoid robots. In: Proceedings of the IEEE International Conference on Robotics and Automation, 2002, ICRA'02, vol. 2, pp. 1398–1403. IEEE (2002)
2. Ijspeert, A.J., Nakanishi, J., Schaal, S.: Learning attractor landscapes for learning motor primitives. In: Advances in Neural Information Processing Systems, pp. 1547–1554 (2003)
3. Schaal, S.: Dynamic movement primitives-a framework for motor control in humans and humanoid robotics. In: Adaptive Motion of Animals and Machines, pp. 261–280. Springer (2006)
4. S. Schaal, P. Mohajerian, A. Ijspeert, Dynamics systems versus optimal control—a unifying view. In: Cisek, P., Drew, T., Kalaska, J.F. (eds.) Computational Neuroscience: Theoretical Insights into Brain Function, vol. 165 of Progress in Brain Research, pp. 425–445. Elsevier (2007)

5. Pastor, P., Hoffmann, H., Asfour, T., Schaal, S.: Learning and generalization of motor skills by learning from demonstration. In: IEEE International Conference on Robotics and Automation, 2009. ICRA'09, pp. 763–768. IEEE (2009)
6. Ijspeert, A.J., Nakanishi, J., Hoffmann, H., Pastor, P., Schaal, S.: Dynamical movement primitives: learning attractor models for motor behaviors. Neural Comput. **25**(2), 328–373 (2013)
7. Sidiropoulos, A., Doulgeri, Z.: A reversible dynamic movement primitive formulation (2020). arXiv:2010.07708
8. Ude, A., Nemec, B., Petrić, T., Morimoto, J.: Orientation in cartesian space dynamic movement primitives. In: IEEE International Conference on Robotics and Automation (ICRA), 2014, pp. 2997–3004. IEEE (2014)
9. Abu-Dakka, F.J., Kyrki, V.: Geometry-aware dynamic movement primitives. In: 2020 IEEE International Conference on Robotics and Automation (ICRA), pp. 4421–4426. IEEE (2020)
10. Hoffmann, H., Pastor, P., Park, D.-H., Schaal, S.: Biologically-inspired dynamical systems for movement generation: automatic real-time goal adaptation and obstacle avoidance. In: IEEE International Conference on Robotics and Automation, 2009, ICRA'09, pp. 2587–2592. IEEE (2009)
11. Ginesi, M., Sansonetto, N., Fiorini, P.: Overcoming some drawbacks of dynamic movement primitives. Robot. Auton. Syst. **144**, 103844 (2021)
12. Matsubara, T., Hyon, S.-H., Morimoto, J.: Learning stylistic dynamic movement primitives from multiple demonstrations. In: IEEE/RSJ International Conference on Intelligent Robots and Systems (IROS), 2010, pp. 1277–1283. Citeseer (2010)
13. Matsubara, T., Hyon, S.-H., Morimoto, J.: Learning parametric dynamic movement primitives from multiple demonstrations. Neural Netw. **24**(5), 493–500 (2011)
14. Paraschos, A., Daniel, C., Peters, J.R., Neumann, G.: Probabilistic movement primitives. In: Advances in neural information processing systems, pp. 2616–2624 (2013)
15. Huang, Y., Rozo, L., Silvério, J., Caldwell, D.G.: Kernelized movement primitives. Int. J. Robot. Res. **38**(7), 833–852 (2019)
16. Calinon, S.: A tutorial on task-parameterized movement learning and retrieval. Intel. Serv. Robot. **9**(1), 1–29 (2016)
17. Kutta, W.: Beitrag zur naherungsweisen integration totaler differentialgleichungen. Z. Math. Phys. **46**, 435–453 (1901)
18. Butcher, J.C., Wanner, G.: Runge-kutta methods: some historical notes. Appl. Numer. Math. **22**(1–3), 113–151 (1996)
19. Park, D.-H., Hoffmann, H., Pastor, P., Schaal, S.: Movement reproduction and obstacle avoidance with dynamic movement primitives and potential fields. In: 8th IEEE-RAS International Conference on Humanoid Robots, 2008. Humanoids 2008, pp. 91–98. IEEE (2008)
20. Hwang, Y.K., Ahuja, N., et al.: A potential field approach to path planning. IEEE Trans. Robot. Autom. **8**(1), 23–32 (1992)
21. Quinlan, S., Khatib, O.: Elastic bands: connecting path planning and control. In: 1993 Proceedings IEEE International Conference on Robotics and Automation, pp. 802–807. IEEE (1993)
22. Y. Wang and G. S. Chirikjian, "A new potential field method for robot path planning," in *Proceedings 2000 ICRA. Millennium Conference. IEEE International Conference on Robotics and Automation. Symposia Proceedings (Cat. No. 00CH37065)*, vol. 2, pp. 977–982, IEEE, 2000
23. Brock, O., Khatib, O.: Elastic strips: a framework for motion generation in human environments. The Int. J. Robot. Res. **21**(12), 1031–1052 (2002)
24. Khatib, O.: Real-time obstacle avoidance for manipulators and mobile robots. In: Proceedings. 1985 IEEE International Conference on Robotics and Automation, vol. 2, pp. 500–505. IEEE (1985)
25. M. Ginesi, D. Meli, A. Calanca, D. Dall'Alba, N. Sansonetto, P. Fiorini, Dynamic movement primitives: volumetric obstacle avoidance. In: 2019 19th International Conference on Advanced Robotics (ICAR), pp. 234–239, Dec. 2019

26. Ginesi, M., Meli, D., Roberti, A., Sansonetto, N., Fiorini, P.: Dynamic movement primitives: Volumetric obstacle avoidance using dynamic potential functions. J. Intell. Robot. Syst. **101**, 79 (2021)
27. Volpe, R.: Real and artificial forces in the control of manipulators: theory and experiments. Ph.D. thesis, Ph.D. thesis, Carnegie Mellon University, Department of Physics (1990)
28. Ginesi, M., Meli, D., Roberti, A., Sansonetto, N., Fiorini, P.: Autonomous task planning and situation awareness in robotic surgery. In: IEEE/RSJ International Conference on Intelligent Robots and Systems, pp. 3144–3150. IEEE (2020)
29. Abonyi, J., Babuska, R., Szeifert, F.: "Modified gath-geva fuzzy clustering for identification of takagi-sugeno fuzzy models. IEEE Trans. Syst. Man Cybern. Part B (Cybernetics) **32**(5), 612–621 (2002)
30. Lioutikov, R., Neumann, G., Maeda, G., Peters, J.: Probabilistic segmentation applied to an assembly task. In: 2015 IEEE-RAS 15th International Conference on Humanoid Robots (Humanoids), pp. 533–540. IEEE (2015)
31. Murali, A., Garg, A., Krishnan, S., Pokorny, F., Abbeel, P., Darrell, T., Goldberg, K.: TSC-DL: unsupervised trajectory segmentation of multi-modal surgical demonstrations with deep learning. In: 2016 IEEE International Conference on Robotics and Automation (ICRA) (2016)
32. Despinoy, F., Bouget, D., Forestier, G., Penet, C., Zemiti, N., Poignet, P., Jannin, P.: Unsupervised trajectory segmentation for surgical gesture recognition in robotic training. IEEE Trans. Biomed. Eng. **63**(6), 1280–1291 (2016)
33. Lioutikov, R., Neumann, G., Maeda, G., Peters, J.: Learning movement primitive libraries through probabilistic segmentation. Int. J. Robot. Res. **36**(8), 879–894 (2017)
34. Krishnan, S., Garg, A., Patil, S., Lea, C., Hager, G., Abbeel, P., Goldberg, K.: Transition state clustering: unsupervised surgical trajectory segmentation for robot learning. Int. J. Robot. Res. **36**(13–14), 1595–1618 (2017)
35. Soares Júnior, A., Moreno, B.N., Times, V.C., Matwin, S., Cabral, L.D.A.F.: Grasp-uts: an algorithm for unsupervised trajectory segmentation. Int. J. Geograph. Inf. Sci. **29**(1), 46–68 (2015)
36. Chiappa, S., Peters, J.R.: Movement extraction by detecting dynamics switches and repetitions. In: Advances in Neural Information Processing Systems, pp. 388–396 (2010)
37. Meier, F., Theodorou, E., Stulp, F., Schaal, S.: Movement segmentation using a primitive library. In: 2011 IEEE/RSJ International Conference on Intelligent Robots and Systems (IROS), pp. 3407–3412. IEEE (2011)
38. Calinon, S., D'halluin, F., Sauser, E.L., Caldwell, D.G., Billard, A.G.: Learning and reproduction of gestures by imitation. IEEE Robot. Autom. Mag. **17**, 44–54 (2010)
39. Visser, I.: Seven things to remember about hidden Markov models: a tutorial on Markovian models for time series. J. Math. Psychol. **55**(6), 403–415 (2011)
40. Vakanski, A., Mantegh, I., Irish, A., Janabi-Sharifi, F.: Trajectory learning for robot programming by demonstration using hidden Markov model and dynamic time warping. IEEE Trans. Syst. Man Cybern. Part B (Cybernetics) **42**(4), 1039–1052 (2012)
41. Juang, B.-H., Rabiner, L.: Mixture autoregressive hidden Markov models for speech signals. IEEE Trans. Acoust. Speech Signal Process. **33**(6), 1404–1413 (1985)
42. Ephraim, Y., Roberts, W.J.: Revisiting autoregressive hidden Markov modeling of speech signals. IEEE Signal Process. Lett. **12**(2), 166–169 (2005)
43. Kroemer, O., Van Hoof, H. Neumann, G., Peters, J.: Learning to predict phases of manipulation tasks as hidden states. In: 2014 IEEE International Conference on Robotics and Automation (ICRA), pp. 4009–4014. IEEE (2014)
44. Guan, X., Raich, R., Wong, W.-K.: Efficient multi-instance learning for activity recognition from time series data using an auto-regressive hidden Markov model. In: International Conference on Machine Learning, pp. 2330–2339 (2016)
45. Bishop, C.M., Nasrabadi, N.M.: Pattern Recognition and Machine Learning, vol. 4, no. 4, p. 738. Springer, New York (2006)
46. Viterbi, A.: Error bounds for convolutional codes and an asymptotically optimum decoding algorithm. IEEE Trans. Inf. Theory **13**(2), 260–269 (1967)

47. Forney, G.D.: The viterbi algorithm. Proc. IEEE, **61**(3), 268–278 (2005)
48. Ginesi, M., Fiorini, P.: Learning of Surgical Gestures for Robotic Minimally Invasive Surgery Using Dynamic Movement Primitives and Latent Variable Models. Ph.D. thesis, University of Verona, Department of Computer Science (2021)
49. Ginesi, M., Fiorini, P.: Generalization of auto-regressive hidden Markov models to non-linear dynamics and unit quaternion observation space. IEEE Robot. Autom. Lett. **8**(9), 5847–5853 (2023)
50. Gao, Y., Vedula, S.S., Reiley, C.E., Ahmidi, N., Varadarajan, B., Lin, H.C., Tao, L., Zappella, L., Béjar, B., Yuh, D.D., Chen, C.C.G.: September. Jhu-isi gesture and skill assessment working set (jigsaws): A surgical activity dataset for human motion modeling. In: MICCAI Workshop: M2cai, vol. 3, No. 2014, p. 3 (2014)
51. Ivchenko, G., Honov, S.: On the Jaccard similarity test. J. Math. Sci. **88**, 789–794 (1998)
52. Maška, M., Ulman, V., Svoboda, D., Matula, P., Matula, P., Ederra, C., Urbiola, A., España, T., Venkatesan, S., Balak, D.M., et al.: A benchmark for comparison of cell tracking algorithms. Bioinformatics **30**(11), 1609–1617 (2014)
53. Rousseeuw, P.J.: Silhouettes: a graphical aid to the interpretation and validation of cluster analysis. J. Comput. Appl. Math. **20**, 53–65 (1987)
54. Fard, M., Ameri, S., Chinnam, R., Ellis, R.: Soft boundary approach for unsupervised gesture segmentation in robotic-assisted surgery. IEEE Robot. Autom. Lett. **2**(1), 171–178 (2016)

Simulation and Autonomy

Eleonora Tagliabue

Abstract This chapter presents a novel viewpoint on the relation between simulation and autonomy, in which simulation is a tool for learning. Section 1 describes the main methods used to simulate the properties of deformable objects, such as those in anatomical environments. Section 2 introduces the use of simulation to generate data for machine learning methods. Section 3 summarizes the methods described in the chapter and is the introduction to the applications of simulations described in the following chapters.

The complexity and uncertainty of the environment make the development of an Autonomous Robotic Surgical System (ARSS) a challenging task, since it requires to consider many different aspects. For example, the definition of the intervention plan and its instantiation on a specific patient already introduce some major difficulties. First of all, it is necessary to identify the sequence of actions needed to complete the desired surgical task in general terms. This requires the integration of both a-priori knowledge from textbooks and the experience, actions and reasoning of multiple surgeons, that can be only learnt from data of real interventions. Once the surgical plan is defined, it must be adjusted to cope with the current patient, according to his/her specific clinical situation and geometric and mechanical properties.

Even though a patient-specific intervention plan is available, the ARSS must be capable of adapting it during execution based on current situation, since the anatomical environment might behave differently from what expected from pre-operative knowledge. To cope with such an uncertain environment, it is key to incorporate strategies for real-time situation awareness, reasoning and control, that allow prompt reaction and online replanning in response to unknown or unexpected situations.

Automating a process in an environment as critical as the surgical one, where errors can be deadly, also requires the availability of an integrated framework that can be used for both the design, test and validation of the intervention plan in the pre-

E. Tagliabue (✉)
Department of Computer Science, University of Verona, Verona, Italy
e-mail: eleonora.tagliabue@zeiss.com

Carl Zeiss AG, Oberkochen, Germany

P. Fiorini (ed.), *Towards Autonomous Robotic Surgery*, Springer Tracts in Advanced Robotics 161, https://doi.org/10.1007/978-3-032-04247-7_6

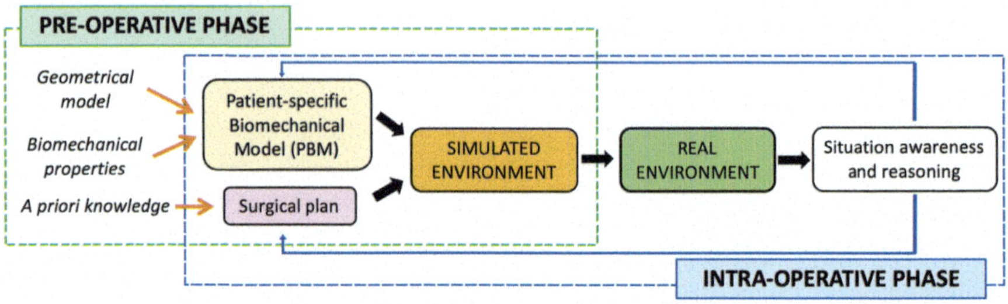

Fig. 1 In an ARSS, a PBM is instantiated pre-operatively with patient-specific geometry and biomechanical properties. Such model is employed to initialize the simulation environment where the surgical plan is verified in the pre-operative phase. In the intra-operative phase, both the PBM and the surgical plan are adjusted depending on the current surgical situation

operative phase, and the control and monitoring of task execution intra-operatively, handling environmental uncertainties.

A great support to the autonomous execution of surgical actions by an ARSS can be provided by the availability of a simulation of the anatomical environment. Such simulation is based on a Patient-specific Biomechanical Model (PBM), which is created in a pre-operative phase from geometry and physical properties of the surgical areas extracted from each patient diagnostic images and/or initialized with values from the literature (Fig. 1).

First of all, simulation represents a test bench where to *design and verify* the surgical plan before its actual execution on the real system. This step is essential in safety-critical scenarios as surgery, since it allows to optimize the plan accounting for each patient's characteristics, and test it before execution to visualize possible problems, identify any major errors and predict potentially critical situations. Robotic actions verification is also required while the intervention is taking place, especially when actions replanning is needed. In order to guarantee that the intra-operative verification is reliable, it is essential that the simulation continuously represents an up-to-date replica of the current surgical situation. The pre-operative PBM should therefore be continuously updated to reflect all the changes introduced by the surgical manipulations based on real data. Figure 1 highlights the role of simulation for surgical plan verification for an ARSS.

The availability of an accurate simulation of the anatomical environment can support the ARSS via the *generation of realistic*—and even patient-specific—*data* that can be used for learning purposes. This is very important since the complexity of both the environment and the cause-effect flow governing surgical actions make ML algorithms ideal for learning tasks, but they are challenged by the impracticality to acquire real world data in the medical field. In fact, such data are generally difficult to get due to the technical, ethical and privacy issues involved in data collection process. By providing a way to generate large amounts of realistic data, computer simulation allows to compensate for this limitation. Generated data can also be exploited for the design of novel data-driven models or methods that might be more informative or more efficient than traditional approaches and can assist the ARSS during task execution.

Furthermore, simulation can *provide* the ARSS *with critical information* during task execution. It can guide the ARSS towards the structures of interest, which might be hidden from the partial view available intra-operatively, or warn it in case it approaches critical regions which might be not directly recognizable on intra-operative images. It can complement information from real sensors, for example estimating the interaction forces between instruments and tissues when direct force measurement systems are not available, as is the case of most current surgical robotic systems [1]. Moreover, since simulation represents the ARSS internal knowledge of the environment, a continuous monitoring of the discrepancy between the simulated and the real scenarios allows to assess if the execution on the real setting is coherent with what the ARSS expects based on its internal knowledge, and adopt specific strategies to accommodate safety in case it is not.

1 Deformable Models for Surgical Simulation

Modelling and simulation of the deformable behavior of the anatomy can support surgical applications in several ways.

After reviewing the main challenges involved in realistic surgical simulation in Sect. 1.1, this chapter provides an overview of the main categories of deformable models for surgical simulation, highlighting their advantages and disadvantages. We first discuss the preferred modelling strategy for applications requiring high simulation accuracy, which relies on a mathematical description of soft tissues behavior through the laws of continuum mechanics (Sect. 1.2). However, this kind of simulations generally suffer from high computational cost. When high solution speed is required, some simplifications are usually introduced into the physics of the environment, in order to achieve a simulation which is at least physically plausible. This class of methods, referred to as heuristic models, will be described in Sect. 1.4. Finally, we present how machine learning techniques can be exploited to predict tissue deformations in Sect. 1.8.

1.1 Challenges of Surgical Simulation

In all the mentioned applications, it would be desirable to rely on a deformation model which represents real tissues behavior in an accurate way, while requiring minimal computation time and staying numerically stable. However, these factors have conflicting computational requirements. Reaching high accuracy levels generally implies usage of complex nonlinear models, which in turns means higher computational cost and higher probability of numerical instability. On the other hand, model simplifications can be introduced to minimize computation time whenever performance is the main factor of interest. Simultaneously meeting all these requirements is very difficult, especially with increasing complexity of the simulation. As a consequence, a variety of models have been proposed to approximate the behavior of soft tissues, optimized in different ways to meet the specific needs of the application they address [2].

Challenge of Patient-Specific Simulations

The first main challenge of surgical simulation is the proper representation of the manipulated tissues, to achieve an accurate modelling of their behavior. With the only exception of training simulators, which can rely on anatomical models extracted from available datasets [3] and approximated deformation properties, all the other mentioned applications require patient-specific model parametrization to reach clinically acceptable precision.

The first step for personalized simulation is the reliance on *organ geometry* from actual patient's data (Fig. 2). The 3D model of the anatomy of interest is generally constructed starting from pre-operative volumetric images such as computerized tomography (CT) or magnetic resonance imaging (MRI). These imaging techniques provide a 3D view of the patient's internal anatomy, where the different structures can be identified and labelled with a process called segmentation. Although several attempts have been made towards automating the segmentation task [4], they are extremely context-dependent, still leaving manual segmentation as the most widely applicable and reliable approach. Afterwards, a 3D surface model of the tissues is generated from the segmentation mask, commonly relying on the marching cubes algorithm [5]. In some approaches, like ChainMail (Sect. 1.7), the generated 3D surface already represents the input to the simulation. However, many simulation approaches also require the discretization of the volume enclosed within the gen-

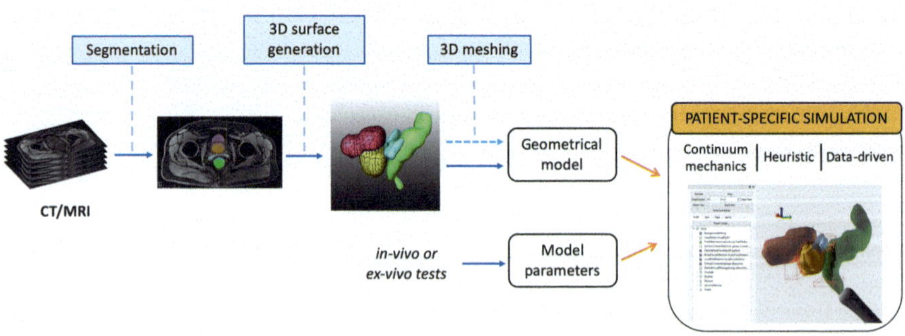

Fig. 2 General workflow for patient-specific simulation. A geometrical model of the anatomy is obtained from segmentation of the patient's volumetric images (CT or MRI) and subsequent 3D surface generation. The obtained surface might be eventually meshed into a full 3D volume, as required by some simulation approaches. Either in-vivo or ex-vivo tests are performed to identify model parameters describing the deformable behavior of the anatomy. The geometrical model and the model parameters initialize the simulation environment, which can be based on different analytical models

erated surface into elementary entities, such as tetrahedrons or hexahedrons, in a process called 3D meshing. Tetrahedral elements are the preferred ones for the discretization of anatomical shapes, since they can easily represent irregular geometries with sufficient detail. The 3D meshing process is generally automated, and relies on Delaunay triangulation [6]. The accuracy of mesh-based simulations depends on the both the number and the regularity of the generated elements, which in turns is influenced by the quality of the starting surface.

Overall, the generation of a good geometrical model is essential for reliable simulations, but it requires extensive manual processing which is both time consuming and subject-dependent, thus representing a first challenge in the generation of patient-specific simulations. Moreover, it is clear that all the inaccuracies in the model generation phase will introduce uncertainties in the physics quantities predicted by simulations [7].

The generation of a reliable patient-specific simulation requires the selection of the most suitable *analytical model* to describe the complex anatomical behavior. This represents an additional challenge since tissues behavior is usually characterized by non-linear material laws, often including heterogeneity (i.e., the presence of multiple materials with different mechanical properties) and anisotropy (i.e., materials showing different mechanical properties in different directions). Existing models can be classified in three main categories. The first category contains models that describe anatomical behavior through the laws of continuum mechanics, which can be solved using ad hoc numerical techniques. The second category consists of heuristic methods, which rely on simplified models of soft tissues geometry with specific constraints that allow to simulate elastic properties. Finally, the third category rely on machine learning techniques to represent tissues behavior. These three categories of models will be investigated in the following Sections.

The choice of the model influences the set of *model parameters* that describe tissues behavior. Model parameters, which include both material properties and boundary conditions, have to be careful selected ideally accounting for patient-specific characteristics. To this end, tissues mechanical properties can be determined through ex-vivo and/or in-vivo measurements. Ex-vivo measurements are obviously easier to perform since there are fewer constraints on the working space for the experimental setup, and conditions can be made more repetitive. However, material properties have proven to vary substantially from the true in-vivo properties, making these experiments less accurate for realistic modelling [8]. In-vivo experiments provide more realistic data, but conditions are less stable and boundary conditions for modelling a lot more difficult to define. By providing information about organs internal composition, tissues biomechanical properties might be inferred from traditional medical imaging techniques (CTs or MRIs). However, there is not an established relationship between tissue composition and their mechanical behavior. Elastography-based imaging has the potential to provide a direct estimate of organ stiffness, by measuring how acoustic strain waves propagate into the tissues [9, 10]. Such techiques still rely on ad-hoc setups and are not easily usable in the standard clinical environments.

Challenge of Interactive Simulations

The computation time required by the simulation is another critical issue. Applications like intra-operative guidance and surgical simulation require high solution speeds, compatible with the required update rates for smooth visual and (potentially) haptic feedback. The update rate required for visual feedback, that allows the human sensory system to achieve continuous motion of the environment, is in the range 20–60 Hz. In case haptics is also present, stable and smooth kinestetic sensation are guaranteed by an update rate between 300 and 1 kHz [11]. Being able to meet such strict time requirements becomes more and more challenging with increasing complexity of the simulation, for example if the organ mechanical behavior is described by nonlinear laws, if the interactions among multiple organs need to be accounted for, or if challenging surgical actions must be modelled, such as cutting and suturing, which involve topological changes. Computation of the numerical solution to the complex non-linear equations that accurately describe the behavior of soft tissues can be very expensive in these cases, thus not compatible with real-time performances. Applications where simulation interactivity is a fundamental requirement usually rely on modelling assumptions to simplify the deformation models or on numerical methods that approximate the exact solution, leaving accuracy aside for the sake of rapidity.

Challenge of Stable Simulations

An additional challenge of simulations involving deformable objects is represented by simulation stability. This property is desirable in all applications, since instability means a diverging solution, which is thus invalid and not usable. Visually, when a simulation becomes unstable, the modelled object "explodes", due to undesired movement of the mesh vertices caused by the propagation of errors in the numerical methods governing the resolution of the equation system. In these cases, small perturbations in the input produce large variations in the obtained deformations.

Guaranteeing simulation stability is particularly challenging when the equation system to solve is stiff. In these kinds of systems, the upper bound of the time step is constrained by stability rather than accuracy requirements. This is generally the case in surgical simulations, where the objects to model are described by non-linear material laws, with anisotropic, heterogeneous and nearly-incompressible properties, which can generate ill-conditioned problems. While solving stiff systems, numerical integration schemes (i.e., those used to advance the simulation in time) might require impractically small time steps to guarantee stability. This happens, for example, with explicit integration schemes [2]. On the other hand, implicit methods allow to use larger time steps while remaining stable, but the equation system to solve at each time step is slightly more complex [12]. Several advanced integration schemes have been proposed to guarantee a convergent solution, i.e. simulation stability, to any kind of input. Schemes with this property are said to be unconditionally stable. However, they obviously come at the expense of an increased computational cost.

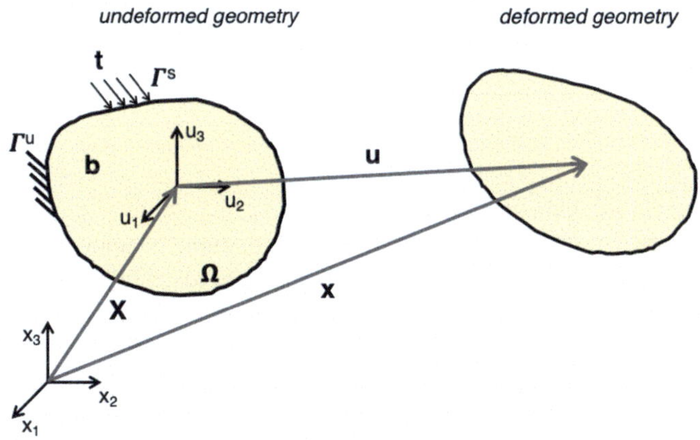

Fig. 3 A body defined over the domain Ω, subject to a body force **b**, surface traction **t** and boundary conditions on Γ, passes from its undeformed configuration **X** to a deformed configuration **x**

1.2 Continuum Mechanics Methods

The deformable behavior of soft tissues can be described with the laws of continuum mechanics. Each point in the undeformed reference configuration **X** is mapped to its corresponding point in the deformed configuration **x** (Fig. 3) through the deformation gradient **F** [13]:

$$\mathbf{F} = \frac{\partial \mathbf{x}}{\partial \mathbf{X}} = \mathbf{I} + \frac{\partial \mathbf{u}}{\partial \mathbf{X}} \tag{1}$$

where $\mathbf{u} = \mathbf{x} - \mathbf{X}$ is the displacement vector.

If a body defined over the domain Ω is in *static* equilibrium under an applied body force **b** (Fig. 3), imposing the balance of linear momentum leads to:

$$\nabla \cdot \boldsymbol{\sigma} + \mathbf{b} = 0 \quad in \quad \Omega \tag{2}$$

where $\nabla \cdot \boldsymbol{\sigma}$ represents the divergence of the Cauchy stress $\boldsymbol{\sigma}$. The Cauchy stress $\boldsymbol{\sigma}$ is a measure of the internal state of stress of the solid, which is related to surface tractions **t** via $\boldsymbol{\sigma}\mathbf{n} = \mathbf{t}$, where **n** is the outward unit normal to the surface.

Whereas, if the body is not in static equilibrium, its behavior is described by the dynamics laws of motion (Newton's second law). In this case, Eq. (2) must be extended to include the contribution of the inertia term, leading to:

$$\nabla \cdot \boldsymbol{\sigma} + \mathbf{b} = \rho \ddot{\mathbf{u}} \quad in \quad \Omega \tag{3}$$

where ρ is the object density. An additional term representing a damping force can be present.

Equations (2) and (3) are subject to some conditions on the boundary Γ of the object:

$$\begin{cases} \mathbf{u} = 0 \quad \text{on} \quad \Gamma_u \\ \boldsymbol{\sigma}\mathbf{n} = \mathbf{t} \quad \text{on} \quad \Gamma_s \end{cases} \tag{4}$$

where Γ_u and Γ_s are defined such that $\Gamma = \Gamma_u \cup \Gamma_s$.

Regardless of being in a static or dynamic situation, computation of realistic organ deformations using the continuum mechanics approach relies on the definition of the physical laws governing the mechanical response of the tissues to the applied sollicitations. Such laws are called constitutive laws and contribute to the definition of the internal forces. In particular, they put in relation the tissue stress, represented by $\boldsymbol{\sigma}$, to the tissue strain, described by the Green strain tensor $\mathbf{E}$, defined as:

$$\mathbf{E} = \frac{1}{2}(\nabla\mathbf{u} + \nabla\mathbf{u}^\top + \nabla\mathbf{u}\nabla\mathbf{u}^\top) \tag{5}$$

being $\mathbf{u}$ the displacement (i.e., the difference between the positions in the deformed and undeformed configurations).

Several different constitutive relations have been suggested in the literature, ranging from a linear law to very complex mathematical expressions [8, 14]. For elastic solids, the Cauchy stress is linearly related to the Green strain tensor by the elasticity matrix $\mathbf{D}$:

$$\boldsymbol{\sigma} = \mathbf{D} : \mathbf{E} \tag{6}$$

where ":" represents a contraction operation (i.e., $\sigma_{ij} = D_{ijkl}\epsilon_{kl}$ following Einstein summation convention[1]). In the elastic scenario, material behavior is fully described by only 2 characteristic constants: the Young's modulus E and Poisson's ratio ν. The simplest type of elastic materials are linear elastic materials, which are described by a linear relationship also between strain and displacement (i.e., neglecting the second order term in Eq. (5)). Although the linear elastic formulation is often preferred due to its computational convenience, it is not capable of handling large deformations correctly, thus it is not always adequate to describe tissues deformation [12].

A common way to describe more complex material behaviors is by means of a strain energy density function W. A material is called hyperelastic if W exists and the relationship between $\boldsymbol{\sigma}$ and $\mathbf{E}$ is obtained from:

$$\mathbf{S} = \frac{\partial W}{\partial \mathbf{E}} \tag{7}$$

$$\boldsymbol{\sigma} = J^{-1}\mathbf{F}\frac{\partial W}{\partial \mathbf{E}}\mathbf{F}^T \tag{8}$$

[1] According to Einstein summation convention, when an index is repeated twice in a single term, it implies summation of that term over the range of the repeated index, e.g. $\mathbf{u} = u_j\mathbf{e_j} = u_1\mathbf{e}_1 + u_2\mathbf{e}_2 + u_3\mathbf{e}_3$, where $\mathbf{e} = [\mathbf{e}_1, \mathbf{e}_2, \mathbf{e}_3]$ represents a basis vector in 3D.

where **S** is the second Piola-Kirchhoff stress, **F** is the deformation gradient in Eq. (1) and J is the determinant of **F** [13].

The simplest hyperelastic formulation is the St. Venant–Kirchhoff, which represents an elastic material able to handle large displacements, since it uses the full Green strain tensor of Eq. (5). The strain density function describing the St. Venant-Kirchhoff material is given by:

$$W(\mathbf{E}) = \frac{\lambda}{2}[tr(\mathbf{E})]^2 + \mu[tr(\mathbf{E}^2)] \tag{9}$$

where tr indicates the trace of the tensor, λ and μ are the Lamé constants, and are uniquely related to the Young's modulus E and Poisson's ratio ν via

$$\lambda = \frac{\nu E}{(1+\nu)(1-2\nu)} \qquad \mu = \frac{E}{2(1+\nu)} \tag{10}$$

Other popular constitutive models are the Neo-Hookean [15] and Ogden [16] model. In these cases, W is defined using the three principal stretches $\lambda_1, \lambda_2, \lambda_3$ (i.e., the three eigenvalues of the deformation gradient). The strain energy function for a Neo-Hookean material is defined as:

$$W(\lambda_1, \lambda_2, \lambda_3) = A(\lambda_1^2 + \lambda_2^2 + \lambda_3^2 - 3) \tag{11}$$

where A is a material constant, linked to μ by $A = \frac{\mu}{2}$.

The Ogden model has been widely used in rubber-like tissue modelling and it is described by:

$$W(\lambda_1, \lambda_2, \lambda_3) = \sum_{i+1}^{N} \frac{\mu_i}{\alpha_i}(\lambda_1 + \lambda_2 + \lambda_3 - 3) \tag{12}$$

where N, μ_i and α_i are material parameters, which must be fitted experimentally.

The system of equations describing the behavior of deformable objects through continuum mechanics laws can include four main types of nonlinearities:

1. *Geometric nonlinearity*: nonlinearity between strain **E** and displacement **u**;
2. *Material nonlinearity*: nonlinearity between stress $\boldsymbol{\sigma}$ and strain **E**;
3. *Force nonlinearity*: nonlinearity between force $\boldsymbol{b}$ and stress $\boldsymbol{\sigma}$ (when applied force depends on deformation);
4. *Kinematic nonlinearity*: nonlinearity between prescribed displacements (boundary conditions) and displacement **u**.

Continuum mechanics laws cannot be solved analytically, thus requiring numerical solution schemes [13].

1.3 The Finite Element Method

The preferred numerical scheme to solve continuum mechanics laws relies on the Finite Element (FE) method [13].

The FE method converts the system of partial differential equations describing the dynamic equilibrium motion equation Eq. (3) into a system of algebraic equations which can be solved numerically, after discretizing the domain both in space and time. Geometric discretization of the domain Ω is achieved by creating tissue 3D meshes, which describe the soft body as composed of elementary volumetric components (usually tetrahedral or hexahedral elements). The continuous solution $\mathbf{u}$ at any point in space is obtained by interpolating the values of the discretized displacements $\mathbf{u}_n$ at the element nodes using shape functions ϕ^n (i.e., polynomial functions that are generally linear or quadratic) [17]:

$$\mathbf{u} = \sum_{n=1}^{N_n} \phi^n \mathbf{u}_n \tag{13}$$

where N_n is the total number of nodes in the mesh. Each node n iin the mesh s associated to a shape function ϕ^n, which must have local support and piecewise continuous. By discretizing Eq. (3) with the FE method, we obtain this discrete problem on each element e:

$$-\mathbf{K}_e\mathbf{u}_e + \mathbf{f}^{ext} = \mathbf{M}_e\ddot{\mathbf{u}}_e \tag{14}$$

where $\mathbf{K}_e$ is the element stiffness matrix, $\mathbf{M}_e$ is the element mass matrix and $\mathbf{f}^{ext}$ is the external force applied to element e. The minus symbol in front of the stiffness matrix is added to explicitly formulate the equation as difference between external and intenal forces (making it more intuitive). If damping is present, the additional term $-\mathbf{C}_e\dot{\mathbf{u}}_e$ appears on the left handside of Eq. (14), where $\mathbf{C}_e$ is the element damping matrix. Global mass, stiffness and damping matrices of the system can be assembled from elementary ones, leading to a global system of equations that can be written in the form:

$$\mathbf{f}(\mathbf{x}, \mathbf{v}) = \mathbf{Ma} \tag{15}$$

with $\mathbf{a} = \ddot{\mathbf{u}}$, $\mathbf{v} = \dot{\mathbf{u}}$, $\mathbf{x} = \mathbf{u}$, and $\mathbf{f}(\mathbf{x}, \mathbf{v})$ represents the net force applied to the object (difference between external and internal forces $\mathbf{f}^{ext} - \mathbf{Cv} - \mathbf{Kx}$).

A time integration scheme (implicit, explicit or other variants) is then used to discretize the problem over time, allowing to formulate the above Eq. (15) as a linear system. The obtained set of linear equations can then be solved using either direct or iterative solvers. Direct solvers compute the solution exactly, either calculating the actual inverse or a factorization of the system matrix. Although these methods are often too costly, some optimized libraries exist that allow to parallelize these operations on CPU [18]. On the other hand, iterative solvers such as the conjugate gradient (CG) produce a sequence of approximate solutions approaching the exact one [19]. These methods can be very fast especially if they are tuned to stop when acceptable accuracy is reached, even if it is before convergence. However, they can converge slowly for ill-conditioned problems.

By relying on a physics-based description of soft tissues behavior, FE-based approaches can simulate anatomical responses to mechanical stimuli with high precision, given that a reliable constitutive model of tissue behavior and its mechanical parameters are available. For this reason, the FE method represents the preferred approach to model the deformable anatomy [20]. Solution accuracy increases with finer domain discretization (i.e., higher number of elements), but at the cost of increased computational load. As a consequence, FE models allow to achieve highly accurate results whenever computation efficiency is not a major concern, e.g. deformable image registration in applications where a computation time up to several minutes is compatible with the clinical workflow [21–23].

In order to employ FE models in applications with more stringent time constraints, various techniques have been proposed to simplify their computational complexity. Some of them have focused on optimizing the solving process, proposing numerical solution approaches like matrix condensation [24] or pre-computing some quantities, as in [25]. The Total Lagrangian Explicit Dynamics (TLED) [26] reduces the computational load by precomputation of spatial derivatives and eliminating the need of iteratively solving a large system of equations. As an example, simulations based on the TLED formulation have demonstrated high efficiency in the context of image registration for neurosurgery [27]. However, the solution is only stable under very small time steps due to the use of explicit time integration. An improved version of TLED, which relies on direct Jacobian (DJ-TLED), has been recently proposed and demonstrated to achieve a significant speedup with respect to standard TLED on simulation of brain deformations [28]. Another optimized approach is the Multiplicative Jacobian Energy Decomposition (MJED) [29], which relies on decomposition of the strain energy into simple terms that can be precomputed.

One of the most popular modeling choice to obtain clinically acceptable accuracy levels while guaranteeing computational efficiency is to model soft tissues relying on the corotational formulation of linear elasticity. The corotational model takes advantage of the computationally efficient linear elastic formulation even to model large deformations, without introducing ghost forces [30, 31]. This formulation has been extensively used to model soft tissues in applications like intra-operative image guidance, e.g. in liver surgery [32–35], brain surgery [36] and needle-based procedures [37–40].

Some other works have accelerated the solving process by implementing the solvers on the Graphic Processing Unit (GPU), whose high number of cores allows to obtain significant speedups on computationally demanding problems [41–44]. For example, NiftySim is a finite element toolkit that provides GPU-based implementation of TLED approach for high-performance biomechanical simulation [42]. However, in addition to requiring specific hardware, not all approaches are suitable for parallel computing on the GPU.

Alternatives to the Standard Finite Element Method

In addition to the optimized solution processes or formulations of the standard FE method mentioned above, some alternative approaches have been proposed to cope with the main limitations of FE models.

A possible strategy to lower the simulation time required by FE-based approaches is through Model Order Reduction (MOR) techniques [45]. The basic idea behind MOR is to reduce the number of degrees of freedom for the calculation of the solution by first creating a database of models obtained by precomputing the tissue response to different conditions and/or loads in an offline step; in the online phase, the solution to the current applied load is obtained by interpolating among the saved precomputed modes. The most popular MOR approach is Proper Orthogonal Decomposition (POD), where the solution to a high-dimensional problem is encoded as a linear combination of few basis vectors defining the precomputed modes that best describes the behavior [46, 47]. The higher the number of modes considered to compute the solution, the higher the accuracy, but the higher the computational load as well. Although POD has been successfully used to achieve efficient simulations of non linear materials [48], it is not always able to capture complex non linear behavior of anatomical tissues [49]. A generalization of POD which is better suited for the simulation of hyperelastic materials is represented by proper generalized decomposition, where the solution is expressed as the sum of separable functions representing general solutions to the problem, thus does not rely on knowledge of complete-model solutions [50].

Other approaches have been proposed to avoid the 3D meshing process required by the standard FE method. In addition to being a time-consuming and tedious process, obtaining a high quality 3D mesh is very difficult due to the complex shape of anatomical organs, but it is essential to guarantee the accuracy of the results. Moreover, even when a high quality mesh is available, large deformations may lead to element distortion and, in turns, failure of the solution method.

The Boundary Element Method (BEM) is a numerical solution approach that deduces volume deformations from deformations at the surface of the object, thus allowing both to skip the 3D mesh generation process (only surface discretization is needed) and providing fast solution speeds [51]. However, since the internal behavior is not explicitly modelled, this approach only works for isotropic and homogeneous objects, preventing from its use in simulations involving topology modifications (e.g., cuts). The most popular application of BEM in surgery is for virtual simulators [51, 52].

Meshless methods represent a class of methods where the domain is discretized by a set of particles filling the volume of interest [53]. State variables at a given point are approximated by interpolating and weigthing variable values at neighbouring particles. However, some meshelss approaches still rely on grids of background cells for numerical integration [54, 55], thus not completely eliminating the finite element layer. Whereas, other approaches like smooth particle hydrodynamics interpolate the variables of interest directly on particles using a smoothing kernel, without the need of any background grid [56]. In general, the simplicity of meshless methods and their capability to handle changes of topology without remeshing are the main reasons for their employment for surgical simulation [54, 57]. However, the use of non linear materials might lower the computational performances, making meshless methods not always suitable for applications requiring fast update rates. Moreover, since they all rely on explicit time integration schemes, very small time steps are required for robust solution, which is a limitation in interactive scenarios.

1.4 Heuristic Methods

Although modelling and simulation of anatomical deformations is traditionally performed using the FE method to reach high accuracy levels, solving continuum mechanics laws is generally too computationally expensive for certain applications. Heuristic methods introduce modelling assumptions that simplify the formulation to obtain more efficient methods, but sacrificing accuracy.

1.5 Mass Spring Models

Mass Spring Models (MSMs) consist of a set of masses distributed throughout a body and linked by a network of springs, as shown in Fig. 4. Deformation dynamics is governed by Newton's second law. Therefore, the position of the mass points is obtained by balancing the contributions of internal and external forces:

$$\mathbf{Ma} + \mathbf{Cv} + \mathbf{K}(\mathbf{x} - \mathbf{x}_0) = \mathbf{f}_{\mathbf{ext}} \tag{16}$$

where $\mathbf{a}, \mathbf{v}, \mathbf{x}$ are, respectively, the acceleration, velocity and position each mass point, and $\mathbf{x}_0$ is the spring rest length. $\mathbf{M}$ is the mass matrix that contains the values of the point masses, while $\mathbf{C}$ and $\mathbf{K}$ are the damping and the stiffness matrices respectively, defining the damping and stiffness coefficients that describe the springs connecting each point to the points in its neighborhood. $\mathbf{f}_{ext}$ represents the external

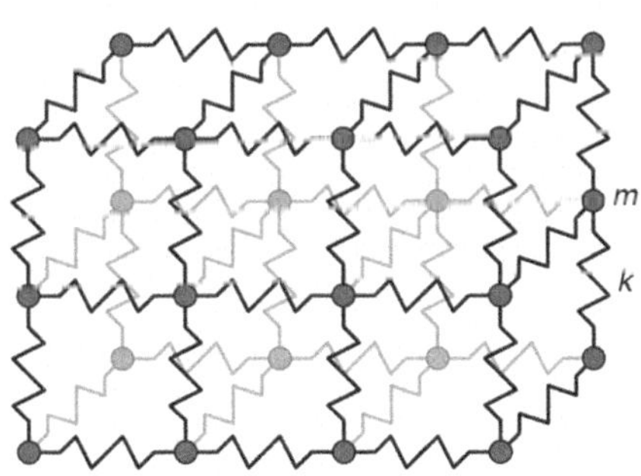

Fig. 4 In MSMs, the object is modelled as an ensemble of lumped masses *m* connected via a network of springs *k* [58]. Image from [12]

forces contribution. A time integration scheme is then used to discretize the problem in time, allowing to formulate the equation above as a linear system, which can eventually be solved exploiting numerical methods.

MSMs have been widely used for their easy implementation and their high speed. In fact, MSMs do not need to preprocess all elements to provide an estimate of the global deformations like FEM, thus being much faster and able to simulate large deformations in near real time. One of the main issues of using this approach is that MSMs parameters are not directly related to tissues mechanical properties. Moreover, they are influenced by the distribution of the mass points and the arrangement of the springs. As a consequence, specific optimization methods are needed to tune model parameters for a given mesh to realistically approximate certain global mechanical behaviors [59, 60]. Enhanced versions of MSMs have been proposed to model sophisticated behaviors, for example by introducing nonlinear springs or using hybrid models [61]. However, only few of these approaches have been validated against real data, and simulation accuracy highly depends on the appropriateness of the employed optimizaion process. Owing to this, MSMs have been mainly used for medical training simulators, whose main requirement is computational efficiency, while accepting visually plausible deformable behavior [62–64]. Furthermore, MSMs are advantageous to model complex tasks which involve topology modifications, such as cutting or suturing, since they can be implemented by simply removing or adding connections between vertices [65]. However, due to recent research advancements in computer graphics and computing architectures, the usage of MSMs for surgical simulation is likely to be superseded by other deformable models that are more physically realistic, while also having competing efficiency [12].

1.6 Position Based Dynamics

Position Based Dynamics (PBD) is a simulation approach that computes the time evolution of a dynamic system by directly updating positions, as first described by Müller et al. in [66]. Simulated objects are discretized as sets of particles, described by their positions $\mathbf{p}_i$ and velocities $\mathbf{v}_i$, subject to a set of positional constraints $C_j(\mathbf{p}_1, \ldots, \mathbf{p}_n) \succ 0$ (symbol $\succ$ denotes either = or $\geq$). In the PBD approach, deformation calculation becomes a constraint-function optimization problem. The simulation workflow starts with a prediction step in which simplectic Euler integration is performed to guess new particle positions and velocities. Then, non-linear Gauss-Seidel solver is used to find the correction $\Delta\mathbf{p}$ to apply to the estimated positions in an iterative fashion, so that each constraint equation (after linearization) is individually satisfied:

$$C(\mathbf{p} + \Delta\mathbf{p}) \approx C(\mathbf{p}) + \nabla C(\mathbf{p})\Delta\mathbf{p} \succ 0 \tag{17}$$

Since the resulting system is under-determined, the position update $\Delta\mathbf{p}$ is constrained to ensure the preservation of linear and angular momenta, which corresponds to forcing $\Delta\mathbf{p}$ to lie in the direction of the constraint gradient ∇C. The position update

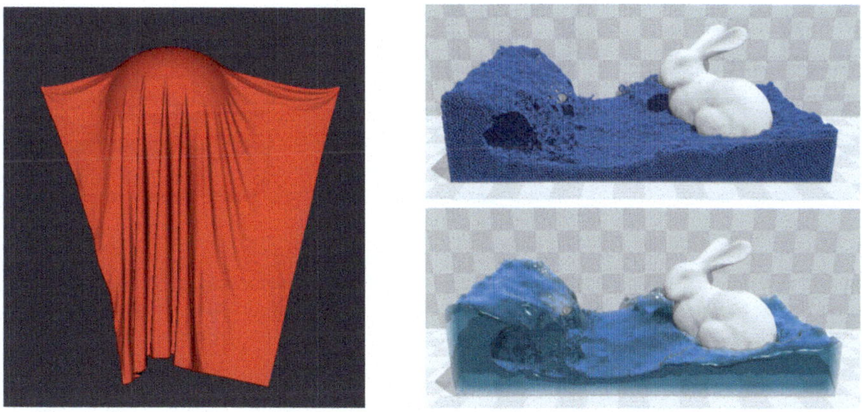

(a) (b)

Fig. 5 Simulation of **a** cloth and **b** fluid using the PBD method, relying on different constraints. Images taken from [67]

is further weighted by the inverse of the mass matrix **M** and multiplied by a parameter $k \in [0, 1]$ which represents the stiffness of the constraint:

$$\Delta\mathbf{p} = k\lambda\mathbf{M}^{-1}\nabla C(\mathbf{p})^T \tag{18}$$

The Lagrange multiplier λ which solves Eq. (17) is thus unique and given by:

$$\lambda = \frac{C(\mathbf{p})}{\nabla C(\mathbf{p})\mathbf{M}^{-1}\nabla C(\mathbf{p})^T} \tag{19}$$

Finally, computed $\Delta\mathbf{p}$ are used to correct both the positions and the velocities. Different types of properties and behaviors can be simulated with PBD by implementing specific constraints and appropriately manipulating modelling parameters [67] (Fig. 5).

By directly updating particle positions, the PBD approach has the potential of achieving a better trade-off between accuracy and computation time with respect to methods based on continuum mechanics. In addition to improving computation performances, most of the constraints do not require the availability of a 3D mesh, but particles are generally placed in space to fill a surface-delimited volume. Further advantages of using particles to discretize objects emerge when topological modifications need to be modelled, since all element-related issues such as element inversion and distortion are avoided. Like all the heuristic models, the main difficulty PBD has to face is the choice of the model parameters, which lack of any connection with real mechanical properties.

Although the PBD approach has been mainly applied in computer graphic fields, the enhanced speed, controllability and unconditional stability of this method are

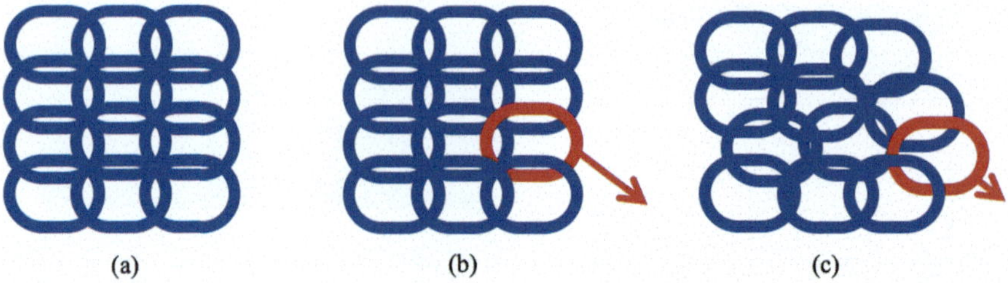

Fig. 6 In ChainMail, the object is composed of a series of chain elements (**a**); as soon as an element moves due to an external input (**b**), the neighbouring elements move in turns to satisfy geometric constraints (**c**)

its most appealing features for its application to medical simulation as well, where interactions between multiple organs and tools have to be modelled and solved in real-time [67]. The most popular exploitation of the PBD concept in the medical field has been in the development of training simulators for surgical procedures involving dissection, exploiting the capability of PBD methods to handle topological changes involved in such tasks maintaining real-time interactive performance [68, 69]. Some other works have focused on the achievement of particular types of deformations by coupling the PBD formulation with mass-spring models [70, 71] or for the simulation of knot tying procedure [72]. Camara et al. employed the PBD scheme to create a patient-specific biomechanical model of the kidney for the real-time simulation of intra-operative US images [73]. Some recent works have demonstrated that, whenever an ad-hoc parameter optimization strategy is designed, PBD-based models can achieve accuracy levels that make them suitable for surgical planning, for example in the context of kidney surgery [74], neurosurgery [75] and general laparoscopy [76].

1.7 Chain Mail

In the Chain Mail approach, the deformable object is discretized into a set of uniformly spaced elements, called *chain elements*, that are linked to each other as the links of a chain (Fig. 6) [77]. Each chain element enforces a bounding region for its neighboring chain elements. Volume deformations are obtained by adjusting the position of the chain elements while respecting the geometric constraints imposed by the neighbouring elements. After position adjustment, a relaxation scheme is employed to minimize the the internal energy of the system, proportional to the displacement of the elements with respect to each other, until convergence. The chain-like structure guarantees the propagation of the deformations over the entire volume. Several works have proposed to extend the basic Chain Mail algorithm to model additional features, such heterogeneity, volume conservation or force-displacement relationship [12]. Similarly to PBD, due to its reliance only on position adjustments to obtain a volumetric deformation, Chain Mail is characterized by high computational efficiency, being able to handle deformations of large volumetric datasets [78, 79]. Advanced interactions can be easily modelled by removing or adding elements [80]. Generation of a 3D mesh is not required with this approach, since the volume is filled with regularly spaced chain elements, thus simplifying the model generation pipeline. However, its main drawback lies again in the selection of the parameters governing the geometric constraints (e.g., the margin of free mobility between the links) to achieve a realistic behavior. Owing to these features, Chain Mail models have been successfully employed in virtual surgery simulators, e.g. for prostate brachytherapy [81], endoscopy [82] and knee arthroscopy [83].

1.8 Machine Learning Based Methods

Recently, Machine Learning (ML) has started to revolutionize several fields (vision, language processing, image recognition, genomics) due to the availability of larger and larger databases and the acceleration provided by powerful GPUs. ML comprises all those methods able to approximate a relationship between some input data and the output without any mathematical formulation of the problem, learning it directly from data. In general, ML approaches learn a function f that maps an input vector $\mathbf{x}$ to an output vector $\mathbf{y}$. The function depends on some parameters θ that are learnt from a huge amount of ground truth data during the so called training phase, such that:

$$f(\mathbf{x}, \theta) = \mathbf{y} \tag{20}$$

Then, in the inference phase, the learnt set of parameters θ is used to predict the value of $\mathbf{y}$ given a new observation $\mathbf{x}$. In general, ML based methods can achieve high inferring speed, which makes them useful for many applications where the prediction speed is a critical parameter.

Some attempts that exploit learning methods to estimate the deformation of biological tissues have been made. By implicitly encoding soft tissue mechanical behavior in the trained ML models, they proved successful to predict the entire 3D organ deformation starting either by applied surface forces [84–86] or by surface displacements [87–91]. The greatest advantage of employing ML algorithms to simulate tissues deformation is the significant computational gain achieved with respect to the FE method, as highlighted in the recent survey by [92].

One of the main challenges of using a ML model to predict anatomical deformations is that its accuracy highly depends on the quality and on the amount of data used to train it. In an ideal scenario, such a model would be trained with an infinite amount of real patient-specific noise-free data, which is in practice not possible since acquiring large amounts of volumetric deformations of an organ is a challenging problem. As a consequence, most of the works which rely on ML to predict tissue deformations have trained their models using data generated with finite element simulations [92]. This approach has many advantages. First of all, being based on continuum mechanics theory, synthetic data generated with this strategy are highly realistic. Moreover, they allow to avoid all the ethical and legal issues connected with data acquisition on human subjects. Also, such data are automatically annotated and they can be augmented directly at simulation setup phase by using different parameter settings. Data generated with the FE method have been used by Lorente et al. to train several regression models that approximate the mechanical behavior of the liver during breathing [89]. Martinez et al. [93] have investigated the capability of tree-based methods to estimate breast deformation due to compression between biopsy plates. They have trained the proposed methods on different patient geometries but with very specific FE simulation representative of the scenario of interest, without including any randomness in the dataset. Neural networks have been used by Tonutti and Rechowicz to predict the displacement of brain tumors and of rib cage surface respectively, starting from the acting forces [85, 86]. However, both these works do not predict whole volume deformation but only surface displacements. Being trained with simulated data from a single geometry, the generated ML algorithm acts as a patient-specific model. However, this implies that network re-training is required for every new patient. Methods based on NNs have been also used to predict tissue deformations in augmented surgery. Morooka et al. have trained a NN to predict liver deformations for a given input force [84]. In their model, they have used Principal Component Analysis (PCA) to compress the size of the deformation modes, which allows to reduce the number of neurons of the output layer, thus the training time. Other works have estimated liver deformations from the known displacement of a partial surface [87, 88, 90, 94, 95]. Among these, the works of Pfeiffer et al. are able to generalize to new patients since models have been trained on several different random geometries of the organs [87, 95].

From all these works, it has emerged that the main advantage of using neural networks to predict anatomical deformations relies on a prediction speed in the order of few milliseconds, which is not affected by the complexity of the model used to generate the dataset. The high inferring speed makes this method useful for many applications such as surgical navigation and real-time simulation.

2 Simulation as a Tool for Learning

Automating a surgical intervention is an extremely complex task, due to the many different actions that are required to complete a procedure. For this reason, the research trend in autonomous surgery has broken down the problem and focused on the automation of individual tasks taking place during surgery. Following the definition of [96], tasks are sequences of activities which aim at a specific surgical objective and is recurrent in many different procedures, e.g. tissue dissection, suturing and knot tying. One of the challenges when attempting to automate surgical actions is that they all involve the interaction with the soft anatomical environment, thus requiring the development of control strategies that can cope with such dynamic behavior. For example, a common task in surgery is Tissue Retraction (TR), which requires the manipulation of soft tissues in order to expose a hidden region of interest.

TR is performed during robot assisted nephrectomy procedures, where the surgeon has to interact with the highly deformable pararenal adipose tissue which covers the kidney in order to have access to the underlying tumor.

Some works have attempted to automate TR with standard motion control algorithms. For example, Nagy et al. have proposed to automate TR using soft computing methods [97]. In [98], authors have proposed a trajectory planner for TR based on coordinates extracted directly from the intra-operative image feed. Both these works have automated TR relying on pre-defined movement sequences without considering tissues dynamics, posing some doubts about its possible exploitation in realistic anatomical environments. In [99, 100], authors employ standard path planning methods to execute an optimal plan for the task generated within a biomechanical simulation in the pre-operative phase, in this way accounting for the deformation properties of the anatomy. However, all these approaches rely hand-crafted control policies, which make the execution of complex non-linear trajectories and behaviors challenging.

Most of the prior works concerning the automation of actions involving soft tissues manipulation rely on Learning from Demonstrations (LfD), where a task is learnt by imitating expert behavior [101–104]. LfD is a preferred approach since it allows to learn proper interaction with deformable tissues without the need to explicitly model of their behavior. In addition, it does not require to explicitly design policies. However, the robustness of learned tasks to changes in the initial conditions or in the environment is strongly affected by the amount and variety of expert demonstrations provided to the system [105]. Collecting a dataset with a vast repertoire of trajectories from multiple experts and varying initial conditions is impractical and often unfeasible in clinical settings. Moreover, with LfD the robot can only become as good as the human's demonstrations, but there is no additional information for improving the learnt behavior.

Deep Reinforcement Learning (DRL) has shown promising results in the automation of robotic tasks like object manipulation and pick-and-place tasks, without the need to design ad-hoc control strategies [106]. In DRL, the component which makes decisions about the action to take is called agent. A DRL agent reaches robust performance after it has explored a huge amount of possible policy options, which requires a large number of interactions with the environment, many of which fail with unsafe behavior [107]. Although safe learning methods have been proposed, their exploitation in the surgical robotic field remains limited, due to the impracticality to acquire many training trials from real surgical robotic systems [108]. For this reason, existing works based on DRL learn surgical tasks in simulated environments, to enable the many trial and error attempts required to train agents in safe and controlled settings [109–112]. One of the main challenges when training in simulation is that the *reality gap* (i.e., the discrepancy between the simulated and real environments) must be kept as low as possible to enable successful deployment of the learnt policies in the real world, in what is called *sim-to-real* approach [113]. In the context of RMIS, this means that the simulation should account for both deformable properties of the anatomy and the interaction with the surgical tools. This is the main limitation of *dVRL*, a simulation framework to train DRL agents for surgical tasks proposed by

Richter et al. [114], which is based on VREP and OpenAI Gym, and supports only rigid objects. Because of the reality gap, simulation-learnt behaviors have been transferred to the real surgical robotic system only for simplified geometries [110]. Only recently, Xu et al. have proposed *SurRoL*, a simulation-based platform for DRL that can simulate deformable objects and is interfaced with the dVRK [115]. *SurRoL* has shown promise for successful transfer of behaviors learnt in simulation to the real world.

Recent research has proposed to combine LfD and DRL with the aim of exploiting the strength of both approaches and overcome their respective drawbacks [116]. In particular, demonstrations can be used to guide the exploration done during learning, reducing the time required to find an improved control policy, which may depart from the demonstrated behavior. A promising strategy is represented by Generative Adversarial Imitation Learning (GAIL) [117], which has been successfully applied to endovascular manipulators but never used in RMIS [118].

Simulation can play a key role to support the process of learning surgical tasks. By providing a realistic replica of the real scenario, simulation represents an exceptional resource for two reasons. First of all, it allows to perform the large amount of trial and error attempts required by learning-based methods in controlled settings, enabling the exploitation of state-of-the-art approaches without the need to access the real surgical systems, which is both impractical (sometimes unfeasible) and risky. Second, it provides an environment where to test the learnt behavior before its exploitation on the real robotic system, allowing to predict potentially unsafe or dangerous situations and prevent from their execution in the real world. One of our main contributions is the development of a modular framework called *UnityFlexML* that provides an interface between a realistic simulation of deformable anatomy, the surgical robotic system and learning-based methods, which will be introduced in chapter "Learning Tissue Retraction in Simulation". We show that the developed framework is suitable for both prototyping and testing two different learning approaches: a standard DRL method requiring multiple interactions with the environment and an approach that combines LfD and DRL, on the automation of a soft tissue retraction task. Finally, we demonstrate that the learnt policies can be successfully transferred to the real system, thanks to the high level of realism achieved by the simulation environment.

3 Conclusion

Several different methods have been proposed to simulate the deformable behavior of the soft anatomical tissues, each achieving a different trade-off between accuracy, computation efficiency and numerical stability. Although it would be ideal to satisfy all these requirements, such a model does not exist due to the complexity to model the anatomical environment. Therefore, the choice of the approach to use depends on the specific requirements of the application of interest. In this chapter, we have provided an overview of the main deformable models available for surgical simulation, providing some example applications.

Methods based on continuum mechanics rely on numerical methods to directly solve the physics equations describing tissues deformations. The most popular solution process exploits the finite element method, where the global tissue behavior is obtained by assembling the response of elementary components in which the tissue is discretized. Although methods based on continuum mechanics can model very complex behaviors, e.g. non linear materials, heterogeneous tissues and anisotropy, numerical solution of such complex equations via the finite element method is computationally expensive and cannot take place in real time. As a consequence, these methods have been generally used for applications where the real-time performance is not a strict requirement. Even though advanced and optimized formulations have been proposed, the improved computational performance is generally achieved by sacrificing the accuracy to some extent.

On the other hand, heuristic methods rely on simplified models that provide optimized computational performance, but they cannot be easily extended to represent all the possible mechanical behaviors of tissues. This modelling approach suffers from ambiguity in specification of model parameters to reproduce tissues mechanical behavior, since a well-defined relationship between model parameters and material constitutive law does not exist. This means that an ad-hoc optimization process is always required to tune model parameters such that an acceptable level of accuracy is achieved. However, whenever reliable parameters are selected, these models can achieve reasonable levels of realism. Due to the simplicity of the models and the fact that they do not generally rely on 3D meshes, this category of methods has been mainly employed for virtual training simulators, which involve topological changes.

The last category of methods takes advantage of machine learning to predict tissue deformations. In fact, a trained ML algorithm significantly reduces the time required to provide an estimate of tissue deformed state starting directly from data, avoiding the computationally expensive resolution of complex system of equations. In order to cope with the lack of real tissue deformation data, the majority of works that predict tissue deformations with ML have relied on training datasets generated with finite element simulations. ML algorithms have proved able to learn complex deformable behaviors reaching the same level of accuracy of the biomechanical simulations used to generate the data while obtaining considerable time gains, passing from minutes (required for the finite element method) to milliseconds (when using ML). Despite being used mainly for applications with strict time requirements such as augmented reality, this approach seems particularly promising and applicable to a wide variety of applications.

References

1. Haouchine, N., Kuang, W., Cotin, S., Yip, M.: Vision-based force feedback estimation for robot-assisted surgery using instrument-constrained biomechanical three-dimensional maps. IEEE Robot. Autom. Lett. **3**(3), 2160–2165 (2018)
2. Meier, U., López, O., Monserrat, C., Juan, M.C., Alcaniz, M.: Real-time deformable models for surgery simulation: a survey. Comput. Methods Programs Biomed. **77**(3), 183–197 (2005)
3. Ackerman, M.J.: The visible human project: a resource for education. Acad. Med.: J. Assoc. Am. Med. Coll. **74**(6), 667–670 (1999)
4. Milletari, F., Navab, N., Ahmadi, S.-A.: V-net: fully convolutional neural networks for volumetric medical image segmentation. In: 2016 Fourth International Conference on 3D Vision (3DV), pp. 565–571. IEEE (2016)
5. Lorensen, W.E., Cline, H.E.: Marching cubes: a high resolution 3S surface construction algorithm. ACM Siggraph Comput. Graph. **21**(4), 163–169 (1987)
6. Golias, N., Dutton, R.: Delaunay triangulation and 3D adaptive mesh generation. Finite Elem. Anal. Des. **25**(3–4), 331–341 (1997)
7. Krygier, M.C., LaBonte, T., Martinez, C., Norris, C., Sharma, K., Collins, L.N., Mukherjee, P.P., Roberts, S.A.: Quantifying the unknown impact of segmentation uncertainty on image-based simulations. Nat. Commun. **12**(1), 1–11 (2021)
8. Fung, Y.-C., et al.: Mechanical Properties of Living Tissues, vol. 547. Springer, Berlin (1993)
9. Sigrist, R.M., Liau, J., El Kaffas, A., Chammas, M.C., Willmann, J.K.: Ultrasound elastography: review of techniques and clinical applications. Theranostics **7**(5), 1303 (2017)
10. Mariappan, Y.K., Glaser, K.J., Ehman, R.L.: Magnetic resonance elastography: a review. Clin. Anat. **23**(5), 497–511 (2010)
11. Delingette, H.: Toward realistic soft-tissue modeling in medical simulation. Proc. IEEE **86**(3), 512–523 (1998)
12. Zhang, J., Zhong, Y., Gu, C.: Deformable models for surgical simulation: a survey. IEEE Rev. Biomed. Eng. **11**, 143–164 (2018)
13. Kim, N.-H.: Introduction to Nonlinear Finite Element Analysis. Springer Science & Business Media (2014)
14. Freutel, M., Schmidt, H., Dürselen, L., Ignatius, A., Galbusera, F.: Finite element modeling of soft tissues: material models, tissue interaction and challenges. Clin. Biomech. **29**(4), 363–372 (2014)
15. Ogden, R.W.: Non-linear Elastic Deformations. Courier Corporation (1997)
16. Ogden, R.W.: Large deformation isotropic elasticity–on the correlation of theory and experiment for incompressible rubberlike solids. Proc. R. Soc. London. A. Math. Phys. Sci. **326**(1567), 565–584 (1972)
17. Bedrosian, G.: Shape functions and integration formulas for three-dimensional finite element analysis. Int. J. Numer. Meth. Eng. **35**(1), 95–108 (1992)
18. Schenk, O., Gärtner, K.: Solving unsymmetric sparse systems of linear equations with PARDISO. Futur. Gener. Comput. Syst. **20**(3), 475–487 (2004)
19. Shewchuk, J.R., et al.: An introduction to the conjugate gradient method without the agonizing pain (1994)
20. Bro-Nielsen, M.: Finite element modeling in surgery simulation. Proc. IEEE **86**(3), 490–503 (1998)
21. Brock, K., Sharpe, M., Dawson, L., Kim, S., Jaffray, D.: Accuracy of finite element model-based multi-organ deformable image registration. Med. Phys. **32**(6) Part 1, 1647–1659 (2005)
22. Schnabel, J.A., Tanner, C., Castellano-Smith, A.D., Degenhard, A., Leach, M.O., Hose, D.R., Hill, D.L., Hawkes, D.J.: Validation of nonrigid image registration using finite-element methods: application to breast MR images. IEEE Trans. Med. Imaging **22**(2), 238–247 (2003)
23. Morin, F., Courtecuisse, H., Reinertsen, I., Le Lann, F., Palombi, O., Payan, Y., Chabanas, M.: Brain-shift compensation using intraoperative ultrasound and constraint-based biomechanical simulation. Med. Image Anal. **40**, 133–153 (2017)

24. Bro-Nielsen, M., Cotin, S., Real-time volumetric deformable models for surgery simulation using finite elements and condensation. In: Computer Graphics Forum, vol. 15, pp. 57–66, Wiley Online Library (1996)
25. Cotin, S., Delingette, H., Ayache, N.: Real-time elastic deformations of soft tissues for surgery simulation. IEEE Trans. Visual Comput. Graph. **5**(1), 62–73 (1999)
26. Miller, K., Joldes, G., Lance, D., Wittek, A.: Total Lagrangian explicit dynamics finite element algorithm for computing soft tissue deformation. Commun. Numer. Methods Eng. **23**(2), 121–134 (2007)
27. Garlapati, R.R., Roy, A., Joldes, G.R., Wittek, A., Mostayed, A., Doyle, B., Warfield, S.K., Kikinis, R., Knuckey, N., Bunt, S., et al.: More accurate neuronavigation data provided by biomechanical modeling instead of rigid registration. J. Neurosurg. **120**(6), 1477–1483 (2014)
28. Zhang, J.: A direct Jacobian total Lagrangian explicit dynamics finite element algorithm for real-time simulation of hyperelastic materials. Int. J. Numer. Meth. Eng. **122**(20), 5744–5772 (2021)
29. Marchesseau, S., Heimann, T., Chatelin, S., Willinger, R., Delingette, H.: Multiplicative Jacobian energy decomposition method for fast porous visco-hyperelastic soft tissue model. In: MICCAI, pp. 235–242. Springer, Berlin (2010)
30. Müller, M., Dorsey, J., McMillan, L., Jagnow, R., Cutler, B.: Stable real-time deformations. In: Proceedings of the 2002 ACM SIGGRAPH/Eurographics symposium on Computer Animation, pp. 49–54 (2002)
31. Felippa, C.A., Haugen, B.: A unified formulation of small-strain corotational finite elements: I. theory. Comput. Methods Appl. Mech. Eng. **194**(21–24), 2285–2335 (2005)
32. Haouchine, N., Dequidt, J., Peterlik, I., Kerrien, E., Berger, M.-O., Cotin, S.: Image-guided simulation of heterogeneous tissue deformation for augmented reality during hepatic surgery. In: 2013 IEEE International Symposium on Mixed and Augmented Reality (ISMAR), pp. 199–208. IEEE (2013)
33. Plantefève, R., Peterlik, I., Haouchine, N., Cotin, S.: Patient-specific biomechanical modeling for guidance during minimally-invasive hepatic surgery. Ann. Biomed. Eng. **44**(1), 139–153 (2016)
34. Peterlík, I., Courtecuisse, H., Rohling, R., Abolmaesumi, P., Nguan, C., Cotin, S., Salcudean, S.: Fast elastic registration of soft tissues under large deformations. Med. Image Anal. **45**, 24–40 (2018)
35. Golse, N., Petit, A., Lewin, M., Vibert, E., Cotin, S.: Augmented reality during open liver surgery using a markerless non-rigid registration system. J. Gastrointest. Surg. **25**(3), 662–671 (2021)
36. Haouchine, N., Juvekar, P., Wells III, W.M., Cotin, S., Golby, A., Frisken, S.: Deformation aware augmented reality for craniotomy using 3D/2D non-rigid registration of cortical vessels. In: Conference on Medical Image Computing and Computer-Assisted Intervention, pp. 735–744. Springer, Berlin (2020)
37. Baksic, P., Courtecuisse, H., Bayle, B.: Shared control strategy for needle insertion into deformable tissue using inverse finite element simulation. In: ICRA 2021-International Conference on Robotics and Automation (2021)
38. Hamzé, N., Peterlík, I., Cotin, S., Essert, C.: Preoperative trajectory planning for percutaneous procedures in deformable environments. Comput. Med. Imaging Graph. **47**, 16–28 (2016)
39. Moreira, P., Peterlik, I., Herink, M., Duriez, C., Cotin, S., Misra, S.: Modelling prostate deformation: sofa versus experiments. Prostate **17**(83), 1 (2013)
40. Goksel, O., Sapchuk, K., Salcudean, S.E.: Haptic simulator for prostate brachytherapy with simulated needle and probe interaction. IEEE Trans. Haptics **4**(3), 188–198 (2011)
41. Allard, J., Courtecuisse, H., Faure, F.: Implicit fem solver on GPU for interactive deformation simulation. In: GPU Computing Gems Jade Edition, pp. 281–294, Elsevier (2012)
42. Johnsen, S.F., Taylor, Z.A., Clarkson, M.J., Hipwell, J., Modat, M., Eiben, B., Han, L., Hu, Y., Mertzanidou, T., Hawkes, D.J., et al.: NiftySim: a GPU-based nonlinear finite element package for simulation of soft tissue biomechanics. Int. J. Comput. Assist. Radiol. Surg. **10**(7), 1077–1095 (2015)

43. Courtecuisse, H., Allard, J., Kerfriden, P., Bordas, S.P., Cotin, S., Duriez, C.: Real-time simulation of contact and cutting of heterogeneous soft-tissues. Med. Image Anal. **18**(2), 394–410 (2014)
44. Hipwell, J.H., Vavourakis, V., Han, L., Mertzanidou, T., Eiben, B., Hawkes, D.J.: A review of biomechanically informed breast image registration. Phys. Med. Biol. **61**(2), R1 (2016)
45. Cueto, E., Chinesta, F.: Real time simulation for computational surgery: a review. Adv. Model. Simul. Eng. Sci. **1**(1), 1–18 (2014)
46. Niroomandi, S., Alfaro, I., Cueto, E., Chinesta, F.: Real-time deformable models of non-linear tissues by model reduction techniques. Comput. Methods Programs Biomed. **91**(3), 223–231 (2008)
47. Niroomandi, S., Alfaro, I., Cueto, E., Chinesta, F.: Accounting for large deformations in real-time simulations of soft tissues based on reduced-order models. Comput. Methods Programs Biomed. **105**(1), 1–12 (2012)
48. Niroomandi, S., Alfaro, I., Cueto, E., Chinesta, F.: Model order reduction for hyperelastic materials. Int. J. Numer. Meth. Eng. **81**(9), 1180–1206 (2010)
49. Bhattacharjee, S., Matouš, K.: A nonlinear manifold-based reduced order model for multiscale analysis of heterogeneous hyperelastic materials. J. Comput. Phys. **313**, 635–653 (2016)
50. Niroomandi, S., González, D., Alfaro, I., Bordeu, F., Leygue, A., Cueto, E., Chinesta, F.: Real-time simulation of biological soft tissues: a PGD approach. Int. J. Numer. Methods Biomed. Eng. **29**(5), 586–600 (2013)
51. Monserrat, C., Meier, U., Alcaniz, M., Chinesta, F., Juan, M.C.: A new approach for the real-time simulation of tissue deformations in surgery simulation. Comput. Methods Programs Biomed. **64**(2), 77–85 (2001)
52. Wang, P., Becker, A., Jones, I., Glover, A., Benford, S., Greenhalgh, C., Vloeberghs, M.: Virtual reality simulation of surgery with haptic feedback based on the boundary element method. Comput. Struct. **85**(7–8), 331–339 (2007)
53. Doblaré, M., Cueto, E., Calvo, B., Martínez, M., Garcia, J., Cegonino, J.: On the employ of meshless methods in biomechanics. Comput. Methods Appl. Mech. Eng. **194**(6–8), 801–821 (2005)
54. Horton, A., Wittek, A., Joldes, G.R., Miller, K.: A meshless total Lagrangian explicit dynamics algorithm for surgical simulation. Int. J. Numer. Methods Biomed. Eng. **26**(8), 977–998 (2010)
55. Zhang, G., Wittek, A., Joldes, G., Jin, X., Miller, K.: A three-dimensional nonlinear meshfree algorithm for simulating mechanical responses of soft tissue. Eng. Anal. Bound. Elem. **42**, 60–66 (2014)
56. Palyanov, A., Khayrulin, S., Larson, S.D.: Application of smoothed particle hydrodynamics to modeling mechanisms of biological tissue. Adv. Eng. Softw. **98**, 1–11 (2016)
57. Miller, K., Horton, A., Joldes, G., Wittek, A.: Beyond finite elements: a comprehensive, patient-specific neurosurgical simulation utilizing a meshless method. J. Biomech. **45**(15), 2698–2701 (2012)
58. Gibson, S.F., Mirtich, B.: A survey of deformable modeling in computer graphics. Technical Report, Citeseer (1997)
59. Zerbato, D., Galvan, S., Fiorini, P.: Calibration of mass spring models for organ simulations. In: 2007 IEEE/RSJ International Conference on Intelligent Robots and Systems, pp. 370–375. IEEE (2007)
60. Lloyd, B., Székely, G., Harders, M.: Identification of spring parameters for deformable object simulation. IEEE Trans. Vis. Comput. Graph. **13**(5), 1081–1094 (2007)
61. Omar, M.N., Zhong, Y.: A review of mass spring method improvements for modeling soft tissue deformation. Hum.-Cent. Technol. Better Tomorrow, pp. 203–215 (2022)
62. Dehghani Ashkezari, H., Mirbagheri, A., Behzadipour, S., Farahmand, F.: A mass-spring-damper model for real time simulation of the frictional grasping interactions between surgical tools and large organs. Sci. Iran. **22**(5), 1833–1841 (2015)
63. Harders, M., Hutter, R., Rutz, A., Niederer, P., Székely, G.: Comparing a simplified fem approach with the mass-spring model for surgery simulation. In: Studies in Health Technology and Informatics, pp. 103–109 (2003)

64. Kühnapfel, U., Cakmak, H.K., Maaß, H.: Endoscopic surgery training using virtual reality and deformable tissue simulation. Comput. Graph. **24**(5), 671–682 (2000)
65. Zhang, Y., Yuan, Z., Ding, Y., Zhao, J., Duan, Z., Sun, M.: Real time simulation of tissue cutting based on GPU and CUDA for surgical training. In: 2010 International Conference on Biomedical Engineering and Computer Science, pp. 1–4. IEEE (2010)
66. Müller, M., Heidelberger, B., Teschner, M., Gross, M.: Meshless deformations based on shape matching. In: ACM Transactions on Graphics (TOG), vol. 24, pp. 471–478. ACM (2005)
67. Bender, J., Müller, M., Macklin, M.: A survey on position based dynamics. In: EUROGRAPHICS 2017 Tutorials (2017)
68. Berndt, I., Torchelsen, R., Maciel, A.: Efficient surgical cutting with position-based dynamics. IEEE Comput. Graph. Appl. **38**(3), 24–31 (2017)
69. Pan, J., Bai, J., Zhao, X., Hao, A., Qin, H.: Real-time haptic manipulation and cutting of hybrid soft tissue models by extended position-based dynamics. Comput. Animat. Virtual Worlds **26**(3–4), 321–335 (2015)
70. Wang, Y., Xiong, Y., Xu, K., Tan, K., Guo, G.: A mass-spring model for surface mesh deformation based on shape matching. GRAPHITE **6**, 375–380 (2006)
71. Xu, L., Lu, Y., Liu, Q.: Integrating viscoelastic mass spring dampers into position-based dynamics to simulate soft tissue deformation in real time. R. Soc. Open Sci. **5**(2), 171587 (2018)
72. Kubiak, B., Pietroni, N., Ganovelli, F., Fratarcangeli, M.: A robust method for real-time thread simulation. In: Proceedings of the 2007 ACM Symposium on Virtual Reality Software and Technology, pp. 85–88. ACM (2007)
73. Camara, M., Mayer, E., Darzi, A., Pratt, P.: Simulation of patient-specific deformable ultrasound imaging in real time. In: Imaging for Patient-Customized Simulations and Systems for Point-of-Care Ultrasound, pp. 11–18. Springer, Berlin (2017)
74. Camara, M., Mayer, E., Darzi, A., Pratt, P.: Soft tissue deformation for surgical simulation: a position-based dynamics approach. Int. J. Comput. Assist. Radiol. Surg. **11**(6), 919–928 (2016)
75. Segato, A., Di Vece, C., Zucchelli, S., Di Marzo, M., Wendler, T., Azampour, M.F., Galvan, S., Secoli, R., De Momi, E.: Position-based dynamics simulator of brain deformations for path planning and intra-operative control in keyhole neurosurgery. IEEE Robot. Autom. Lett. (2021)
76. Dawda, S., Camara, M., Pratt, P., Vale, J., Darzi, A., Mayer, E.: Patient-specific simulation of pneumoperitoneum for laparoscopic surgical planning. J. Med. Syst. **43**(10), 1–9 (2019)
77. Gibson, S.F.: 3D chainmail: a fast algorithm for deforming volumetric objects. In: Proceedings of the 1997 Symposium on Interactive 3D Graphics, pp. 149–ff (1997)
78. Aguilera, A.R., León, A., Arroyo, G., Mantas, J.M.: SP-chainmail: a GPU-based sparse parallel chainmail algorithm for deforming medical volumes. J. Supercomput. **71**, 3482–3499 (2015)
79. Fortmeier, D., Mastmeyer, A., Handels, H.: Image-based palpation simulation with soft tissue deformations using chainmail on the GPU. In: Bildverarbeitung für die Medizin, pp. 140–145. Springer, Berlin (2013)
80. Frisken-Gibson, S.F.: Using linked volumes to model object collisions, deformation, cutting, carving, and joining. IEEE Trans. Visual Comput. Graph. **5**(4), 333–348 (1999)
81. Wang, X., Fenster, A.: A virtual reality based 3d real-time interactive brachytherapy simulation of needle insertion and seed implantation. In: 2004 2nd IEEE International Symposium on Biomedical Imaging: Nano to Macro (IEEE Cat No. 04EX821), pp. 280–283. IEEE (2004)
82. Neubauer, D.-I.A.: A ChainMail algorithm for direct volume deformation in virtual endoscopy applications. Ph.D. thesis (2005)
83. Gibson, S., Samosky, J., Mor, A., Fyock, C., Grimson, E., Kanade, T., Kikinis, R., Lauer, H., McKenzie, N., Nakajima, S., et al.: Simulating arthroscopic knee surgery using volumetric object representations, real-time volume rendering and haptic feedback. In: CVRMed-MRCAS'97, pp. 367–378. Springer, Berlin (1997)

84. Morooka, K., Chen, X., Kurazume, R., Uchida, S., Hara, K., Iwashita, Y.: Hashizume, M.: Real-time nonlinear fem with neural network for simulating soft organ model deformation. In: MICCAI, pp. 742–749. Springer, Berlin (2008)
85. Tonutti, M., Gras, G., Yang, G.-Z.: A machine learning approach for real-time modelling of tissue deformation in image-guided neurosurgery. Artif. Intell. Med. **80**, 39–47 (2017)
86. Rechowicz, K.J., McKenzie, F.D.: Development and validation methodology of the NUSS procedure surgical planner. SIMULATION **89**(12), 1474–1488 (2013)
87. Pfeiffer, M., Riediger, C., Weitz, J., Speidel, S.: Learning soft tissue behavior of organs for surgical navigation with convolutional neural networks. Int. J. Comput. Assist. Radiol. Surg. 1–9 (2019)
88. Brunet, J.-N., Mendizabal, A., Petit, A., Golse, N., Vibert, E., Cotin, S.: Physics-based deep neural network for augmented reality during liver surgery. In: International Conference on Medical Image Computing and Computer-Assisted Intervention, pp. 137–145. Springer, Berlin (2019)
89. Lorente, D., Martínez-Martínez, F., Rupérez, M.J., Lago, M., Martínez-Sober, M., Escandell-Montero, P., Martínez-Martínez, J.M., Martínez-Sanchis, S., Serrano-López, A.J., Monserrat, C., et al.: A framework for modelling the biomechanical behaviour of the human liver during breathing in real time using machine learning. Expert Syst. Appl. **71**, 342–357 (2017)
90. Mendizabal, A., Tagliabue, E., Hoellinger, T., Brunet, J.-N., Nikolaev, S., Cotin, S.: Data-driven simulation for augmented surgery. Dev. Nov. Approaches Biomech. Metamaterials **132**, 71–96 (2020)
91. Mendizabal, A., Tagliabue, E., Brunet, J.-N., Dall'Alba, D., Fiorini, P., Cotin, S.: Physics-based deep neural network for real-time lesion tracking in ultrasound-guided breast biopsy. In: Computational Biomechanics for Medicine Workshop MICCAI (2019)
92. Phellan, R., Hachem, B., Clin, J., Mac-Thiong, J.-M., Duong, L.: Real-time biomechanics using the finite element method and machine learning: review and perspective. Med. Phys. **48**(1), 7–18 (2021)
93. Martínez-Martínez, F., Rupérez-Moreno, M.J., Martínez-Sober, M., et al.: A finite element-based machine learning approach for modeling the mechanical behavior of the breast tissues under compression in real-time. Comput. Biol. Med. **90**, 116–124 (2017)
94. Yamamoto, U., Nakao, M., Ohzeki, M., Matsuda, T.: Deformation estimation of an elastic object by partial observation using a neural network (2017). arXiv:1711.10157
95. Pfeiffer, M., Riediger, C., Leger, S., Kühn, J.-P., Seppelt, D., Hoffmann, R.-T., Weitz, J., Speidel, S.: Non-rigid volume to surface registration using a data-driven biomechanical model, pp. 724–734 (2020)
96. Lalys, F., Jannin, P.: Surgical process modeling: a review. Int. J. CARS **9**(3), 495–511 (2014)
97. Nagy, T.D., Takács, M., Rudas, I.J., Haidegger, T.: Surgical subtask automation-soft tissue retraction. in: 2018 IEEE 16th World Symposium on Applied Machine Intelligence and Informatics (SAMI), pp. 55–60. IEEE (2018)
98. Attanasio, A., Scaglioni, B., Leonetti, M., Frangi, A.F., Cross, W., Biyani, C.S., Valdastri, P.: Autonomous tissue retraction in robotic assisted minimally invasive surgery-a feasibility study. IEEE Robot. Autom. Lett. **5**(4), 6528–6535 (2020)
99. Patil, S., Alterovitz, R.: Toward automated tissue retraction in robot-assisted surgery. In: 2010 IEEE International Conference on Robotics and Automation, pp. 2088–2094. IEEE (2010)
100. Jansen, R., Hauser, K., Chentanez, N., et al.: Surgical retraction of non-uniform deformable layers of tissue: 2D robot grasping and path planning. In: 2009 IEEE/RSJ International Conference on Intelligent Robots and Systems, pp. 4092–4097. IEEE (2009)
101. Schulman, J., Gupta, A., Venkatesan, S., Tayson-Frederick, M., Abbeel, P.: A case study of trajectory transfer through non-rigid registration for a simplified suturing scenario. In: 2013 IEEE/RSJ International Conference on Intelligent Robots and Systems, pp. 4111–4117. IEEE (2013)
102. Osa, T., Harada, K., Sugita, N., Mitsuishi, M.: Trajectory planning under different initial conditions for surgical task automation by learning from demonstration. In: 2014 IEEE International Conference on Robotics and Automation (ICRA), pp. 6507–6513. IEEE (2014)

103. Murali, A., Sen, S., Kehoe, B., Garg, A., McFarland, S., Patil, S., Boyd, W.D., Lim, S., Abbeel, P., Goldberg, K.: Learning by observation for surgical subtasks: multilateral cutting of 3D viscoelastic and 2D orthotropic tissue phantoms. In: 2015 IEEE International Conference on Robotics and Automation (ICRA), pp. 1202–1209. IEEE (2015)
104. Su, H., Mariani, A., Ovur, S.E., Menciassi, A., Ferrigno, G., De Momi, E.: Toward teaching by demonstration for robot-assisted minimally invasive surgery. In: IEEE Transactions on Automation Science and Engineering (2021)
105. Hussein, A., Gaber, M.M., Elyan, E., Jayne, C.: Imitation learning: a survey of learning methods. ACM Comput. Surv. (CSUR) **50**(2), 1–35 (2017)
106. Kober, J., Bagnell, J.A., Peters, J.: Reinforcement learning in robotics: a survey. Int. J. Robot. Res. **32**(11), 1238–1274 (2013)
107. Garcıa, J., Fernández, F.: A comprehensive survey on safe reinforcement learning. J. Mach. Learn. Res. **16**(1), 1437–1480 (2015)
108. Cheng, R., Orosz, G., Murray, R.M., Burdick, J.W.: End-to-end safe reinforcement learning through barrier functions for safety-critical continuous control tasks. In: Proceedings of the AAAI Conference on Artificial Intelligence, vol. 33, pp. 3387–3395 (2019)
109. Nguyen, N.D., Nguyen, T., Nahavandi, S., Bhatti, A., Guest, G.: Manipulating soft tissues by deep reinforcement learning for autonomous robotic surgery. In: 2019 IEEE International Systems Conference (SysCon), pp. 1–7. IEEE (2019)
110. Thananjeyan, B., Garg, A., Krishnan, S., Chen, C., Miller, L., Goldberg, K.: Multilateral surgical pattern cutting in 2D orthotropic gauze with deep reinforcement learning policies for tensioning. In: 2017 IEEE International Conference on Robotics and Automation (ICRA), pp. 2371–2378. IEEE (2017)
111. Shin, C., Ferguson, P.W., Pedram, S.A., et al.: Autonomous tissue manipulation via surgical robot using learning based model predictive control. In: 2019 International Conference on Robotics and Automation (ICRA), pp. 3875–3881. IEEE (2019)
112. Pedram, S.A., Ferguson, P.W., Shin, C., Mehta, A., Dutson, E.P., Alambeigi, F., et al.: Toward synergic learning for autonomous manipulation of deformable tissues via surgical robots: an approximate q- approach. In: 2020 8th IEEE RAS/EMBS Int. Conf. for Biomedical Robotics and Biomechatronics (BioRob), pp. 878–884. IEEE (2019)
113. Boeing, A., Bräunl, T.: Leveraging multiple simulators for crossing the reality gap. In: 2012 12th International Conference on Control Automation Robotics & Vision (ICARCV), pp. 1113–1119. IEEE (2012)
114. Richter, F., Orosco, R.K., Yip, M.C.: Open-sourced reinforcement learning environments for surgical robotics (2019). arXiv:1903.02090
115. Xu, J., Li, B., Lu, B., Liu, Y.-H., Dou, Q., Heng, P.-A.: SurRol: an open-source reinforcement learning centered and DVRX compatible platform for surgical robot learning. In: 2021 IEEE/RSJ International Conference on Intelligent Robots and Systems (IROS). IEEE (2021)
116. Nair, A., McGrew, B., Andrychowicz, M., Zaremba, W., Abbeel, P.: Overcoming exploration in reinforcement learning with demonstrations. In: 2018 IEEE International Conference on Robotics and Automation (ICRA), pp. 6292–6299. IEEE (2018)
117. Ho, J., Ermon, S.: Generative adversarial imitation learning. In: Advances in Neural Information Processing Systems, pp. 4565–457 (2016)
118. Chi, W., Dagnino, G., Kwok, T.M., Nguyen, A., Kundrat, D., Abdelaziz, M.E., Riga, C., Bicknell, C., Yang, G.-Z.: Collaborative robot-assisted endovascular catheterization with generative adversarial imitation learning. In: 2020 IEEE International Conference on Robotics and Automation (ICRA), pp. 2414–2420. IEEE (2020)

Plan Instantiation, Simulation and Execution

The first part of the book presented some of the challenges facing the design of an autonomous system especially in the areas of knowledge extraction, representation and task planning. The first part summarized the results achieved:

- Textbook analysis and procedural knowledge extraction and representation in Chapter "Learning Surgical Procedures from Text".
- A logical framework for task planning and learning in Chapter "Surgical Task Planning and Learning".
- The development of a pipeline of text to planning in Chapter "Towards Surgical Task Planning from Text".
- Extraction of surgical motion primitive and task structure from data in Chapter "Learning Surgical Gestures from Data".
- Simulation as a tool for knowledge representation, learning and task verification in Chapter "Simulation and Autonomy".

The second part of the book presents how these concepts are integrated to demonstrate some basic robotic capabilities. The first Chapter "Situation Awareness in Autonomous Surgical Robots: Calibration and Medical SLAM" describes how the plans are grounded in the current anatomical environment and how their execution is monitored. The new hand-eye calibration proposed achieves a much higher accuracy in position estimation than the state of the art, and a new anatomical SLAM algorithm permits monitoring accurately the task execution.

Then, Chapter "The Cognitive Architecture" describes the software architecture proposed for the experiments that includes a parallel simulation as a real-time task supervisor. This architecture supports the experimental verification of autonomous tissue retraction described in Chapter "Autonomous Tissue Retraction with DEFRAS", and Chapter "Learning Tissue Retraction in Simulation" describes the experimental results of tissue retraction and different aspects of the use of simulation in autonomous robotic tasks. In Chapter "The Cognitive Architecture" we address also the issue of human interpretation of a task, introducing the need of common sense reasoning in surgical planning.

Chapter "New Hardware: Design, Models and Analysis" describes the new hardware developed to overcome some of the limitations of current robotic systems. The first section in the eleventh chapter describes a model that could account for needle deflection, thus improving the accuracy of percutaneous interventions. The second section in the eleventh chapter describes a novel sensing approach to identify tissues and detect non-homogeneous masses, such as tumors, hidden from the surface. Finally, the third section in the eleventh chapter describes and characterizes a novel force and torque sensor that could measure the interaction forces with the tissues and support haptic feedback.

Situation Awareness in Autonomous Surgical Robots: Calibration and Medical SLAM

Andrea Roberti

Abstract One of the main challenges for computer-assisted surgery (CAS) is to determine the intra-operative morphology and motion of soft-tissues. This information is prerequisite to the registration of multi-modal patient-specific data for enhancing the surgeon's navigation capabilities by observing beyond exposed tissue surfaces and for providing intelligent control of robotic-assisted instruments. In minimally invasive surgery (MIS), optical techniques are an increasingly attractive approach for in vivo 3D reconstruction of the soft-tissue surface geometry. This chapter addresses the evolution of the computer vision necessary to achieve surgical autonomy, through the study of the anatomical environment, exploring the technology present and what is needed to analyze the scene. The issue of hand-eye calibration is then addressed, aligning the vision system and the robot into a unified reference frame, thereby enhancing the precision of the surgical work plan. This chapter delves into the integration of vision and calibration within the context of 3D reconstruction. In minimally invasive surgery (MIS), simultaneous localization and mapping (SLAM) can be employed to determine the pose of the endoscopic camera and construct a 3D model of the tissue surface. Another crucial aspect for MIS is maintaining real-time awareness of the positions of surgical tools relative to the surgical camera and the underlying anatomy.

1 Introduction

This chapter explores the evolution of computer vision in the surgical domain. It begins with an examination of the sensors available in robotics, followed by the calibration of these sensors with the robot, and ultimately covers the reconstruction of an unknown environment.

The first section analyzes the sensors used in robotic surgery, discussing their advantages and disadvantages, which highlight the need for new technology to enhance the accuracy of environmental reconstruction.

A. Roberti (✉)
Department of Engineering for Innovation Medicine, University of Verona, Verona, Italy
e-mail: andrea.roberti@univr.it

P. Fiorini (ed.), *Towards Autonomous Robotic Surgery*, Springer Tracts in Advanced Robotics 161, https://doi.org/10.1007/978-3-032-04247-7_7

The second section focuses on developing a calibration procedure adaptable to all types of sensors, offering improved accuracy in the workspace compared to current state-of-the-art methods.

A major challenge in autonomous robotic surgery is the unpredictability of the anatomical environment and its intra-operative behavior, which varies with each patient. Therefore, the third section integrates previous work to develop a new Simultaneous Localization and Mapping (SLAM) algorithm that allow adapting an existing anatomical model to a changed anatomy. This involves registering pre-operative images to the 3D reconstruction, distinguishing dynamic from static features, and adapting an existing SLAM algorithm to a dynamic environment.

2 Vision Sensors

This section describes all the vision sensors available in a robotic system, starting with an explanation of how the cameras operate and then comparing the various sensors. The section highlights the strengths and weaknesses of each sensor type, culminating in the introduction of the new endoscope model developed for Robotic-assisted Minimally Invasive Surgery (R-MIS).

2.1 Image Acquisition

An imaging apparatus works by collecting the light reflected from the objects in the scene and creating a two-dimensional image. If we want to use the image to obtain information on the scene, we must study the nature of this process. The most common types of cameras are shown in Fig. 1 and briefly compared in the Table 1.

The simplest geometric model of image formation is the pinhole camera, represented in Fig. 2. This is the same principle that was used in the Renaissance darkroom. Let M be a point of the scene, with coordinates (X, Y, Z) and let M' be his projec-

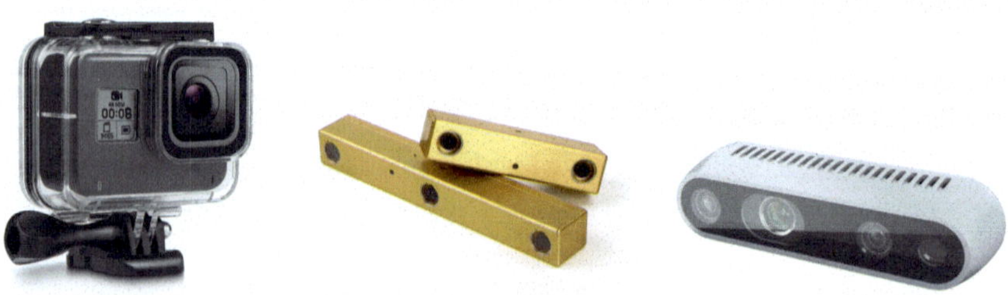

(a) Monocular (b) Stereo (c) RGB-D

Fig. 1 Most common sensors available

Table 1 A comparison of the sensors

Sensor	Advantages	Drawbacks
Monocular	Smallest	Scale is unobservable
	Lowest power consumption	Scale drift
	Lowest cost	3D only from multi-view
	Minimal calibration	No mapping under pure rotations
Stereo	3D from one stereo frame	More processing per frame
		Extrinsic calibration
RGB-D	Directly provide dense depth map	Active sensor
	Dense maps	Only indoors
	3D metric system	Complex calibration
		Power consumption

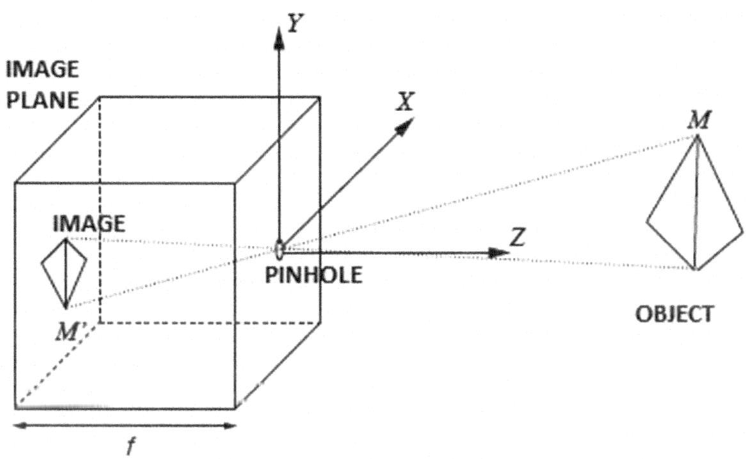

Fig. 2 Formation of the image in the pinhole camera

tion on the image plane, with coordinates (X', Y', Z'). If f is the distance of the projection center from the image plane (focal distance), then from the similarity of the triangles we obtain:

$$\frac{-X'}{f} = \frac{X}{Z} \; and \; \frac{-Y'}{f} = \frac{Y}{Z} \tag{1}$$

then,

$$X' = \frac{-fX}{Z} \qquad Y' = \frac{-fY}{Z} \qquad Z' = -f \tag{2}$$

Note that the image is inverted with respect to the scene, both right-left than above-below, as indicated by the minus sign. These equations define the process of image formation that takes the name of perspective projection. We can model the projection perspective by placing the image plane in front of the projection center, thus eliminating the negative sign. The division by Z is responsible for the foreshortening effect, so the size of the image of an object varies according to its distance from the observer.

2.2 Monocular Camera

Monocular cameras are the most common devices, we use them every day with our smartphone and there are many types and resolutions. These cameras are mainly composed of the image sensor and lens. We assume that the camera can be accurately modeled as a pinhole camera, once the lens distortion has been removed, so that a $3D$ point $X_c \in \mathbb{R}^3$ in the camera coordinate reference system C is projected into $2D$ pixel coordinates x with the projection function $\pi_m : \mathbb{R}^3 \rightarrow \mathbb{R}^2$:

$$x = \pi_m(X_c) = \begin{bmatrix} f_x \frac{X}{Z} + c_x \\ f_y \frac{Y}{Z} + c_y \end{bmatrix} \tag{3}$$

$$X_c = [X, Y, Z]^T, \qquad x = [u, v]^T$$

where f_x and f_y are the horizontal and vertical focal lengths, and c_x and c_y the horizontal and vertical coordinates of the principal point. These are intrinsic calibration parameters that can be computed from several images of a known calibration pattern. The camera coordinate system C has its origin at the optical center and follows the standard directives for its transform: the Z axis is looking forward, the X axis points to the right and the Y axis points downwards. The projection function π assumes no distortion introduced by the lens. Well known software and libraries like Matlab [1] or OpenCV [2] include toolboxes for camera calibration, including distortion.

2.3 Stereo Camera

Stereo cameras consist of two rigidly connected cameras. Ideally both cameras are hardware synchronized so that image capturing is triggered at the same time. Depth can be estimated from just one stereo frame through the stereopsis, which is the process that allows obtaining information of the three-dimensional structure from a pair of images, coming from two cameras that view a scene from different locations. The distance between the two cameras, known as the baseline b, along with focal length and image resolution of the cameras, determines the depth range at which depth estimation is accurate. We can identify two subproblems: computation of correspondences and triangulation. The first consists of coupling points in the two images that are the projections of the same point of the scene on the image plane of the two cameras. These points are called *conjugate points*. Given these premises, the positions of the points in the scene that are projected on the two image planes can be reconstructed once we know the couplings between the points of the two images, the reciprocal position of the cameras with respect to each other, and the intrinsic parameters of the cameras. This triangulation process requires the calibration of the stereo system, i.e. the calculation of the intrinsic parameters and the reciprocal position (extrinsic parameters) of the cameras. In order to facilitate stereo matching, images are typically rectified, removing distortion and rotations, so that the epipolar lines are horizontal, i.e. a pixel in the left image lies on the same row of the corresponding pixel in the right image. The projection function for a rectified stereo camera $\pi_s : \mathbb{R}^3 \rightarrow \mathbb{R}^3$:

$$x = \pi_s(X_c) = \begin{bmatrix} f_x \frac{X}{Z} + c_x \\ f_y \frac{Y}{Z} + c_y \\ f_x \frac{X-b}{Z} + c_x \end{bmatrix} \tag{4}$$

$$X_c = [X, Y, Z]^T, \qquad x = [u_L, v_L, u_R]^T$$

where (u_L, v_L) are the coordinates in the left image and u_R is the horizontal coordinate in the right image. The vertical coordinate in both images is the same for each point, and we assume that both cameras have the same intrinsic parameters after rectification. The theory of depth from stereo has been the subject to many publications and book, for example [3, 4].

2.4 RGB-D Camera

RGB-D cameras are the combination of a monocular RGB camera and a depth sensor, based on structured light or time of flight. The measured depth can be registered into a depth map with 1 : 1 pixel correspondences to the RGB image, after the extrinsic calibration between the camera and the depth sensor. The main advantage of this camera is that for every pixel in the image we know its depth value without the need to perform a stereo matching as in the case of the stereo camera. However, their use is restricted to indoors and the depth range is limited [5].

2.5 Endoscope

An endoscope is a long, thin, flexible or rigid tube that has a light and camera at its distal end. Images of the inside of a body are shown on a television screen. Such a device could provide minimally invasive access to sections that are accessible only through invasive approaches. Conventional endoscopes are highly flexible devices for minimally invasive inspection in interior lumens and cavities, such as the stomach, colon, urinary tract, respiratory tract, etc. These medical imaging devices are available in many sizes to suit different purposes. Different types of endoscope cameras are used for different areas of the body. Upper endoscopes, bronchoscopes, colonoscopes, sigmoidoscopes, and many other endoscopes are named for the areas where they are used. Endoscope cameras are important pieces of medical equipment. They are versatile enough to be used both as diagnostic and treatment instruments. These cameras provide visual imaging as a mean to replace unnecessary or exploratory surgery. With the availability of several options, doctors can choose the best endoscope for each area of the body. The introduction of the stereo endoscope has played an important role in video $3D$ laparoscopy system, providing stereo view to the surgeon. Earlier endoscopic stereo cameras consisted of parallel optical paths bringing the images to a pair of cameras at the proximal end of the endoscope [6]. Current 3D endoscopes are called *chip of tip* camera [7] since they consist of two complementary metal-oxide-semiconductor (CMOS) camera modules mounted on the distal end of the endoscope, which provide the real-time stereo view to the surgeon. Because the small distance between the two camera chips does not match the human intra-eye distance, some software processing is carried out so that the surgeon viewing the two images on the stereo visor, or on a 3D screen, has a realistic three-dimensional view of the anatomic site. Stereo vision helps the Robotic Minimally Invasive Surgery (R-MIS) because it provides the depth perception necessary to move the instruments without damaging the patient tissues. Currently, all surgical robotic systems on the market are teleoperated by a main surgeon from a separate console [8–10], while an assistant surgeon directly operates next to the patient with laparoscopic tools. This setup helps the main surgeon in smoothing his/her movements and increasing their precision through motion scaling, while also reducing both the required physical and cognitive effort to perform the operation. On the other hand, having no direct contact with the patient visual perception of the anatomical environment becomes a crucial point in such systems.

The next step forward in R-MIS is expected to come with an autonomous robot that can either perform some routine operations on its own or assist the main surgeon during an intervention [11–14]. The introduction of degrees of autonomy requires systems with advanced capabilities in perception as well as in reasoning, motion planning and physical interaction.

3 Hand-Eye Calibration

Autonomy in robotic systems requires advanced perception, reasoning, and motion planning capabilities, as emphasized in recent studies [11, 12]. Improved medical imaging and vision techniques have notably enhanced the performance of robotic surgical systems in various clinical scenarios, including orthopedics and neurosurgery [15]. Vision systems can extract pre-operative and intra-operative information from computed tomography (CT) [16], magnetic resonance imaging (MRI), and ultrasound to plan tool trajectories and support surgeons' decision-making. However, image-guided interventions necessitate precise calibration to align the poses of robots, instruments, and anatomical structures within a common reference frame.

For a robot to accurately estimate the 3D position and orientation of an object relative to its base using a video camera, it must determine the relative positions and orientations between the robot's hand and base, the camera and the hand, and the object and the camera. This requires the calibration of the robot, the robot eye-to-hand system, and the camera, typically involving complex nonlinear optimization, specialized setups, and expert skills.

D robotic hand-eye calibration involves calculating the relative 3D position and orientation between the camera and the robot gripper in an eye-on-hand configuration, where the camera is rigidly attached to the robot gripper. The camera may be grasped by the gripper or securely fastened to it. Specifically, this task entails determining the relative rotation and translation (homogeneous transformation) between two coordinate frames: one centered at the camera lens and the other at the robot gripper. The gripper coordinate frame is centered on the robot manipulator's last link and must have sufficient degrees of freedom to rotate the camera around two different axes while keeping it focused on a stationary calibration object, ensuring a unique and accurate 3D geometric relationship between the camera and the gripper.

3.1 *Theory of Calibration*

Hand-eye calibration has been widely studied within the robotics literature [17]. The most common way to describe the hand-eye calibration problem is using the homogeneous transformation matrix as:

$$AX = XB \tag{5}$$

where A and B are known homogeneous matrices, and X is the unknown transformation between the robot coordinate frame and camera coordinate frame. For each homogeneous matrix, it is in the form of

$$\begin{bmatrix} R & t \\ 0 & 1 \end{bmatrix} \tag{6}$$

where R is a 3×3 rotational matrix, and t is a 3×1 translational vector. Thus, we can expand (5) as

$$\begin{bmatrix} R_A & t_A \\ 0 & 1 \end{bmatrix} \begin{bmatrix} R_x & t_x \\ 0 & 1 \end{bmatrix} = \begin{bmatrix} R_x & t_x \\ 0 & 1 \end{bmatrix} \begin{bmatrix} R_B & t_B \\ 0 & 1 \end{bmatrix} \tag{7}$$

where R_A, R_X and R_B are the rotational matrix parts of A, X and B, and t_A, t_X and t_B are the translational parts, respectively. Equation (7) can be further simplified as:

$$\begin{bmatrix} R_A R_X & R_A t_X + t_A \\ 0 & 1 \end{bmatrix} = \begin{bmatrix} R_X R_B & R_X t_B + t_X \\ 0 & 1 \end{bmatrix} \tag{8}$$

The purpose of hand-eye calibration is to find R_X and t_X given j pair of A_i and the corresponding B_i, where $i = 1, 2 \ldots J$. The majority of the approaches regards the rotation estimation decoupled from the translation estimation. At least two rotations containing motions with nonparallel rotation axes are required to solve the problem [18]. Several approaches have been proposed for the estimation of R_X from (8): using the rotation axis and angle [18, 19], quaternions [20] and canonical representation [21].

3.2 Calibration for Robotic Surgery

In the Autonomous Robotic Surgery (ARS) project described in this book, we proposed a novel calibration method for the surgical robotic scenario using the da Vinci Research Kit (dVRK) and an RGB-D camera. Differently from [22], the accuracy and computational time of our method do not depend on the placement of the calibration board within the workspace. We performed exhaustive experimental validation on relevant use cases for surgery. We separated the calibration of the robotic arms (two Patient-Side Manipulators, PSM1 and PSM2, and an Endoscope Camera Manipulator, ECM) from the hand-eye calibration of the camera. For both calibrations we proposed a three-step method with closed-form solution:

1. touching the reference points on a custom calibration board with the end-effectors of the surgical robot.
2. recognizing the same reference points with the RGB-D camera.
3. mapping the poses reached by the robotic arms in the first step to the 3D points computed in the second step.

The main advantage of the proposed method is the improved accuracy in a 3D metric space, which is increased by a factor of four with respect to the state-of-the-art results with comparable sensors. Moreover, with our method the camera can be mounted on the moving endoscopic arm of the dVRK, overcoming the limitations of a fixed camera.

3.3 Proposed Method

The aim of the calibration procedure was twofold. First, we performed the computation of the rigid transformations $T_{\star}^{w}$ between the common reference frame ($world$)

and the base frame of the arms, $\star \in \{ecm_b, psm_{1b}, psm_{2b}\}$. Second, we estimated the transformation T_{ecm}^{cam} between the camera reference frame and the ECM reference frame. The resulting transformation tree is shown in Fig. 3.

We used a custom calibration board, shown in Fig. 4a, with an ArUco marker in the center of a circumference of 50 mm radius, with several reference dots. We

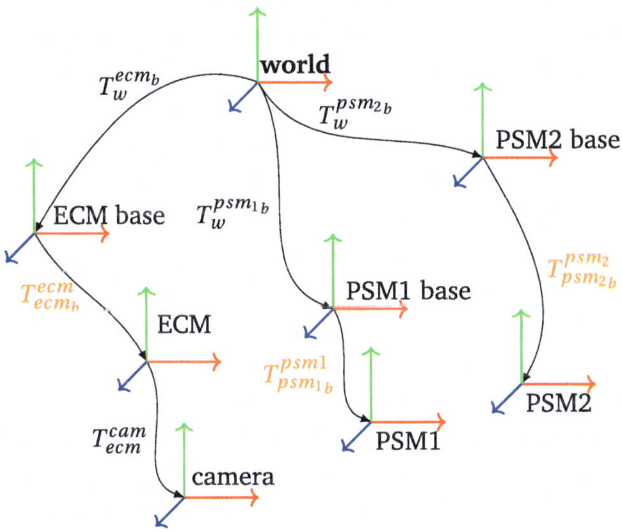

Fig. 3 The reference frames produced by our proposed method (the axes direction of the reference frames are only for visualisation purpose). The orange transformations are known, whereas the black transformations are to be estimated

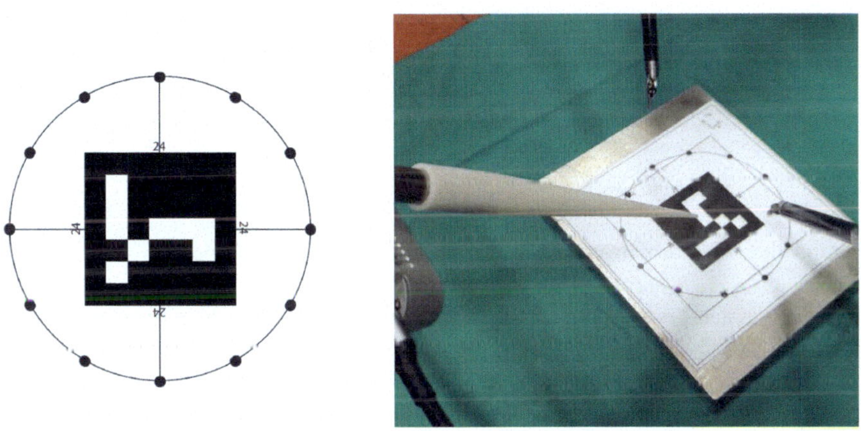

(a) Calibration pattern **(b)** ECM adapter

Fig. 4 The calibration components. **a** the calibration board with the marker, the colored axes represent the common reference frame directions **b** the adapter for the ECM positioning equipped the ECM with the 3D-printed adapter, shown in Fig. 4b. The adapter had a smaller tip than the ECM to guarantee precise positioning on the dots on the board.

The procedure started by positioning the calibration board in the robot workspace. We chose a set of reference points P such that each point $p \in P$ was reachable by the three arms and visible from the camera. The points in P must be symmetric with respect to the center of the board to compute the origin of the common reference frame, and at least three points were needed to estimate the plane coefficients. The best fitting plane was characterized by the centroid of the point set P, $\mathbf{c}$, and the normal vector $\mathbf{n}$. Their optimal estimations were the solution of the optimization problem

$$\{\hat{\mathbf{c}}, \hat{\mathbf{n}}\} = \arg\min_{\mathbf{c},|\mathbf{n}|_2=1} \sum_{i=1}^{n}((\mathbf{p}_i - \mathbf{c})^T \mathbf{n})^2 \tag{9}$$

As in [23] the centroid was estimated by

$$\hat{\mathbf{c}} = \frac{1}{n}\sum_{i=1}^{n}\mathbf{p}_i. \tag{10}$$

The normal vector $\mathbf{n}$ was obtained by factorizing the distance matrix A with Singular Value Decomposition (SVD)

$$A = USV^T = \left[\mathbf{p}_1 - \hat{\mathbf{c}}, \ldots \mathbf{p}_n - \hat{\mathbf{c}}\right] \in \mathbb{R}^{3\times n} \tag{11}$$

and taking the third column of the matrix $U = \left[\mathbf{u}_1\ \mathbf{u}_2\ \mathbf{u}_3\right]$, $\hat{\mathbf{n}} = \mathbf{u}_3$. To generate a common reference frame for all the tools, we implemented the following three main steps:

1. Arm calibration
2. Camera calibration
3. Hand-eye calibration.

3.3.1 Arm Calibration

To find the transformation of the arms' base frame with respect to the common reference frame we recorded the end effector pose of the arms (PSMs and ECM with adapter) on each point in the set P. In order to obtain the ECM effective pose, we removed the known rigid transformation between the adapter and the ECM. On this set, we estimated the best fitting plane using (9). The set P was then augmented by adding a point above the calibration board acquired by moving the arm's end effector. This last point was used to define the desired plane normal direction

$$\mathbf{n}_d = \frac{\mathbf{p}_{n+1} - \mathbf{c}}{|\mathbf{p}_{n+1} - \mathbf{c}|_2}$$

where $\mathbf{p_{n+1}}$ was the last point in the ordered set P, $\mathbf{c}$ was the centroid of P and $| * |_2$ was the vector norm. For each arm, the homogeneous transformation $T_\star^w$ of the common reference with respect to the arm base frame was defined using the direction versors.

$$\mathbf{u} = \text{sign}(\mathbf{n} \cdot \mathbf{n_d})\mathbf{n}$$

$$\mathbf{l} = \mathbf{u} \times \frac{\mathbf{p_1} - \mathbf{c}}{|\mathbf{p_1} - \mathbf{c}|_2}$$

$$\mathbf{f} = \mathbf{l} \times \mathbf{u}$$

and the centroid $\mathbf{c}$,

$$T_\star^w = \begin{bmatrix} \mathbf{f}_x & \mathbf{l}_x & \mathbf{u}_x & \mathbf{c}_x \\ \mathbf{f}_y & \mathbf{l}_y & \mathbf{u}_y & \mathbf{c}_y \\ \mathbf{f}_z & \mathbf{l}_z & \mathbf{u}_z & \mathbf{c}_z \\ 0 & 0 & 0 & 1 \end{bmatrix}$$

3.3.2 Camera Calibration

To find the transformation T_{cam}^w for the RGB-D camera we first detected the center of the ArUco marker on the board with respect to the camera frame. Once we found a camera position that ensured good visibility and a stable pose of the ArUco marker, we aligned the pose on the point cloud generated from the depth map acquired by the RGB-D camera. We used the marker pose and its known radius to generate the pose of every dot in the set P in the marker reference frame, as well as the point above the calibration board that was needed to define the desired plane normal direction.

Once the pose set P was obtained, we found the best fitting plane using (9) and then we built the homogeneous transformation T_{cam}^w between the common reference frame to the camera base frame by adapting the previous approach used for the arms.

3.3.3 Hand-Eye Calibration

The hand-eye calibration problem was formulated using the homogeneous transformation matrices:

$$AX = XB$$

where A and B are known homogeneous matrices representing the frames of the base of the robot and the camera, respectively. The unknown transformation X was between the robot coordinate frame and the camera coordinate frame. Given T_{cam}^w, we could compute X as the relative homogeneous transformation between the end effector of the ECM and the RGB-D base frame:

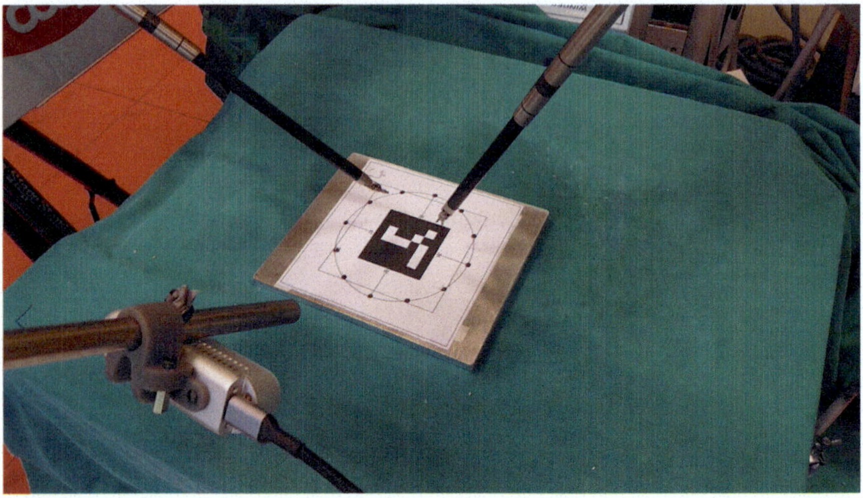

Fig. 5 The proposed setup for calibration, with the RealSense d435, the PSMs and the calibration pattern

Table 2 RealSense d435 specifications

Camera specifications	
Resolution	1280 × 720
Field of view (FOV)	91 × 65 × 100
Frame rate	90 fps
Baseline	50 mm
Z-accuracy	≤2% of the working distance

$$T_{ecm}^{cam} = T_{w}^{cam}(T_{w}^{ecm})^{-1}.$$

3.4 *Experimental Setup*

The validation of the proposed method has been carried out with the dVRK robot shown in Fig. 5.

The stereo endoscope had been augmented with an Intel RealSense d435 RGB-D camera rigidly attached to the endoscope through a 3D printed adapter. The camera specifications are reported in Table 2. The whole calibration method was implemented in the Robot Operating System (ROS) using the Point Cloud Library (PCL) and OpenCV.

The present setup is not compatible with a surgical scenario because of the size of the RGB-D camera. However it is well possible that in the near future small RGB-D cameras could become available and be integrated within the endoscope.

3.5 *Experimental Results*

To experimentally validate our methodology we compared our calibration with Tsai's method [18], which is the current state of the art, in two benchmark tests for surgical robotics:

- Localization and grasping of small targets,
- Dual-arm manipulation

Finally, we evaluated the accuracy of the projection from 2D camera image plane to the 3D workspace.

3.5.1 Localization and Grasping

In the first scenario (Fig. 6) the two PSMs must autonomously grasp a ring placed on the calibration board, in this case on location 2. The RGB-D camera identified the point cloud corresponding to the ring after color and shape segmentation. Points

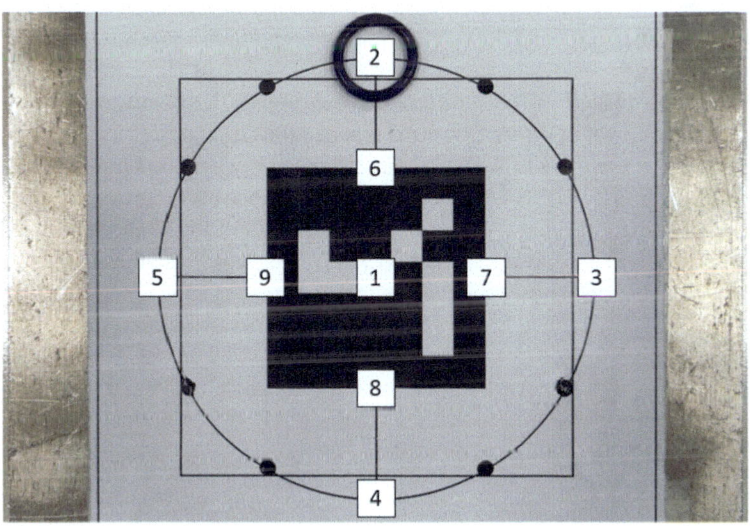

Fig. 6 Setup for the localization and grasping experiment. The numbers on calibration board represents the nine locations used during the experiment. The ring is identified by the camera and then reached by the PSMs

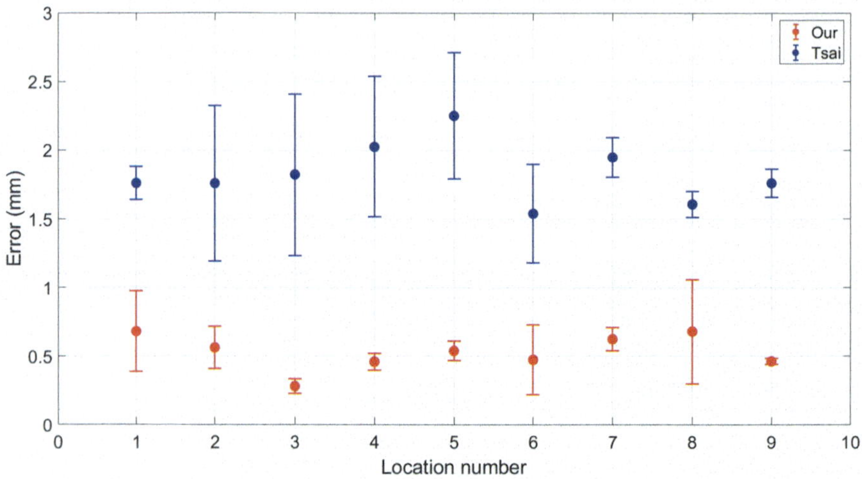

Fig. 7 The measured 3D positioning errors between the robot end effector and the grasping point

Table 3 A comparison of the error in the localization and grasping test

	Max error (mm)	Mean error (mm)	Std dev (mm)
Our method	1.07	0.53	0.15
Tsai [18]	3.17	1.83	0.33

were then transformed from the camera to the common reference frame. The ring had a diameter of 15 mm, and the target point for both PSMs was chosen as the center of the ring.

The ring was placed in the 9 different locations on the board to cover the full $x - y$ plane, as shown in Fig. 6. The arms reached the target points ten times, and for each iteration we computed the Euclidean distance between the target and the final positions of the PSMs. In this way, we estimated the mean accuracy of our calibration procedure on the $x - y$ plane. The results are reported in Fig. 7 and compared with state-of-the-art Tsai's calibration method [18]. It is worth mentioning that errors are comprehensive of the estimated kinematic accuracy of the dVRK: 1.02 mm on average when localizing and reaching fiducial markers [24], with a maximum error of 2.72 mm [25].

Table 3 shows that our method achieves significantly better accuracy 0.53 mm average error against 1.83 mm with Tsai's calibration. The error does not depend on the location of the ring on the $x - y$ plane.

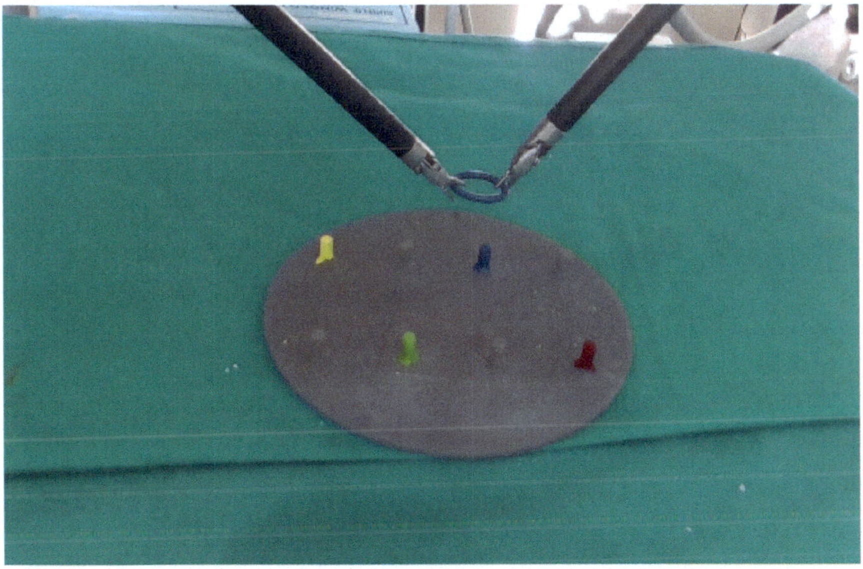

Fig. 8 Dual arm manipulation experiment. The two arms carries a ring while performing circular trajectories through the workspace

3.5.2 Dual Arm Manipulation

In the second scenario (Fig. 8) the PSMs started holding the same ring, and they must execute simultaneous pre-computed circular trajectories with center on the z axis of the common reference frame (45 mm above the calibration board) and radius r ranging from 10 to 40 mm. Circumferences were first defined in the $x - z$ plane of the common reference frame (normal to the calibration board), and then replicated in planes rotated around the z axis with a step of 10deg. In this way we defined a spherical workspace by interpolation between the recorded trajectories. PSMs were commanded with the transformed waypoints in their relative frames. This task validated the accuracy of the transformations between the arms computed with the proposed method. We measured the difference between the trajectories of the two PSMs, and we considered the standard and the maximum deviations from the mean for each radius. In absence of calibration and kinematic errors, the difference between the trajectories would have had null standard deviation.

Figure 9 shows the absolute error through the workspace for spheres with radii 20, 30 and 40 mm, by using the Lambert equal-area cylindrical projection. The workspace has been projected using the Lambert equal-area cylindrical projection, the error is reported in mm. In Fig. 9 the labels refer to: (a) the workspace surface of the sphere with radius 10 mm, (b) the projected surface of the sphere with radius 10 mm, (c) the workspace surface of the sphere with radius 20 mm, (d) the projected surface of the sphere with radius 20 mm, (e) the workspace surface of the sphere with radius 30 mm,

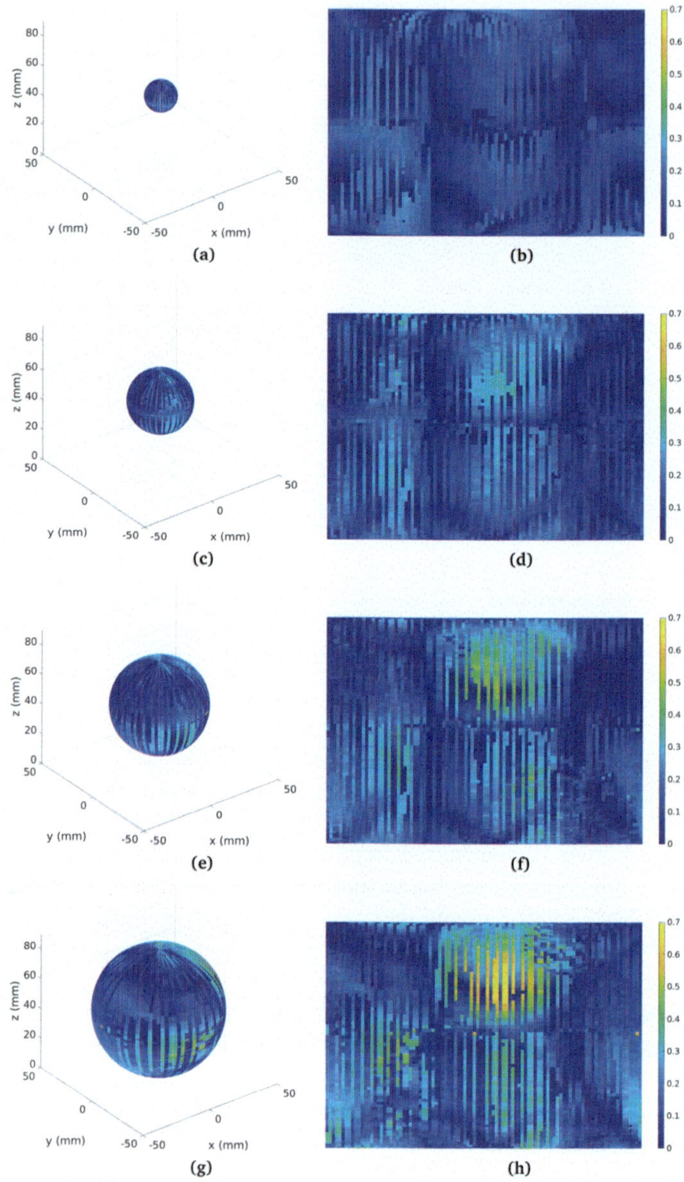

Fig. 9 Absolute error of the dual arm manipulation through the workspace. **a** the workspace surface of the sphere with radius 10 mm, **b** the projected surface of the sphere with radius 10 mm, **c** the workspace surface of the sphere with radius 20 mm, **d** the projected surface of the sphere with radius 20 mm, **e** the workspace surface of the sphere with radius 30 mm, **f** the projected surface of the sphere with radius 30 mm, **g** the workspace surface of the sphere with radius 40 mm, **h** the projected surface of the sphere with radius 40 mm

Table 4 The positioning error between the PSM1 and PSM2 during the dual-arm manipulation experiment

Radius (mm)	Max error (mm)	Mean error (mm)	Std dev (mm)
10	0.61	0.11	0.06
20	0.37	0.13	0.08
30	0.51	0.14	0.10
40	0.62	0.16	0.11

(f) the projected surface of the sphere with radius 30 mm, (g) the workspace surface of the sphere with radius 40 mm, (h) the projected surface of the sphere with radius 40 mm In Table 4 we report the errors for all the spheres. We notice that the mean error increases with the radius of the sphere, as the PSMs move away from the calibration plane. The standard deviation of the error increases with the radius but remains below 0.11 mm, hence the overall error does not change significantly on the surface of the spheres. This ensures good repeatability of motions in the whole workspace. The accuracy of our calibration method in 3D is compatible with the requirements of surgery (the mean error between the arms is below 1 mm, comparable with the known kinematic accuracy of the latest da Vinci models).

3.6 2D/3D Projection

In the last scenario the PSM1, with a colored marker on its tip, executed a spiral-shaped trajectory along the entire workspace. The RGB-D camera identified the marker in the image plane, and the corresponding 3D point could be computed using the depth value. The trajectory started near the origin of the common reference frame and then increased in radius and altitude according to the following parametric equations

$$
\begin{aligned}
x(t) &= \kappa t \cos(\omega t) \\
y(t) &= \kappa t \sin(\omega t) \\
z(t) &= \kappa t
\end{aligned}
$$

where ω is the constant angular speed and $\kappa \in \mathbb{R}$ is a time-scaling factor. The orientation of the end effector was kept fixed towards the camera along the trajectory. We measured the Euclidean error between the points in the trajectory executed by the arm and the re-projected points from the camera image plane. Figure 10 and Table 5 show that the re-projection accuracy with our method significantly outperforms the one reached with Tsai's. In fact, the mean error (4.71 mm) and the maximum error (11.76 mm) are four and two times smaller than the one achieved by

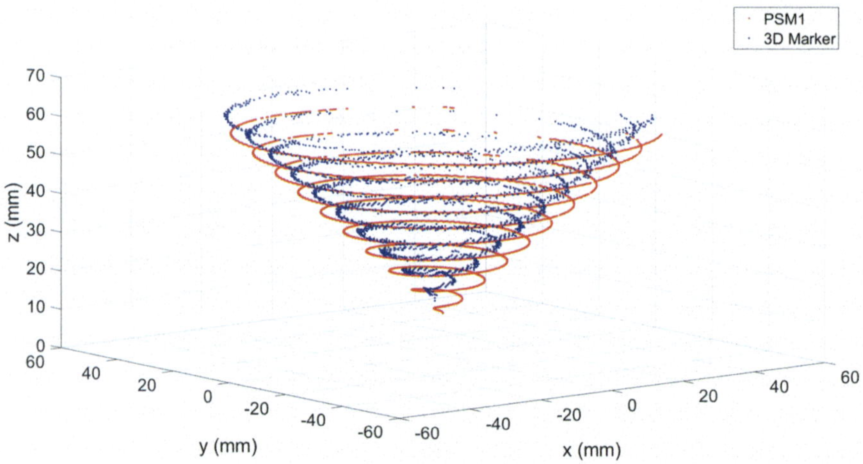

(a)

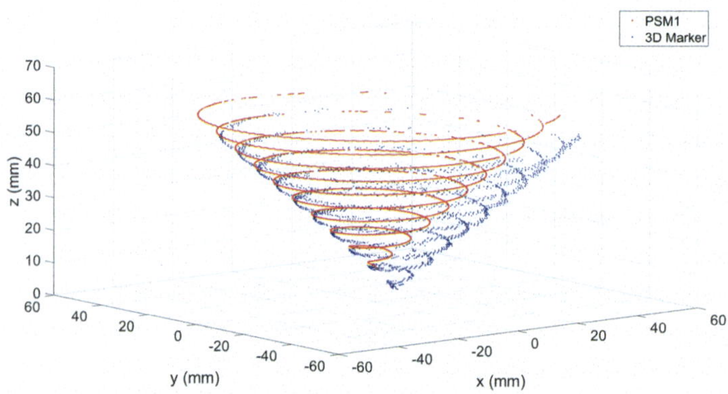

(b)

Fig. 10 Spiral-shaped trajectory executed by the PSM1 with our method in (**a**) and Tsai's method in (**b**). The red trajectory represents the kinematics of the PSM1, while the blue trajectory represents the marker identified in 3D space

Table 5 A comparison of the error between the marker tip trajectory and the measured tip trajectory for the projection test

	Max error (mm)	Mean error (mm)	Std dev (mm)
Our method	11.76	4.71	0.89
Tsai [18]	20.85	16.41	1.21

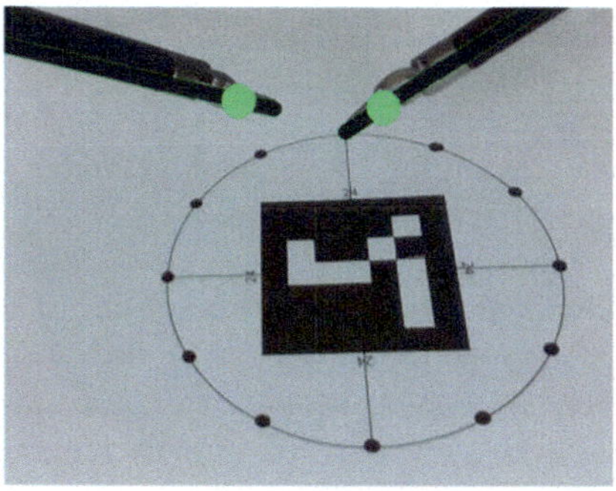

(a) Our method

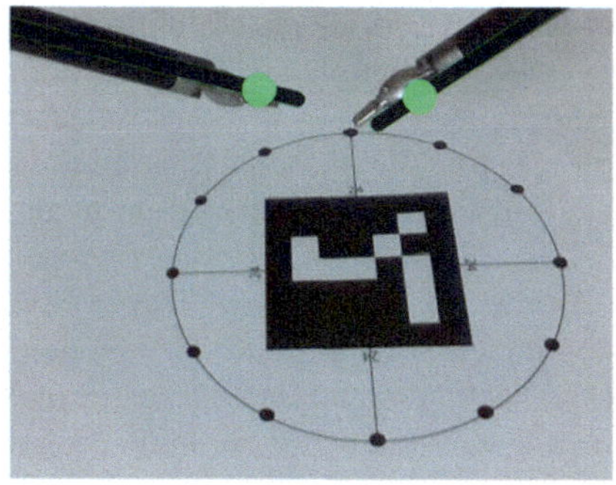

(b) Tsai's method

Fig. 11 An example of re-projection of da Vinci surgical instruments by using kinematic re-projection of the model directly onto camera color image

Tsai's method. It is important to remark that the measured error also includes the marker detection accuracy.

Finally Fig. 11 shows the re-projection of PSMs end effector position onto the camera image plane with both calibration methods. Our method achieves a better re-projection of the 3D instruments.

4 Medical SLAM

Minimally Invasive Surgery (MIS) significantly benefits from pre- and intra-operative image guidance. Despite these advantages, its use in procedures involving substantial tissue deformation, such as cardiovascular, gastrointestinal, and abdominal surgeries, remains limited.

We previously emphasized the importance of a common reference frame for 3D reconstruction, enabling the integration of preoperative and intraoperative data while aligning this information with the results of Simultaneous Localization and Mapping (SLAM). Various methods, including fiducial markers, optical tracking, and intra-operative imaging techniques like ultrasound, MRI, and X-ray fluoroscopy, have been extensively explored. However, leveraging vision techniques based on images from laparoscopes and endoscopes during MIS presents distinct advantages. These techniques avoid the need for additional equipment in an already complex surgical environment.

One of the main challenges in soft-tissue Minimally Invasive Surgery (MIS) is the fast, accurate, and robust acquisition of anatomical data during surgery. For augmented reality (AR) visualization, which overlays subsurface anatomical details onto the laparoscopic video, it is necessary to non-rigidly register intra-operative 3D data with pre-procedural planning images and models. Various tomographic intra-operative imaging modalities, such as ultrasound (US), intra-operative computed tomography (CT), and interventional magnetic resonance imaging (iMRI), have been explored to obtain detailed information about tissue morphology. However, these methods face significant technological challenges, high costs, and risks associated with real-time image acquisition in the surgical theatre or interventional radiology suite, often struggling to provide images with an acceptable signal-to-noise ratio (SNR).

A promising approach in MIS involves 3D reconstruction of soft-tissue surfaces using the endoscope itself. This method interprets the properties and geometry of light reflecting off the surgical site surfaces. Optical techniques for 3D surface reconstruction can be divided into two categories: passive methods, which only require images, and active methods, which require controlled light projected into the environment. Passive methods include stereoscopy, monocular Shape-from-X (SfX) [26], and Simultaneous Localization and Mapping (SLAM) [27]. Active methods are best known for structured light and Time-of-Flight (ToF) techniques [28]. Both active and passive technologies have been successfully applied in various fields, including robotics, and the film and gaming industries.

However, reconstructing patient anatomy for MIS poses specific challenges that remain unsolved. Unlike many applications that focus on the 3D reconstruction of static scenes, MIS methods must cope with dynamic and deformable environments. Additionally, tissue often has homogeneous texture, making the automatic detection of salient features and their matching in different image frames, very difficult.

The detection and matching of features in different frames is essential to localize the surgical instruments in the anatomical environment and make the autonomous surgical robot “aware” of their positions and the available range of motion.

Furthermore, the critical nature of surgery demands high accuracy and robustness to ensure patient safety, which is particularly challenging in the presence of specular highlights, smoke, and blood, all common in MIS procedures. Moreover, new technologies in the operating room must integrate seamlessly into the clinical workflow with minimal setup and calibration times.

In this section, we present how we modified the architecture of ORB-SLAM2 algorithm, which is one of the most used SLAM algorithm in literature, to manage some simple deformations and how to recognize and separate static from dynamic features.

4.1 A Method to Distinguish Static and Dynamic Features

To detect dynamic features in a scene, various methods are employed, which can be broadly categorized into three types:

- Dynamic feature detection based solely on geometric information.
- Dynamic feature detection based solely on semantic information.
- Dynamic feature detection through a naive combination of geometric calculations and semantic information in a loosely coupled manner.

Most existing works on the geometry of multiple images assume that the observed scene is rigid [29, 30]. This rigidity constraint allows the derivation of matching relationships among two or more images, represented by entities like the fundamental matrix.

In the context of semantic segmentation within a surgical environment, deep learning algorithms have faced challenges in delivering satisfactory results. This performance degradation in medical images primarily stems from the complexity of the scene [31, 32]. Typically, researchers work with scenarios where the objects have fixed color structures and shapes, with clear boundaries and interconnected components, making them easier to identify in different images. In contrast, organs in a surgical environment do not maintain fixed shapes, and their boundaries are often unclear. Additionally, the surgical scene is dynamic, constantly changing due to factors like biological motions, bleeding and the presence of smoke. Semantically different organs often share similar colors and textures, further complicating differentiation.

Recent semantic segmentation models predominantly utilize an encoder-decoder architecture. These models comprise two submodules: the encoder, which compresses image information and extracts low-dimensional feature representations, often adapted from standard classification CNN architectures like AlexNet, Inception, and ResNet; and the decoder, which upsamples the features to the original size using deconvolution and produces class probabilities for each pixel via a softmax layer [31, 32].

Fully Convolutional Neural Networks (FCNNs), first introduced for semantic scene segmentation by Long et al. [33], offer several advantages over traditional CNNs. FCNNs lack fully connected layers, significantly reducing the number of parameters. This architecture is scale-independent, allowing the models to accept input images of various sizes, scales, and aspect ratios, unlike conventional CNNs that only accept a fixed input size. This scale independence facilitates domain adaptation and fine-tuning, making FCNNs easier to train on images or video frames of different dimensions.

Ongoing research in semantic segmentation focuses on improving model architecture and refining the loss function to better define the problem at hand. Notably, many approaches have been proposed to enhance FCNN models' performance for semantic segmentation. For instance, U-Net [34], designed specifically for medical images, employs skip connections between the encoder and decoder layers to preserve spatial context. V-Net [35], inspired by U-Net, uses a similar approach but processes volumetric data (3D volumes from multiple frames) instead of 2D images.

In the ARS project, we proposed a semantic registration method for a semi-autonomous surgical robotic system. This approach enhanced the method presented in the previous chapter by incorporating semantically annotated medical images (such as CT, MRI, and PET scans) to improve the reliability of 3D registration in dynamic surgical environments. As illustrated in Fig. 12, we integrated semantic information into the inputs (pre-operational images and the camera image). Our framework registered the anatomical model from a CT scan, enriched with semantic information, to its 3D semantic reconstruction obtained from an RGB-D sensor.

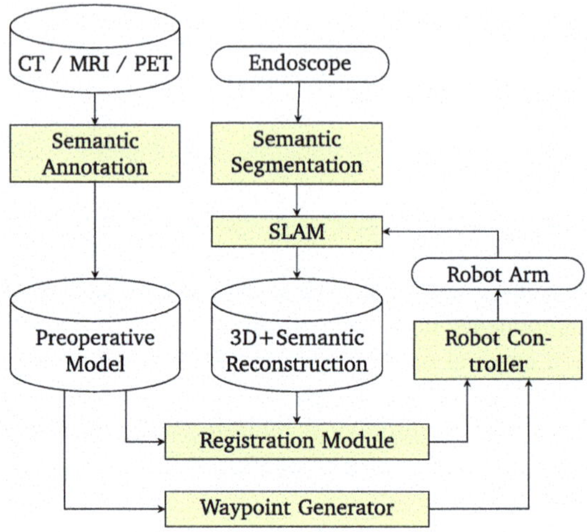

Fig. 12 The revised software architecture: the differences from [16] are in the use of medical images and the real time SLAM preceded by a semantic segmentation module

This process aimed to understand the surgical scene's state, including the nature of events and the current situation in the surgical cavity, aiding various autonomous components during the procedure.

4.2 *Pre-operative Model*

The pre-operative model used in the experimental validation of this work was obtained from a CT scan of the anatomical phantom for robotic assisted radical prostatectomy (RARP). In particular, the semi-automatic segmentation approach provided by Slicer3D [36] was exploited to extract the structures of interest.

Once the model was extracted, we highlighted the structures useful for semantic registration by encoding them with the same color map used for the segmentation, described in Table 6: for our experiments, the most prominent anatomies were the bladder, the connective tissue, and the prostate, whenever visible (Fig. 13).

4.3 *Semantic Segmentation*

We applied the model presented in [37], a Generative Adversarial Network (GAN), to the ARS phantom setup, incorporating replicated anatomical structures along with the catheter, the dVRK system, and the ARS tools. The realistic surgical phantom (developed by ACMIT Gmbh) is composed of a 3D-printed pelvis bone and the following silicone elements: rectum, bladder, urethra, seminal vesicles, vas deferens, and prostate, all immersed in a silicate fat-like foam. The GAN network had the

Table 6 Semantic scene color encoding

Color	Semantic meaning
	Background
	Da Vinci tools
	ARS tools
	Pelvic bone
	Pelvic floor muscle
	Anterior prostatic fat
	Vas deferns and seminal vescicles
	Ureter
	Catheter
	Bladder
	Bladder neck
	Prostate
	Prostate neck
	Urethra

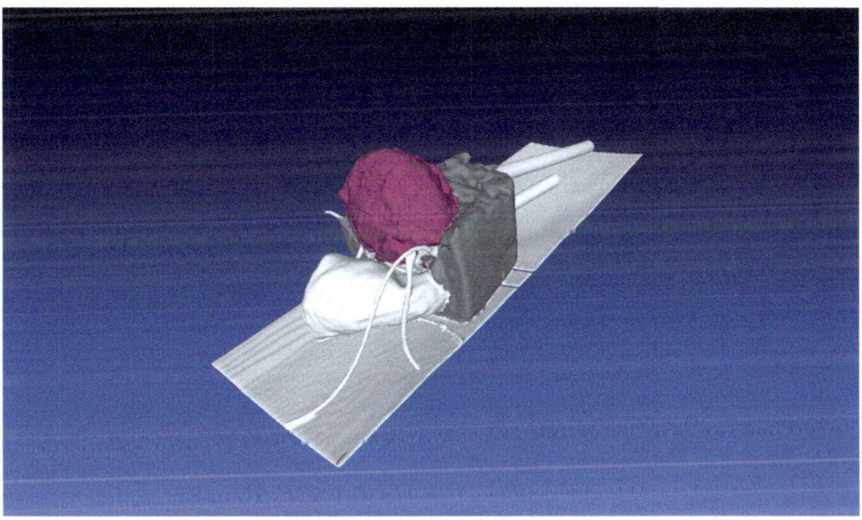

Fig. 13 A pre-operative semantically-segmented model representing the CT anatomical phantom for robotic assisted radical prostatectomy

advantage of requiring very few training samples to achieve high-quality results. In our tests, only 15 labeled images were needed to achieve the desired segmentation output, compared to the thousands typically required for models like U-NET [34]. This efficiency was achieved through a dual network configuration, where two neural networks are used together in a complementary way.

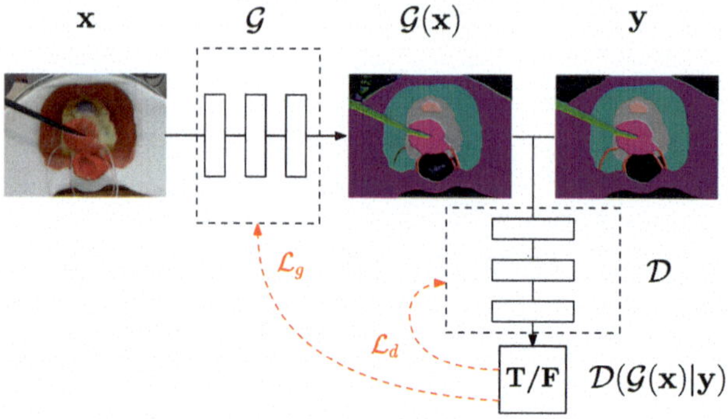

Fig. 14 GAN schematics for network training: the discriminator $\mathcal{D}$ operates as a loss function for both itself and the generator $\mathcal{G}$

The first network, the *Generator* (G), was trained to produce multiple samples of labeled images from the input sample image, typically using a modified U-Net structure. The second network, the *Discriminator* (D), functioned as a loss function to determine whether the generated image resembled the ground truth (Fig. 14 provides a schematic of the network).

The result was a pixel-to-pixel mapping model (hence the name *pix2pix*), where the generator can "fool" the best-trained discriminator, making it capable of segmenting the input image. However, due to the low granularity and pixel-to-pixel nature of the mapping learned by the model, the output required post-processing to remove noise. We applied a median and clustering filter to reduce scattered patches.

Critical structures for the semi-autonomous tasks were color-coded as shown in Table 6. Figure 15 illustrates two examples of scene segmentation acquired from a RealSense® camera and the dVRK endoscope camera perspective (Fig. 15a and c, respectively). The quality of the segmentation is immediately evident, with the dVRK tool clearly discernible, despite a few misidentified spots in the upper-left corner, which are outside the phantom area and easily ignored. Importantly, the bladder is uniformly colored, and the rectum is clearly separated (labeled as "background" since it is irrelevant to prostatectomy operations). The model also identified the *vas deferens* and seminal vesicles acceptably, despite their semi-transparent structure. Additionally, the prostate was correctly identified, as it was not fully covered in fat in this phantom iteration.

The primary drawback of this neural network family was the tendency to generate multiple false positives, influenced by the distinct semantic mappings used during training. This can lead to the false identification of anatomical structures in locations where they typically appeared in the training dataset. For example, the prostate might be identified around the edges of instruments even if it is covered in fat (as seen slightly in Fig. 15d), or the ureters might appear at the bottom of the bladder when not visible. This issue could be easily corrected by adding a single new image to the

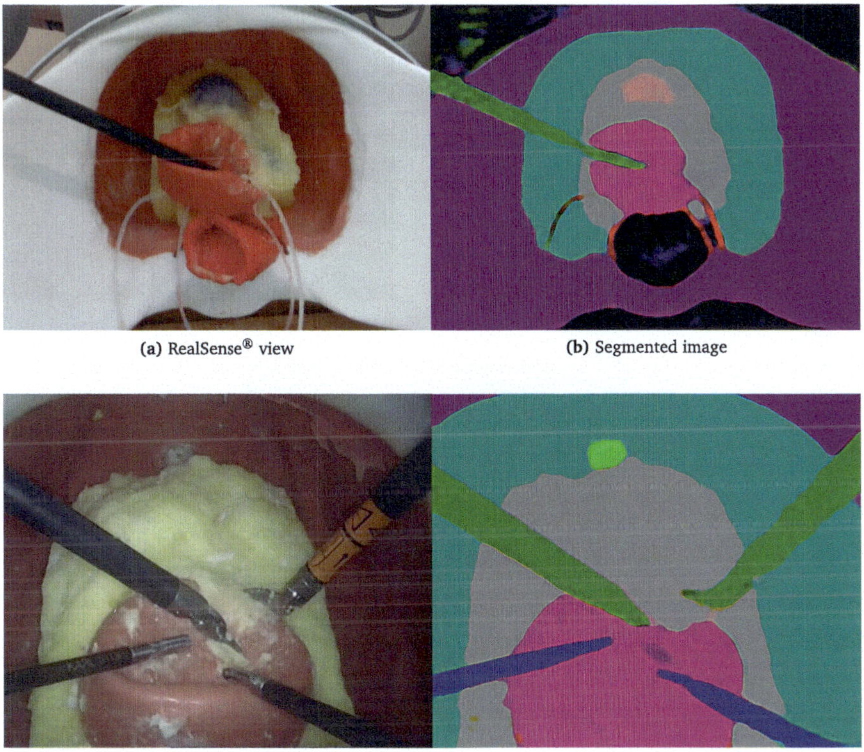

(a) RealSense® view (b) Segmented image

(c) Endoscope view (d) Segmented image

Fig. 15 Examples of real-time semantic segmentation computed over two different cameras: in the first row the RealSense frame and its semantic segmentation; in the second row the Endoscope frame and its semantic segmentation

training dataset and retraining the model, which was quick due to the small dataset size.

4.4 Semantic Monocular SLAM

A fundamental assumption in most current SLAM (Simultaneous Localization and Mapping) approaches is that the environment remains static. However, many real-world scenes, including laparoscopic surgery, involve dynamic objects. In laparoscopic surgery, the most common dynamic objects are the surgical tools and the organ or surface being manipulated. To address this issue, it is essential to identify and exclude these dynamic objects from the static parts of the environment before performing pose estimation.

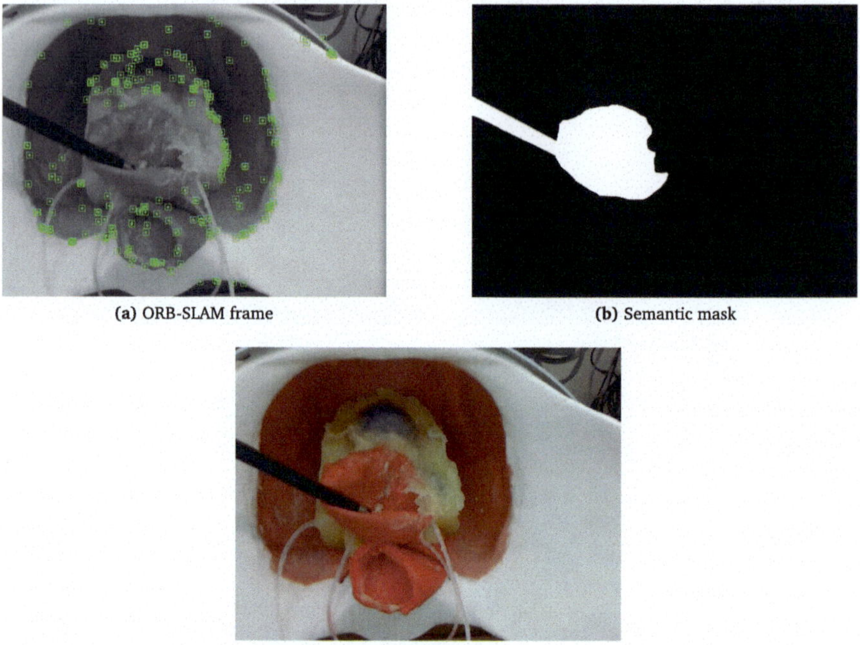

(a) ORB-SLAM frame (b) Semantic mask (c) Original frame

Fig. 16 SLAM process frame acquisition: **a** ORB feature detection after applying the semantic mask; **b** the semantic mask of the bladder and instruments; **c** the original RGB frame

Given the specific surgery being performed, we can predict which organs might move or which surfaces are most deformable. Using semantic segmentation, we can create a mask around these dynamic areas. By assuming that each input frame contains dynamic features, we obtain a mask through binary semantic segmentation. The ORB [38](Oriented FAST and Rotated BRIEF) feature extraction algorithm in the SLAM system can then remove features located within the mask region from the feature sequence, while features in other regions are used for subsequent tracking and mapping. This masking technique prevents feature points from concentrating on dynamic objects, thereby avoiding false extraction and matching.

As illustrated in Fig. 16, the detection of feature points on dynamic objects was effectively excluded using the mask. Figure 16b shows an example of filtering dynamic ORB features by applying semantic segmentation results as masks. In Fig. 16a, the ORB features extracted by the SLAM algorithm excluded the mask, which encompassed the bladder and the surgical instruments. This approach ensured that the SLAM system focused only on static features, improving the accuracy and reliability of pose estimation in dynamic surgical environments.

Compared with the original ORB-SLAM2 algorithm, the feature points on the surface of dynamic objects are eliminated using semantic segmentation, and a higher quality of map construction can be obtained. Figure 17 shows a qualitative reconstruc-

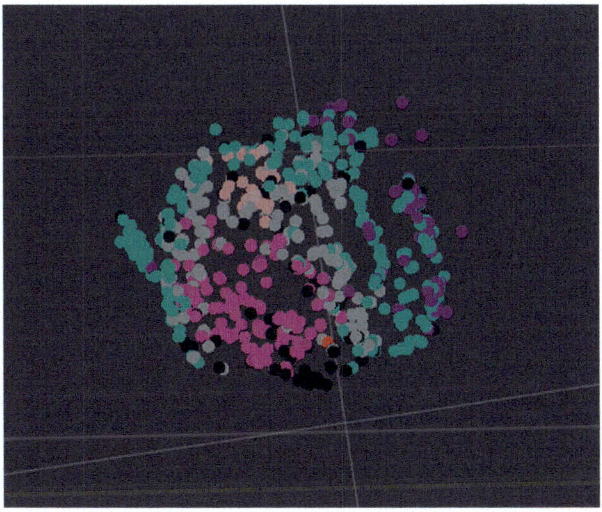

Fig. 17 Sparse point cloud encoded with semantic colors

tion. It shows the sparse point cloud obtained after removing the instruments, with anatomy mapped with semantic colors, following the encoding defined in Table 6.

5 Conclusions

This chapter presented a comprehensive overview of the integration of computer vision and robotics in the context of Autonomous Robotic Surgery (ARS), with a particular focus on enhancing precision and autonomy in Minimally Invasive Surgery (MIS). Starting from the analysis of available imaging sensors and progressing through sensor calibration, 3D reconstruction, and SLAM integration, the chapter outlined a robust framework for enabling surgical robots to navigate complex anatomical environments.

The proposed calibration methodology, specifically developed for the da Vinci Research Kit (dVRK), demonstrated superior accuracy compared to traditional approaches such as Tsai's method. By leveraging a multi step calibration process involving RGB-D cameras, custom calibration tools, and a common reference frame, the system achieved sub-millimeter accuracy in both single and dual-arm robotic manipulation tasks. This level of precision is crucial for maintaining safety and effectiveness in surgical procedures.

Furthermore, the extension of the ORB-SLAM2 algorithm to support semantic segmentation enabled the differentiation of static and dynamic features in surgical scenes. This advancement addresses the inherent challenges of soft-tissue deformation, limited texture, and visual artifacts such as smoke and blood. By incorporating semantic information from pre-operative CT scans and real-time endoscopic images, the system achieved reliable 3D reconstructions necessary for accurate tool tracking and augmented reality visualization.

In summary, this work lays the groundwork for achieving higher degrees of autonomy in robotic surgery by seamlessly integrating vision, calibration, and intelligent mapping techniques. Future developments may focus on real-time implementation within clinical settings, expanding anatomical models for broader surgical applications, and refining segmentation accuracy through continual learning with minimal data.

References

1. Fetić, A., Jurić, D., Osmanković, D.: The procedure of a camera calibration using camera calibration toolbox for MATLAB. In: 2012 Proceedings of the 35th International Convention MIPRO, IEEE, pp. 1752–1757 (2012)
2. Bradski, G., Kaehler, A., et al.: Opencv. Dr. Dobb's J Softw Tools **3**(2) (2000)
3. Jones, G.R., Lee, D., Holliman, N.S., Ezra, D.: Controlling perceived depth in stereoscopic images. In: Stereoscopic Displays and Virtual Reality Systems VIII, vol. 4297, pp. 42–53. SPIE (2001)
4. Kytö, M., Nuutinen, M., Oittinen, P.: Method for measuring stereo camera depth accuracy based on stereoscopic vision. In: Three-Dimensional Imaging, Interaction, and Measurement, vol. 7864, pp. 168–176. SPIE (2011)
5. Zollhöfer, M., Stotko, P., Görlitz, A., Theobalt, C., Nießner, M., Klein, R., Kolb, A.: State of the art on 3D reconstruction with RGB-D cameras. In: Computer Graphics Forum, vol. 37, pp. 625–652. Wiley Online Library (2018)
6. De Groen, P.C.: History of the endoscope [scanning our past]. Proc. IEEE **105**(10), 1987–1995 (2017)
7. Baillie, J.: The endoscope. Gastrointest. Endosc. **65**(6), 886–893 (2007)
8. Palep, J.H.: Robotic assisted minimally invasive surgery. J. Minimal Access Surg. **5**(1), 1 (2009)
9. Yang, G.Z., Cambias, J., Cleary, K., Daimler, E., Drake, J., Dupont, P.E., Hata, N., Kazanzides, P., Martel, S., Patel, R.V., et al.: Medical robotics—regulatory, ethical, and legal considerations for increasing levels of autonomy. Sci. Robot. **2**(4), 8638 (2017)
10. De Rossi, G., Minelli, M., Roin, S., Falezza, F., Sozzi, A., Ferraguti, F., Setti, F., Bonfè, M., Secchi, C. and Muradore, R.: A first evaluation of a multi-modal learning system to control surgical assistant robots via action segmentation. IEEE Trans. Med. Robot. Bionics 1–11 (2021)
11. Fiorini, P., Dall'Alba, D., Ginesi, M., Maris, B., Meli, D., Nakawala, H., Roberti, A.: Challenges of autonomous robotic surgery. In: Hamlyn Symposium on Medical Robotics (HSMR) (2019)
12. De Rossi, G., Minelli, M., Sozzi, A., Piccinelli, N., Ferraguti, F., Setti, F., Bonfè, M., Secchi, C., Muradore, R.: Cognitive robotic architecture for semi-autonomous execution of manipulation tasks in a surgical environment. In: IEEE/RSJ International Conference on Intelligent Robots and Systems (IROS) (2019)
13. Oleari, E., Leporini, A., Trojaniello, D., Sanna, A., Capitanio, U., Dehó, F., Larcher, A., Montorsi, F., Salonia, A., Setti, F. and Muradore, R.: Enhancing surgical process modeling for artificial intelligence development in robotics: the saras case study for minimally invasive procedures. In: International Symposium on Medical Information and Communication Technology (ISMICT) (2019)
14. Muradore, R., Fiorini, P., Akgun, G., Barkana, D.E., Bonfe, M., Boriero, F., Caprara, A., Rossi, G.D., Dodi, R., Elle, O.J., Ferraguti, F., Gasperotti, L., Gassert, R., Mathiassen, K., Handini, D., Lambercy, O., Li, L., Kruusmaa, M., Manurung, A.O., Meruzzi, G., Nguyen,

H.Q.P., Preda, N., Riolfo, G., Ristolainen, A., Sanna, A., Secchi, C., Torsello, M., Yantac, A.E.: Development of a cognitive robotic system for simple surgical tasks. Int. J. Adv. Rob. Syst. **12**(4), 37 (2015)
15. Adebar, T.K., Fletcher, A.E., Okamura, A.M.: 3-d ultrasound-guided robotic needle steering in biological tissue. IEEE Trans. Biomed. Eng. **61**(12), 2899–2910 (2014)
16. Piccinelli, N., Roberti, A., Tagliabue, E., Setti, F., Kronreif, G., Muradore, R., Fiorini, P.: Rigid 3D registration of pre-operative information for semi-autonomous surgery. In: I.S. on Medical Robotics (ed.) 2020 International Symposium on Medical Robotics (2020) - Atlanta (USA) (2020)
17. Shah, M., Eastman, R.D., Hong, T.: An overview of robot-sensor calibration methods for evaluation of perception systems. In: Proceedings of the Workshop on Performance Metrics for Intelligent Systems, pp. 15–20 (2012)
18. Tsai, R.Y., Lenz, R.K., et al.: A new technique for fully autonomous and efficient 3D robotics hand/eye calibration. IEEE Trans. Robot. Autom. **5**(3), 345–358 (1989)
19. Shiu, Y.C., Ahmad, S.: Calibration of wrist-mounted robotic sensors by solving homogeneous transform equations of the form ax = xb. IEEE Trans. Robot. Autom. **5**(1), 16–29 (1989)
20. Chou, J.C., Kamel, M.: Finding the position and orientation of a sensor on a robot manipulator using quaternions. Int. J. Robot. Res. **10**(3), 240–254 (1991)
21. Li, M., Betsis, D.: Head-eye calibration. In: Proceedings of IEEE International Conference on Computer Vision, pp. 40–45. IEEE (1995)
22. Fuchs, S.: Calibration and multipath mitigation for increased accuracy of time-of-flight camera measurements in robotic applications. Ph.D. thesis, Universitätsbibliothek der Technischen Universität Berlin (2012)
23. Gander, W., Hrebicek, J.: Solving Problems in Scientific Computing Using Maple and Matlab®. Springer Science & Business Media (2011)
24. Haidegger, T., Kazanzides, P., Rudas, I., Benyó, B., Benyó, Z.: The importance of accuracy measurement standards for computer-integrated interventional systems . In: EURON GEM Sig Workshop on The Role of Experiments in Robotics Research at IEEE ICRA, pp. 1–6 (2010)
25. Kwartowitz, D.M., Herrell, S.D., Galloway, R.L.: Toward image-guided robotic surgery: determining intrinsic accuracy of the da Vinci robot. Int. J. Comput. Assist. Radiol. Surg. **1**(3), 157–165 (2006)
26. Buelthoff, H.H.: Shape from x: psychophysics and computation (1991)
27. Aulinas, J., Petillot, Y.R., Salvi, J., Lladó, X.: The slam problem: a survey. CCIA **184**(1), 363–371 (2008)
28. May, S., Dröschel, D., Fuchs, S., Holz, D., Nüchter, A.: Robust 3D-mapping with time-of-flight cameras. In: 2009 IEEE/RSJ International Conference on Intelligent Robots and Systems, pp. 1673–1678. IEEE (2009)
29. Bescos, B., Fácil, J.M., Civera, J., Neira, J.: Dynaslam: tracking, mapping, and inpainting in dynamic scenes. IEEE Robot. Autom. Lett. **3**(4), 4076–4083 (2018)
30. Hartley, R., Zisserman, A.: Multiple View Geometry in Computer Vision. Cambridge University Press (2003)
31. Madani, A., Namazi, B., Altieri, M.S., Hashimoto, D.A., Rivera, A.M., Pucher, P.H., Navarrete-Welton, A., Sankaranarayanan, G., Brunt, L.M., Okrainec, A., et al.: Artificial intelligence for intraoperative guidance: using semantic segmentation to identify surgical anatomy during laparoscopic cholecystectomy. Ann. Surg. **276**(2), 363–369 (2022)
32. Liu, H., Zhang, B., Xiang, Y., Hu, Y., Shen, A., Lin, Y.: Adversarial neural networks in medical imaging advancements and challenges in semantic segmentation (2024). arXiv:2410.13099
33. Long, J., Shelhamer, E., Darrell, T.: Fully convolutional networks for semantic segmentation. In: Proceedings of the IEEE Conference on Computer Vision and Pattern Recognition, pp. 3431–3440 (2015)
34. Ronneberger, O., Fischer, P., Brox, T.: U-net: convolutional networks for biomedical image segmentation. In: International Conference on Medical image computing and computer-assisted intervention, pp. 234–241. Springer, Berlin (2015)

35. Milletari, F., Navab, N., Ahmadi, S.-A.: V-net: fully convolutional neural networks for volumetric medical image segmentation. In: 2016 Fourth International Conference on 3D Vision (3DV), pp. 565–571. IEEE (2016)
36. Pieper, S., Halle, M., Kikinis, R.: 3D slicer. In: 2004 2nd IEEE International Symposium on Biomedical Imaging: Nano to Macro (IEEE Cat No. 04EX821), pp. 632–635. IEEE (2004)
37. Isola, P., Zhu, J.-Y., Zhou, T., Efros, A.A.: Image-to-image translation with conditional adversarial networks. In: 2017 IEEE Conference on Computer Vision and Pattern Recognition (CVPR) (2017)
38. Bansal, M., Kumar, M., Kumar, M.: 2D object recognition: a comparative analysis of sift, surf and orb feature descriptors. Multimed. Tools Appl. **80**(12), 18839–18857 (2021)

The Cognitive Architecture

Eleonora Tagliabue and Marco Bombieri

Abstract In this chapter we present the DEFRAS architecture that was used in some of the ARS experiments, based on the integration of task simulation and execution. While in the previous chapters, simulation was used to verify the correctness of a plan or to generate data for machine learning, in Sect. 2 simulation is used as a nominal trace of the task execution to verify that the assumptions about the anatomy and the environment are correct. However, this approach highlighted that textbook knowledge and logical planning are not sufficient to deal with the uncertain and unpredictable anatomical environments. Surgeons in fact rely on their experience to interpret the textbook indications and to adapt them to the specific situations. In Sect. 3 we analyze what it would take to add common sense reasoning to an autonomous surgical robot.

One of the limiting factors for extensive development of autonomous robotic systems is the lack of an established theoretical framework that provides the required features to handle the different aspects and situations that an autonomous system has to face. This is due to the fact that identifying and implementing the required properties for autonomy is extremely challenging, especially when dealing with safety-critical scenarios as surgery, where errors can be deadly. In addition to being a high-risk scenario, surgery is characterized by a particularly complex environment consisting of deformable tissues, whose mechanical properties are only partially known in the pre-operative phase and challenging to measure and model [1]. The diversity and uncertainty of the environments that an ARSS has to face makes it impossible to foresee all possible courses of actions at design stage. For this reason, existing attempts to autonomous execution of surgical tasks have been demonstrated only

E. Tagliabue (✉)
Department of Computer Science, University of Verona, Verona, Italy
e-mail: eleonora.tagliabue@zeiss.com

Carl Zeiss AG, Oberkochen, Germany

M. Bombieri
Department of Computer Science, University of Verona, Verona, Italy

Department of Information Engineering and Computer Science, University of Trento, Trento, Italy

P. Fiorini (ed.), *Towards Autonomous Robotic Surgery*, Springer Tracts in Advanced Robotics 161, https://doi.org/10.1007/978-3-032-04247-7_8

on structured and controlled environments [2], making them still quite far from the applicability to real clinical scenarios.

To make a step forward towards autonomy in real surgical environments, in this chapter we present a framework for autonomous robotic surgery that integrates the main properties that an ARSS should have. To cope with real anatomical environments, we have identified the following specific skills that an ARSS shall integrate:

- it should have *deliberative* capabilities [3], i.e. the capability of *monitoring* the environment through *sensors* while *acting*, in order to *reason* and *plan* a new strategy when the expected behavior does not match reality. Moreover, it must be able to adapt its prior model by *learning* from observations, to cope with the uncertainty of the environment and minimize critical events;
- it should be *informed* from pre-operative anatomical data and expert knowledge about task description and operative constraints, in order to devise a patient-specific strategy for the intervention;
- it should provide *interpretable* plans, which can be easily understood by a supervising surgeon, to guarantee more reliability of the ARSS [1, 4, 5], as required from level 2 of autonomy [6].

In this chapter, we introduce the DEliberative Framework for Robot-Assisted Surgery (DEFRAS) that integrates all the identified skills necessary to cope with uncertain anatomical environments. The framework has a modular structure, thus offering the opportunity to implement each deliberative function individually, specializing each module at algorithmic level depending on the desired task. In this Chapter, we introduce DEFRAS modules and functionalities in general terms, and reason on the need of commonsense for autonomous surgery. A technical description and example of the usage of DEFRAS on a real surgical task will be presented in Chap. 9.

1 Dealing with Uncertainty in Autonomous Robotic Surgery

Before providing the details of the proposed framework, in this section we review recent frameworks for surgical robotic autonomy under uncertainty clarifying our contribution, and we motivate the use of deliberation and logic.

Uncertainty poses challenges to ARSSs relying only on prior models and/or task description [7], and can be related to multiple aspects of a surgical procedure. *Localization uncertainty* includes imprecise localization of the structures of interest or the instruments, due to limitations of available sensors, kinematic models or situation awareness algorithms, and can be addressed with improved mechanics [8] or sensors [9]. *Environmental uncertainty* encompasses the partial knowledge of the anatomical behavior and its unpredictability, which can be tackled with strategies for online model update [10–12]. *Procedural uncertainty* involves understanding of the current and next state in the surgical workflow, which can be improved through filtering of the predictions of the next action [13]. These approaches aim at reducing uncertainty, rather than integrating it in the planning process, so criticisms in real executions might still arise. Some works have tried to deal with uncertainty directly at tool motion planning level, exploiting model predictive control [13, 14]. However, also task-level uncertainty (e.g., wrong plans rising from poor awareness) shall be taken into account. To this aim, full motion parameters can be learnt, either with hidden Markov models [15] or with supervised refinement of finite state machines [16]. However, estimation of task-level parameters with offline learning methods fails to generalize to possible unexperienced situations.

While existing works have attempted either to reduce uncertainty at sensing level or to deal with it at motion/task level, in this chapter we address both aspects by introducing deliberative functions of autonomous agents, as described in [3]. In particular, we integrate specific modules for uncertainty *monitoring* and pre-operative model refinement through online *learning* within a framework for robot-assisted surgery that guarantees interpretability at task level with logic programming and supports online re-planning. Several paradigms for deliberation have been proposed in the field of artificial intelligence, focusing on different aspects of autonomy, e.g. planning (Belief-Desire-Intention model [17], and its implementations [18, 19]) and learning [20]. However, in order to guarantee adaptability to diverse complex tasks, we here focus on the integration and parallel development of different skills for autonomy, which can be improved individually depending on the task of interest. For this reason, our framework builds on the modular architecture and definitions of deliberative functions described in [3], which reports a large number of robotic applications.

In addition to deliberation, an ARSS must provide an interpretable behavior for a human supervisor [4, 5]. Interpretability for autonomous robots can be guaranteed by logic-based reasoning systems [21]. They encode prior concepts and specifications about a robotic domain in a knowledge base, using logic formalism which is easily readable by humans. A logic-based task planner does not encode pre-defined workflows (as finite state machines do); instead, it performs human-like logic inference from knowledge and data from sensors, in order to generate an appropriate workflow for the current situation. Hence, the logic-based approach formally guarantees that specifications encoded in prior knowledge (which may be, e.g., safety constraints in surgery) are satisfied during the execution. In the surgical context, logic formalization has been often implemented with ontologies [22, 23], which are computationally inefficient when knowledge update is needed, as required when operating in unstructured environments [24]. We propose to use non-monotonic logic programming [25], which provides an efficient and interpretable way to describe tasks, permits online revision of incomplete or dynamic information and allows to define safety constraints for planning the execution [26]. All these features are essential in safety-critical scenarios as surgery [27]. Non-monotonic logic programming has been applied in surgery only to automate a standard surgical training task in rigid domain [26].

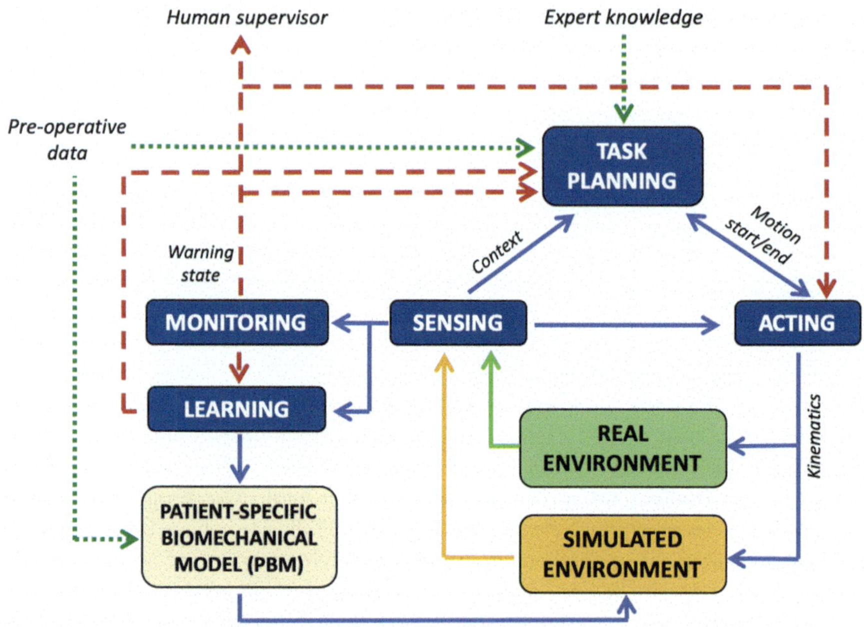

Fig. 1 The architecture of DEFRAS. Deliberative modules are in blue boxes. Green dotted lines represent information exchanged only in the pre-operative phase. Red dashed lines trigger actions only when monitoring threshold/s is exceeded

2 DEFRAS: DEliberative Framework for Robot Assisted Surgery

In this section, we present the modules of our DEliberative Framework for Robot Assisted Surgery (DEFRAS). The framework has been made publicly available at https://gitlab.com/altairLab/tissue_retraction.git (Fig. 1).

Task Planning

A task planning module computes the task plan, i.e. the sequence of actions to solve the task. Actions are elementary operations which correspond to a single motion trajectory or joint-level command, according to the granularity definitions described in [28]. The plan is computed based on available expert procedural knowledge, conveniently expressed in the declarative logic programming formalism of Answer Set Programming (ASP) [29], a non-monotonic logic paradigm which is more computationally efficient and expressive if compared to its main competitor Prolog [30].

An ASP program represents the domain of the task with a *description* $\mathscr{D}$ and a *history* $\mathscr{H}$. $\mathscr{D}$ comprises the alphabet of the task $\mathscr{A}$, defining relevant attributes of the domain, and axioms. Attributes may be *statics*, i.e., domain attributes whose values do not change over time; *fluents*, i.e., domain attributes whose values can be changed; and *actions*. Attributes may be *terms*; *atoms*, i.e. predicates of terms (e.g. $\mathtt{Atom}(\mathtt{T}_1, \ldots, \mathtt{T}_n)$ is an atom with terms $\mathtt{T}_{1,\ldots,n}$ as arguments); and their logical negations. Values of terms are *constants* (either integers or strings). A term whose value is assigned is *ground*, and an atom is ground if its terms are ground. Axioms are logical relations between attributes. Causal rules $\mathtt{A}_h$: $-\mathtt{A}_{b1}, \ldots, \mathtt{A}_{bn}$ define pre-conditions $\mathtt{A}_{b1,\ \ldots,\ bn}$ (*body* of the rule) for grounding the *head* $\mathtt{A}_h$. Logical implications are implemented to define pre-conditions and effects of actions, and constraints (e.g., infeasibility of some actions).

Given the ASP program, an ASP solver returns both the plan and the set of anatomical features which generated it, thus ensuring task-level interpretability of the ARSS.

Sensing

Throughout task execution, the sensing module analyses the state of the robot and the environment, to provide high-level environmental features for task planning. It also communicates target position for each action to the acting module, for motion planning. Moreover, it recognizes whether critical conditions occur, in which cases it triggers task re-planning or motion interruption to prevent risks.

Acting

The acting module controls the execution of each action in the plan at low level. Different motion planning algorithms can be used, depending on the application. The appropriate motion law for each action can be selected from a pre-defined set, as obtained with analytical approaches such as roadmaps, potential fields or cell decomposition [31]. These methods work well when complete representation of the environment is available, as can be extracted, for example, from pre-operative data. However, complex surgical tasks, like tissue suturing or cutting, require enhanced dexterity and bi-manual coordination which might be impossible to encode within hand-crafted control policies. In this cases, trajectories may be generated by imitating expert human demonstrations [16, 32, 33]. Alternative approaches to motion planning can also be integrated, such as those relying on reinforcement learning, which has shown promise to solve challenging robotic planning tasks by trial-and-error, especially when combined with deep neural networks [34], or emerging approaches based on neural planning, e.g. [35].

Monitoring

The monitoring module continuously estimates if the system internal model of the environment, given by a patient-specific simulation initialized with pre-operative information and running in parallel, is coherently representing the actual scenario. To this aim, a metric assessing the level of discrepancy between the real and the simulated environments is computed starting from sensing information. This metric represents the current level of uncertainty that the system has about the environment. Depending on this metric, different warning states are raised, associated with specific strategies at task-motion level which aim at increasing the reliability of the autonomous operation and accommodate safety.

Learning

If the system is in a warning state, the learning module is in charge of updating the ARSS internal model of the environment starting from real observations. Being the system model represented by the simulated PBM, the learning module implements strategies to update PBM parameters from real data, to compensate for environmental uncertainty caused by imprecise parametrization.

Simulated Environment

A Patient-specific Biomechanical Model (PBM) of the anatomical environment is created starting from patient-specific geometry and mechanical properties extracted from pre-operative data, as described in Chap. 6. Such model initializes a simulated environment which is exploited to design a patient-specific task plan accounting for all the information available in the pre-operative phase. Furthermore, the simulation is run in parallel to the real execution in the intra-operative phase and it is continuously updated based on the current robot configuration received from the acting module. At each time step, the simulation represents what the system expects from its interaction with the environment based on the available knowledge, hence it allows to monitor the real world execution (Fig. 1). Moreover, the online simulation can provide complementary information to real sensor data.

Human Supervisor

The context and the plan are continuously monitored by a human supervisor, who can easily interpret the output of the autonomous system thanks to reliance on logic formalism. The presence of the human supervisor is required to guarantee the reliability of the ARSS, following the latest European regulations for high-risk autonomous systems [5].

3 The Need of Commonsense in Next Generation ARSS

While executing a surgical procedure, surgeons do not only rely on their specific medical knowledge, but also on a set of skills that are "obvious" to them and allow to intuitively evaluate and react to the intervention evolution. Such skills belong to what is usually called commonsense, which is essential to carry out an intervention. While general commonsense refers to all the basic concepts about the world and belongs to all human beings, we believe that field-specific commonsense is developed depending on individual experiences within a field of expertise. In surgery, field-specific commonsense is the "glue" knowledge that is not explicitly described in surgical manuals, but it is acquired during the long surgical training. Understanding how to describe, represent and learn this knowledge is paramount to develop robust and reliable Autonomous Robotic Surgical Systems (ARSS). Despite being already discussed in other fields [36], to the best of our knowledge the importance and challenges of commonsense in robotic surgery have not been addressed yet.

Commonsense and Surgery

Our research on ARSSs has shown that automatic extraction of surgical procedures from surgical textbooks does not allow to include the large amount of implicit knowledge that humans use during a task [37]. In the following, we refer to the classification of surgical procedures in phases, steps, actions, and motions by Lalys [38] and, based on the above argument, we propose a preliminary classification of surgical knowledge into four levels:

1. *Procedural knowledge* is the description of the sequence of phases required to perform a procedure, as can be learned from surgical manuals. It does provide general information about the specific steps but it does not specify the parameters of each one, i.e., the physical quantities that instantiate individual actions and motions, such as the motion velocity or the force to be applied.
2. *Surgical commonsense* is a field-specific commonsense and encompasses all those skills surgeons acquire while experiencing (assisting and performing) a specific procedure multiple times. It allows to intuitively define the parameters of each step. It also includes the capability to interpret surgical situations and understand correlations, causes and consequences of actions.
3. *Medical commonsense* is another subset of field-specific commonsense, that is not specific to a single surgical procedure and is acquired during medical studies. It includes the knowledge of basic anatomical concepts (e.g., positions and functions of organs), and sequence of elementary actions to perform standard tasks.
4. *General commonsense* is the commonsense that surgeons have as human beings. It represents the basic knowledge of the world, is acquired while experiencing everyday situations, and helps while inferring meaning and behaviour of things.

To clarify this classification, Fig. 2 describes the suturing phase of a partial nephrectomy intervention. The sentence at the top is taken from a surgical textbook and represents the *procedural knowledge* of the intervention [37]. However, it does neither describe how to assess the conditions of a good suture (*surgical commonsense*), nor it lists the individual steps and actions needed to accomplish it (*medical commonsense*), nor it provides the implicit general knowledge about objects involved in the suture, e.g., a needle is needed, and it must be grasped, inserted and extracted (*general commonsense*). Surgical textbooks alone are not sufficient to fully describe an intervention, and an ARSS must acquire the same level of knowledge listed above to perform the surgical task and to properly handle the situations it will face.

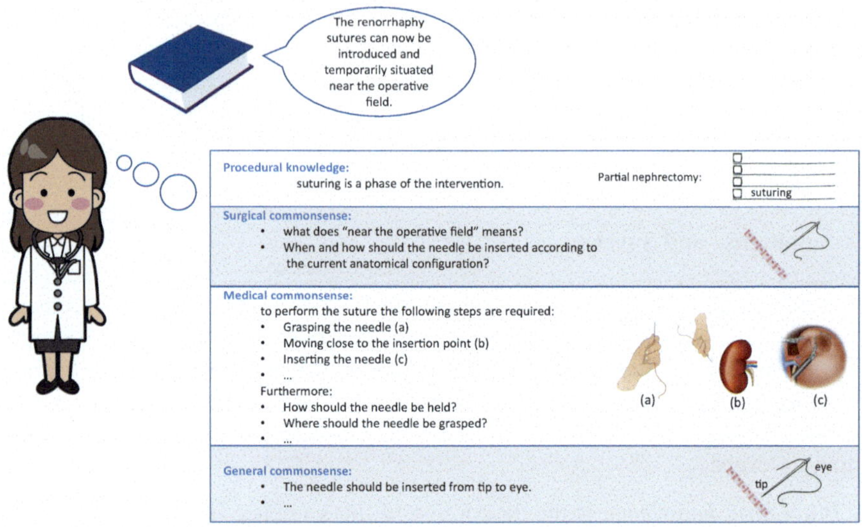

Fig. 2 Procedural knowledge enriched with surgical, medical and general commonsense

Developing ARSS

Depending on its autonomous capabilities, an ARSS can be classified into different levels of autonomy [6]. Different levels of autonomy are obviously associated to different levels of knowledge, and we propose the classification schematized in Fig. 3. In particular, the sophisticated capabilities required to reach high autonomy levels are implicitly connected to the breadth of the required commonsense knowledge.

Current surgical robots are teleoperated systems with some assistive function (level of autonomy 0 and 1), and have no knowledge of the steps to be performed but simply monitor some working variables, such as current levels, maximum speed, and noise suppression. The specific phases and steps of the intervention are determined by the surgeon who directly controls the surgical actions.

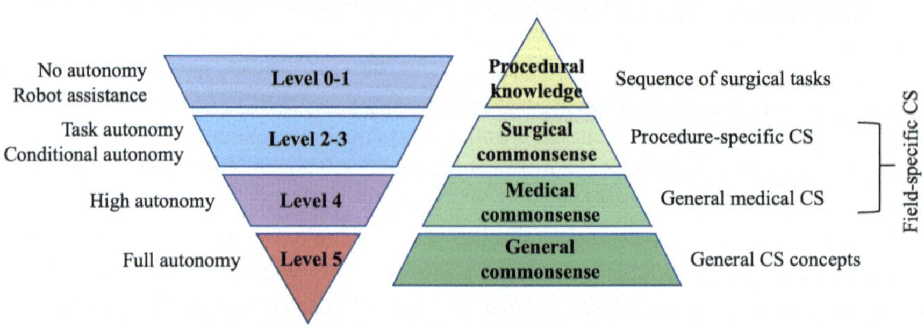

Fig. 3 Mapping between autonomy levels and the required knowledge levels. Higher autonomy requires broader knowledge. "CS" stays for "commonsense"

When a surgical robot is able to execute some individual actions (levels of autonomy 2 and 3, becoming an ARSS), it would require the presence of *surgical commonsense*. In fact, the robot would need to perform some basic reasoning on the patient-specific pathology and anatomy, with the surgeon ready to intervene if needed. Referring to Fig. 2, the robot would have to interpret the "near the operative field", and decide where to insert the needle given the patient anatomy. Some concepts of *medical commonsense* would be needed to give the ARSS more autonomy and connect multiple phases of an intervention. In the example above, the robot would have to know that a suture needs a *surgical* needle, which has to be grasped with a specific orientation for optimal insertion. It has to control motion parameters (force and velocity) during the insertion and it has to know how to close the suture. It is not always easy to identify a sharp division between *surgical commonsense* and *medical commonsense*, since a combination of both is necessary to specialize a well-defined textbook procedure into the real intervention.

To achieve higher autonomy, an ARSS must be able to make autonomous decisions related to the complete procedure. It will generate, select, execute and monitor a surgical plan, adapt it to different anatomies and react to unexpected situations. Enhanced sensing, situation awareness and reasoning technologies are key to achieve such capabilities [1], together with a broader commonsense to properly assess and react to the situation. While *medical commonsense* would allow to reach high autonomy (level 4), fully autonomous systems (level 5) would need the integration of *general commonsense* because decisions would be required that go outside the medical field, such as lifting and moving objects, turning on and off devices and lights, understanding human emotions.

Conclusion

As long as surgical robots maintain assistive role, they can rely on the commonsense of the operating surgeons. As soon as they become aids or surgical colleagues, they must be able to perform commonsense reasoning on their own, making it crucial to understand how to deal with this kind of knowledge. The map between knowledge bases and autonomy levels proposed in this article aims at making the problem more tractable and encourage researchers to fill the scientific and technological gaps related to commonsense knowledge and reasoning.

References

1. Attanasio, A., Scaglioni, B., De Momi, E., Fiorini, P., Valdastri, P.: Autonomy in surgical robotics. Annu. Rev. Control, Robot., Auton. Syst. **4**, 651–679 (2021)
2. D'Ettorre, C., Mariani, A., Stilli, A., Baena, F.R.Y., Valdastri, P., Deguet, Kazanzides, P., Taylor, R.H., Fischer, G.S., DiMaio, S.P., Menciassi, A., Stoyanov, D.: Accelerating surgical robotics research: a review of 10 years with the da Vinci research kit. IEEE Robot. Autom. Mag. **28**(4), 56–78 (2021)

3. Ingrand, F., Ghallab, M.: Deliberation for autonomous robots: a survey. Artif. Intell. **247**, 10–44 (2017)
4. Fiazza, M.-C., Fiorini, P.: Design for interpretability: Meeting the certification challenge for surgical robots. In: 2021 IEEE International Conference on Intelligence and Safety for Robotics, pp. 264–267. IEEE (2021)
5. Regulation of the European parliament and of the council laying down Harmonised rules on artificial intelligence (artificial intelligence act) and amending certain union legislative acts. https://eur-lex.europa.eu/resource.html?uri=cellar:e0649735-a372-11eb-9585-01aa75ed71a1.0001.02/DOC_1&format=PDF, note = Accessed: 11 Aug 2024
6. Yang, G.-Z., Cambias, J., Cleary, K., Daimler, E., Drake, J., Dupont, P.E., Hata, N., Kazanzides, P., Martel, S., Patel, R.V., et al.: Medical robotics—regulatory, ethical, and legal considerations for increasing levels of autonomy. Sci. Robot. **2**(4), 8638 (2017)
7. Nagy, T.D., Haidegger, T.: A DVRK-based framework for surgical subtask automation. In: Acta Polytechnica Hungarica, pp. 61–78 (2019)
8. Sen, S., et al.: Automating multi-throw multilateral surgical suturing with a mechanical needle guide and sequential convex optimization. In: 2016 IEEE International Conference Robotics and Automation (ICRA), pp. 4178–4185. IEEE (2016)
9. Shademan, A., Decker, R.S., Opfermann, J.D., Leonard, S., Krieger, A., Kim, P.C.: Supervised autonomous robotic soft tissue surgery. Sci. Transl. Med. **8**(337) (2016)
10. Wu, J.Y., Kazanzides, P., Unberath, M.: Leveraging vision and kinematics data to improve realism of biomechanic soft tissue simulation for robotic surgery. Int. J Comput. Assist. Radiol. Surg. **15**(5), 811–818 (2020)
11. Liu, F., et al.: Real-to-sim registration of deformable soft tissue with position-based dynamics for surgical robot autonomy. In: The 2021 IEEE International Conference on Robotics and Automation (ICRA), pp. 12328–12334. IEEE (2021)
12. Alambeigi, F., Wang, Z., Hegeman, R., Liu, Y.-H., Armand, M.: A robust data-driven approach for online learning and manipulation of unmodeled 3D heterogeneous compliant objects. IEEE Robot. Autom. Lett. **3**(4), 4140–4147 (2018)
13. De Rossi, G., et al.: Cognitive robotic architecture for semi-autonomous execution of manipulation tasks in a surgical environment. In: 2019 IEEE/RSJ International Conference on Intelligent Robots and Systems (IROS), pp. 7827–7833. IEEE (2019)
14. Kehoe, B., et al.: Autonomous multilateral debridement with the raven surgical robot. In: 2014 IEEE International Conference Robotics and Automation (ICRA), pp. 1432–1439. IEEE (2014)
15. Berthet-Rayne, P., et al.: Hubot: a three state human-robot collaborative framework for bimanual surgical tasks based on learned models. In: 2016 IEEE International Conference Robotics and Automation (ICRA), pp. 715–722 (2016)
16. Murali, A., Sen, S., Kehoe, B., Garg, A., McFarland, S., Patil, S., Boyd, W.D., Lim, S., Abbeel, P., Goldberg, K.: Learning by observation for surgical subtasks: multilateral cutting of 3D viscoelastic and 2D orthotropic tissue phantoms. In: 2015 IEEE International Conference on Robotics and Automation (ICRA), pp. 1202–1209. IEEE (2015)
17. Bratman, M.: Intention, Plans, and Practical Reason. Harvard University Press, Cambridge, MA (1987)
18. Georgeff, M.P., Lansky, A.L.: Reactive reasoning and planning. In: AAAI, vol. 87, pp. 677–682 (1987)
19. Bratman, M.E., et al.: Plans and resource-bounded practical reasoning. Comput. Intell. **4**(3), 349–355 (1988)
20. Bolisani, E., Bratianu, C.: Knowledge strategy planning: an integrated approach to manage uncertainty, turbulence, and dynamics. J. Knowl. Manag. (2017)
21. Tenorth, M., Beetz, M.: KnowRob - a knowledge processing infrastructure for cognition-enabled robots. Int. J. Robot. Res. (IJRR) **32**(5), 566–590 (2013)
22. Nakawala, H., Bianchi, R., Pescatori, L.E., De Cobelli, O., Ferrigno, G., De Momi, E.: "Deep-onto" network for surgical workflow and context recognition. Int. J. Comput. Assist. Radiol. Surg. **14**(4), 685–696 (2019)

23. Katić, D., Wekerle, A.-L., Gärtner, F., Kenngott, H., Müller-Stich, B.P., Dillmann, R., Speidel, S.: Ontology-based prediction of surgical events in laparoscopic surgery. In: Medical Imaging 2013: Image-Guided Procedures, Robotic Interventions, and Modeling, vol. 8671, p. 86711A. International Society for Optics and Photonics (2013)
24. Ginesi, M., Meli, D., Nakawala, H.C., Roberti, A., Fiorini, P.: A knowledge-based framework for task automation in surgery. In: 2019 19th International Conference on Advanced Robotics, pp. 37–42 (2019)
25. Dimopoulos, Y., Nebel, B., Koehler, J.: Encoding planning problems in nonmonotonic logic programs. In: European Conference on Planning, pp. 169–181. Springer, Berlin (1997)
26. Ginesi, M., Meli, D., Roberti, A., Sansonetto, N., Fiorini, P.: Autonomous task planning and situation awareness in robotic surgery. In: IEEE/RSJ International Conference on Intelligent Robots and Systems, pp. 3144–3150. IEEE (2020)
27. Muradore, R., Fiorini, P., Akgun, G., Barkana, D.E., Bonfe, M., Boriero, F., Caprara, A., Rossi, G.D., Dodi, R., Elle, O.J., Ferraguti, F., Gasperotti, L., Gassert, R., Mathiassen, K., Handini, D., Lambercy, O., Li, L., Kruusmaa, M., Manurung, A.O., Meruzzi, G., Nguyen, H.Q.P., Preda, N., Riolfo, G., Ristolainen, A., Sanna, A., Secchi, C., Torsello, M., Yantac, A.E.: Development of a cognitive robotic system for simple surgical tasks. Int. J. Adv. Rob. Syst. **12**(4), 37 (2015)
28. Lalys, F., Jannin, P.: Surgical process modeling: a review. Int. J. CARS **9**(3), 495–511 (2014)
29. Lifschitz, V.: Answer set programming and plan generation. Artif. Intell. **138**(1–2), 39–54 (2002)
30. Colmerauer, A.: An introduction to prolog iii. In: Computational Logic, pp. 37–79. Springer, Berlin (1990)
31. Latombe, J.-C.: Robot motion planning, vol. 124. Springer Science & Business Media (2012)
32. Su, H., Mariani, A., Ovur, S.E., Menciassi, A., Ferrigno, G., De Momi, E.: Toward teaching by demonstration for robot-assisted minimally invasive surgery. IEEE Trans. Autom. Sci. Eng. (2021)
33. Ginesi, M., Meli, D., Roberti, A., Sansonetto, N., Fiorini, P.: Autonomous task planning and situation awareness in robotic surgery. In: International Conference on Intelligent Robots and Systems (IROS), pp. 3144–3150. IEEE (2020)
34. Kober, J., Bagnell, J.A., Peters, J.: Reinforcement learning in robotics: a survey. Int. J. Robot. Res. **32**(11), 1238–1274 (2013)
35. Qureshi, A.H., Miao, Y., Simeonov, A., Yip, M.C.: Motion planning networks: bridging the gap between learning-based and classical motion planners. IEEE Trans. Rob. **37**(1), 48–66 (2020)
36. Davis, E., Marcus, G.: Commonsense reasoning and commonsense knowledge in artificial intelligence. Commun. ACM **58**(9), 92–103 (2015)
37. Bombieri, M., Rospocher, M., Dall'Alba, D., Fiorini, P.: Automatic detection of procedural knowledge in robotic-assisted surgical texts. Int. J. Comput. Assist. Radiol. Surg. **16**(8), 1287–1295 (2021)
38. Lalys, F., Jannin, P.: Surgical process modelling: a review. Int. J. Comput. Assist. Radiol. Surg. **9**(3), 495–511 (2014)

Autonomous Tissue Retraction with DEFRAS

Eleonora Tagliabue

Abstract In this Chapter, we describe the Tissue Retraction (TR) task, which has been selected as representative task to validate DEFRAS (Chapter 9), and we detail its implementation within our framework. The TR task allows to assess the ability of the framework to deal with uncertainty, since it involves interaction with the soft anatomical tissues, whose mechanical properties are generally only approximately known before the intervention. While an initial Patient-specific Biomechanical Model (PBM) can be generated from each patient pre-operative images and data, it may not accurately describe the actual behavior of the tissue, thus requiring intra-operative update. Section 1 describes the implementation of the tissue retraction task, and Sect. 2 presents the simulation and experimental setup that were used. Section 3 discusses the results of the simulations of TR and Sect. 4 presents the experimental validation on the laboratory experimental setup. Section 5 concludes this Chapter.

Previous works for autonomous TR have proposed either to generate the plan by optimizing some metrics [1–5] or to learn the task from human demonstrations [6–8]. However, none of them integrates methods to reason on the current environment and deal with unexpected situations which might occur in real surgery. In this Chapter, we demonstrate how TR can be implemented relying on a deliberative architecture [9, 10].

1 Implementation of Tissue Retraction in DEFRAS

Tissue retraction is a very common surgical task which consists in grasping and retracting soft tissues (e.g., adipose tissue) to expose a hidden Region Of Interest (ROI) (e.g., a tumor) to an intra-operative camera. The tissue is usually attached to surrounding anatomics in correspondence of Attachment Points (APs). In general,

E. Tagliabue (✉)
Department of Computer Science, University of Verona, Verona, Italy
e-mail: eleonora.tagliabue@zeiss.com

Carl Zeiss AG, Oberkochen, Germany

P. Fiorini (ed.), *Towards Autonomous Robotic Surgery*, Springer Tracts in Advanced Robotics 161, https://doi.org/10.1007/978-3-032-04247-7_9

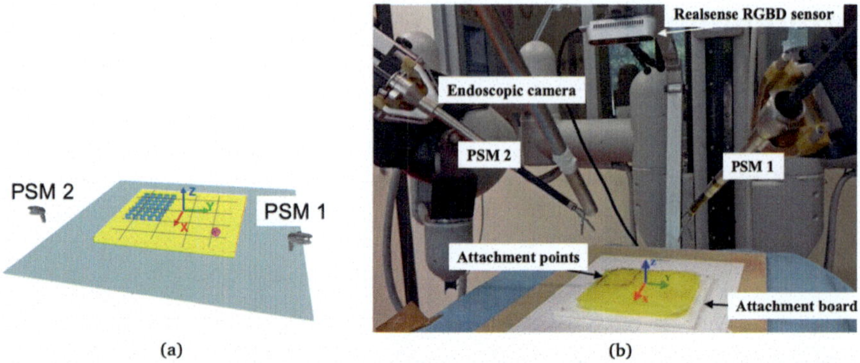

Fig. 1 Experimental setup for autonomous tissue retraction with DEFRAS. The simulated and real scene are calibrated with respect to a common reference frame at the tissue center. **a** Simulated setup. The magenta sphere represents the ROI, while blue dots are the attachment points. Gray lines delineate the discretization for selection of grasping points. **b** Real setup. The attachment board allows to define tissue attachment points. A Realsense RGBD sensor captures the point cloud of the tissue throughout the task

ROI exposure during TR is obtained primarily by pulling up the tissue after grasping. However, this action is not always successful due to kinematic limitations imposed by the anatomical environment and the insertion points of the instruments in the body, which define fixed pivots for the robotic arms. Furthermore, pulling may induce high forces which can damage the tissue. In these cases, alternative actions can be performed, such as moving the tissue in a parallel plane to the tissue surface, either folding it away from the intra-operative camera or possibly towards the ROI.

We create a PBM leveraging on tissue geometric and mechanical properties as well as locations of the ROI and APs obtained from pre-operative data (Fig. 1). Such model is used to initialize a simulation which is exploited to find a patient-specific task plan in the pre-operative phase (see Sect. 1.1 for details). For computational convenience, we subdivide the tissue in small regions, and consider only centers of these regions as possible grasping points. The pre-operative plan is then executed in the real environment with one of the Patient-Side Manipulators (PSMs) of the dVRK.

During execution, the biomechanical simulation is run in parallel, and the state of the real environment is continuously monitored with intra-operative sensors (Fig. 1). When mismatch is identified, the pre-operative plan may become sub-optimal or even infeasible, hence specific strategies to improve the plan shall be implemented and some simulation parameters may be updated. In particular, here we focus on the update of APs. Although the position of APs can be initialized based on anatomical knowledge or statistical information [11, 12], precise definition of APs in surgery can only be obtained interacting with the tissue, as we demonstrated in [9, 13]. The reason why we focus on APs is twofold. First of all, they constitute model boundary conditions, thus represent an important parameter influencing simulation accuracy.

Second, knowledge of APs location is very important in TR to prevent the pulling of highly constrained areas, minimizing the risk of tissue damage.

In addition, the simulation also continuously provides an estimate of the applied force on the tissue, compensating for the lack of force feedback in surgical robotic systems.

1.1 Task Planning

The task planning module computes the best sequence of actions to solve the task, and it encodes task knowledge in the formalism of ASP [14]. Definitions of actions and relevant environmental features are encoded following the generic explanation of Sect. 1. Statics are `block` (from now on `B`), representing a generic region on the tissue with centroid `B`$_C$; and `arm` (from now on `A`), representing the robotic arm (either `psm1` or `psm2`).

Possible actions (for each tool) in the considered task are *reaching a grasping point, opening gripper, grasping, pulling, releasing the tissue* and folding the tissue, either *moving planarly towards the ROI* or *moving away from the intra-operative camera*. Actions are expressed as predicates in plain English as *action(tool, object, property)*.

Fluents are relevant environmental conditions for the task. They include *locations of APs and ROI* with respect to grasping points; critical conditions on the *force exerted on the tissue*; kinematic states of the robot, e.g. whether it is *holding tissue* or the *gripper is open*, or condition of *maximum height* reached above the tissue; *reachability*[1] conditions to define which points can be grasped by which robotic arm; *distance* between blocks. All fluents are defined as *external* atoms, so they can be grounded from the sensing module. Table 1 reports actions and fluents used in the TR task, expressed as atoms with the ASP formalism.

Axioms express logical relations between atoms. For the TR task, we consider axioms representing causal laws, executability constraints, choice rules and optimization statements.

Causal laws define effects of actions on fluents (e.g., `A`'s gripper is closed after grasping, `closed_gripper(A, t) :- grasp(A, B`$_C$`, t-1)`).

Executability constraints specify the set of actions and fluents that cannot hold concurrently (e.g., it is not possible to pull the tissue if the force applied to the tissue exceeds constraints, `:- pull(A, B`$_C$`, t), max_height(A, t)`).

Choice rules specify the environmental pre-conditions which must be satisfied to execute actions. For our task, at most one single action can be executed at each time step. Then, we define a choice rule gathering pre-conditions for actions as `0 {action(t) : pre-cond(t)} 1`, which constrains the cardinality of the set of possible actions returned at each time step between 0 and 1.

Optimization statements define preference in the set of possible actions, in particular for grasping point selection in case the pre-operative plan is not successful

[1] With reference to Fig. 1a, a point on the tissue is reachable by a PSM if it lies on the same side as the PSM with respect to the $x - z$ plane in the common reference system.

Table 1 List of actions and fluents implemented for the TR task with the ASP formalism. B_C is a generic grasping point, A is the robotic arm, t is a discrete time step for temporal reasoning

Actions a	**Description**
reach(A, B_C, t)	A reaches grasping point B_C
grasp(A, B_C, t)	A grasps the tissue in B_C
release(A, t)	A opens the gripper
pull(A, B_C, t)	A pulls B_C
move_ROI(A, B_C, t)	A moves towards the ROI while holding B_C
move_away(A, B_C, t)	A moves away from the camera while holding B_C
Fluents *F*	**Description**
fixed(B, t)	B_C is above APs
above_ROI(B, t)	B_C is above ROI
at(A, B, t)	A is above B_C on tissue
max_force(t)	Critical force is overcome
in_hand(A, B, t)	A holds the tissue in B_C
closed_gripper(A, t)	Gripper of A is closed
max_height(A, t)	A has reached the maximum allowed height
visible_ROI(t)	ROI is visible
reachable(A, B, t)	B_C is reachable by A
distance(B1, B2, X, t)	X is the distance between B_1-B_2

and re-planning is needed. In this case, the best grasping point B_C is chosen as the one which has minimal distance from ROI (to ease its exposure) and maximal distance from APs (to reduce tissue damage). Logic-level optimization allows to easily define a commonsense criterion for evaluating candidate grasping points. However, in order to ensure computational tractability of ASP solving, the set of candidate grasping points must be finite. Hence, the tissue surface is discretized as an $N \times N$ grid, centered above the tissue to grasp. Possible grasping points B_C are defined at the centers of the grid cells.

We finally define the goal of the TR task as the constraint that the ROI must be eventually visible within a predefined percentage (`:- visible_ROI(t)`).

Pre-operative Plan

In the pre-operative phase, all the candidate grasping points are tried in simulated environment to find the optimal patient-specific plan. Considering the goals of our task, we select the plan that maximizes ROI exposure while minimizing tissue exerted force and interaction with it, in order to maximize the economy of motion and reduce the possibility of critical events. To achieve this, DEFRAS is launched after deactivating the monitoring and learning modules. We record plans originated picking all possible grasping points, and we select only plans reaching a minimum visibility of 80%. Among these, we select the 3 plans minimizing the tissue solicitation, i.e. the ones with lowest $F_{\max}$, where $F_{\max}$ is the maximum recorded tissue force over the entire execution. Finally, we choose the optimal plan as the one with the lowest number of actions, thus minimizing interaction with tissue and obtaining the maximum economy of motion.

In case re-planning is needed in the intra-operative phase, a new grasping point is then selected according to the ASP optimization criteria described above.

1.2 Sensing

The sensing module continuously receives the state of the robot and the environment. The state of the robot S_R consists of the position of tools $p_{1,2}$ and opening angles of grippers $j_{1,2}$. The state of the environment S_E includes the point cloud of tissue surface PC_t from the real environment; visual information about the ROI from the intra-operative camera I; the position of the ROI p_{ROI}; the set of known APs PC_{AP}; and the set Σ of mechanical forces at each tissue point from the simulated environment. All the kinematic quantities are referred to the same reference frame after camera-robot calibration. The main tasks of the sensing modules are summarized in Algorithm 1.

Algorithm 1 Sensing module

1: **Input**: S_E, S_R, current action `a`
2: **Output**: Set of context fluents F, target position g, motion rate r, replanning request `replan`, motion rate r
3: **while** not `task_ended` **do**
4: F = compute_fluents(S_E, S_R)
5: `replan`, r = check_failure(F)
6: g = compute_target(a)

Throughout task execution, the sensing module computes the environmental features described at the logic planning level as detailed in Algorithm 2[2] and recognizes whether critical conditions occur (e.g., maximum height of PSMs or critical tissue force are reached). In these cases, the motion of PSMs is interrupted, and the current environmental situation is communicated to the planning module to adapt the flow of execution accordingly. In particular, the function *check_failure* verifies if the maximum arm height has been reached, or the maximum tissue force has exceeded a pre-defined threshold ϵ. In the former case, motion is interrupted and re-planning is triggered. In the latter case, DEFRAS first tries to reduce tissue solicitation by decreasing motion velocity [15]. If this does not bring the applied force below ϵ, motion is interrupted and re-planning is triggered.

Another important function of the sensing module is to compute target positions g for actions of PSMs, with the function *compute_target* in Algorithm 1. The target is needed only for reaching the tissue, moving away from camera and moving towards ROI.

[2] Time `t` is omitted in Algorithm 2 because it is assigned at ASP level.

1.3 Acting

The acting module selects the appropriate motion law for each action from a predefined set, similarly to [16]. Some actions (*reaching tissue, moving away from camera* and *moving towards ROI*) are executed after also the target position g is received from the sensing module. Gripper actions are simple joint commands, while *pulling* is a motion of 10 mm along z axis. We consider only linear trajectories, keeping a fixed orientation at the end-effector for the sake of simplicity, as in [17]. This does not represent a limitation for our initial evaluation on a controlled setup. However, more sophisticated motion laws can be employed (Sect. 2). The acting module executes trajectories at the rate r specified by the sensing (Sect. 1.2) and monitoring modules (Sect. 1.4).

Algorithm 2 Compute_fluents

Input: $S_E = \{PC_t, PC_{AP}, p_{ROI}, I, \Sigma\}$, $S_R = \{j_{1,2}, p_{1,2}\}$
Output: Set of context fluents F
Init: $F = \emptyset$, S_B = discretize(PC_t) ▷ *S_B is the set of regions* B *on the tissue*
for B $\in S_B$ **do**
  $j = argmin_{i=\{1,2\}} ||y_i - y_{B_C}||_1$ ▷ *Reachability with respect to $x - z$ plane*
  F.append(`reachable(A`$_j$`, B)`)
  if $\exists p \in PC_{AP}$: $p \in$ B **then** ▷ *B is a fixed block*
    F.append(`fixed(B)`)
  if $p_{ROI} \in$ B **then** ▷ *ROI under block* B
    F.append(`above_ROI(B)`)
  for B$_2 \in S_B$ **do** ▷ *Distance between centroids of blocks*
    F.append(`distance(B, B`$_2$`, X)`)
if compute_visibility(I) > 80% **then** ▷ *ROI visibility*
  F.append(`visible_ROI`)
for $i \in \{1, 2\}$ **do**
  if j_i <20° **then** ▷ *Gripper state*
    F.append(`closed_gripper(A`$_i$`)`)
  for B $\in S_B$ **do**
    if $p_i \in$ B **then** ▷ *Arm location*
      F.append(`at(A`$_i$`, B)`)
      if j_i <20° **then** ▷ *Tissue grasped*
        F.append(`in_hand(A`$_i$`, B)`)
    if $p_i[2] > 50mm$ **then** ▷ *Max height reached*
      F.append(`max_height(A`$_i$`)`)
    if $max\Sigma > \epsilon$ **then** ▷ *Max force reached*
      F.append(`max_force(A`$_i$`)`)
  return F

1.4 Monitoring

The monitoring module continuously receives PC_t and the point cloud of the simulated tissue PC_s from the sensing module, and computes a discrepancy metric μ, chosen as the median Euclidean distance of closest points between PC_t and PC_s. The distance is normalized with respect to its rest value (i.e., before grasping occurs) to compensate for offsets induced by registration error and sensor noise. Inspired from recent works as [18], the monitoring module considers 3 thresholds δ_1, δ_2, δ_3 (empirically set to 2, 4 and 6 mm) to classify the warning state of the system (Algorithm 3). In particular, when $\mu > \delta_1$ (Line 10) the motion velocity is reduced for caution, to minimize the risk of applying excessive forces [15] and to allow prompt capturing of eventual higher levels of discrepancy. If δ_2 is exceeded (Line 12), motion is interrupted and re-planning is asked at task planning level, meaning that probably the environmental conditions have significantly changed. In both these warning states, the learning module is triggered to update environmental knowledge exploiting data from sensors. Overcoming δ_3 (Line 14) results in interruption of DEFRAS and human intervention is required because either the current situation is too anomalous or the environmental model is inadequate.

Algorithm 3 Monitoring module

1: **Input**: PC_t, PC_s, motion rate r, `grasped_tissue`
2: **Output**: Warning state s, motion rate r, trigger learning `learn`
3: **Init**: $d_{rest} = []$
4: **while** not `task_ended` **do**
5:     **while** not `grasped_tissue` **do**
6:         d_{rest}.append($||PC_t - PC_s||_2$)
7:     $d_{rest} = \text{mean}(d_{rest})$
8:     $d = ||PC_t - PC_s||_2$
9:     $\mu = d - d_{rest}$
10:     **if** $\delta_1 < \mu \leq \delta_2$ **then**
11:         **return** $s = 1; r = \frac{r}{2}$; `learn=True`
12:     **else if** $\delta_2 < \mu \leq \delta_3$ **then**
13:         **return** $s = 2; r = 0$; `learn=True`
14:     **else if** $\mu > \delta_3$ **then**
15:         **return** $s = 3; r = 0$; `learn=False`
16:     **else**
17:         **return** $s = 0; r = r$; `learn=False`

1.5 Learning

As motivated in Sect. 1, in this work we focus on the intra-operative update of APs whenever required by the monitoring module. Update relies on BA-Net, the deep neural network which predicts APs starting from the tissue pre-operative geometry and the current observed PC_t, presented in [13]. This method has proved suitable for intra-operative model refinement, requiring a very low inference time and even improving biomechanical model accuracy. To improve the robustness to sensor noise, we consider the intersection among the latest 30 predictions provided by BA-Net as new estimate of APs. The new estimate of APs is used on the one hand by the task planning module to update its knowledge of the regions to avoid, in case of grasp re-planning. On the other hand, it is exploited to refine the PBM which drives the simulated environment, thus improving its overall reliability (in particular of the force estimate).

1.6 Simulated Environment

To obtain a physically accurate result, we model the deformable behavior of anatomical tissues exploiting continuum mechanics laws, solved with the finite element (FE) method (see Chap. 6, Sect. 2). The choice of a physics-based method allows to continuously estimate forces exerted on the tissue, compensating for the lack of force feedback in surgical robotic systems. Monitoring of the applied forces is crucial in our task to avoid unnecessary tissue damage. The deformable tissue is modelled as a linear elastic material with Young's modulus 3 kPa and Poisson ratio 0.45, a common modelling choice for adipose tissues [19], which are often responsible of hiding structures of interest during real surgery [20]. In order to handle large deformations while guaranteeing the computational efficiency required to run the simulation in parallel to the real execution, we rely on the corotational formulation of linear elasticity [21] provided by the SOFA framework [22]. In the considered simulation environment, grasping is implemented by constraining the tissue points closest to the simulated PSM (distance below a small threshold, 5 mm in our task) to follow PSM motion, similarly to [1]. Grasping is activated or released based on commands received from the acting module. Current implementation does not consider the possibility of slippage or breaking contacts between the tool and the tissue, that might happen during real retraction.

2 Autonomous Tissue Retraction with DEFRAS

Experiments are conducted both in simulated and real environments to assess the capability of DEFRAS to successfully accomplish the TR task, coping with inaccurate parametrization of the available model of the environment from pre-operative information [13].

2.1 Experimental Setup

We consider the problem of retracting a thin layer of soft tissue ($120 \times 120 \times 5$ mm) to expose a ROI to the endoscopic camera, which is placed at the main surgical viewpoint (Fig. 1). The task is executed on the dVRK, whose PSMs are equipped with ProGrasp® surgical grasping tools (Fig. 1b). The ROI is considered exposed if at least 80% of its surface is visible from the endoscope. For monitoring purposes, we continuously capture the tissue point cloud PC_t with an additional Intel® Realsense D435 RGBD sensor, placed opposite to the endoscope to maximize tissue visibility during manipulation. The RGBD sensor, endoscopic camera and the PSMs are calibrated with respect to a common reference frame placed at the center of the tissue (Fig. 1), using the methodology described in [23]. The simulated environment is aligned to the same reference frame and a simulated RGBD sensor, placed in the same position as the real one, provides the point cloud of the simulated tissue PC_s.

2.1.1 FRAS: Framework for Robot-Assisted Surgery

At this point, it is worth introducing a base version of the framework, called FRAS [10], where:

- grasping point is always chosen following the heuristic used by DEFRAS in case of intra-operative re-planning, as described in Sect. 1.1. This means that FRAS does not rely on any pre-operative plan;
- neither the monitoring or the learning modules are activated.

FRAS is used to assess the values of some metrics that are independent from the monitoring and learning modules. For example, FRAS is used to identify a reasonable value for the force threshold ϵ (see Sect. 1.2). We consider 17 pre-operative configurations of tissue, each one with different locations for APs and ROI. For each pre-operative configuration we launch FRAS only in simulation, ignoring also force measurements. We compute plans for all possible grasping points under these conditions, and we record the estimated forces from the simulation. We obtain a median force $F_m = 0.15N$ among all 425 executions. F_m is chosen to represent the typical force on the tissue in the considered setup, hence we set $\epsilon = 2 \cdot F_m = 0.3N$.

Furthermore, FRAS is used as a comparison to assess the role of monitoring and learning modules, as well as the utility of the pre-operative plan.

2.2 Validation of DEFRAS in Simulation

The capability of DEFRAS to cope with uncertain environmental parameters has been initially assessed in simulation. Experiments in simulation allow to evaluate the performance of the framework excluding possible inaccuracies arising from the presence of real sensor noise. We design 8 pre-operative scenarios, each characterized by a different configuration of APs (red outlines in Fig. 2) extracted as random surface patches following the same approach presented in [13]. For each pre-operative scenario, we generate optimal plans following the strategy described in Sect. 1.1.

Each pre-operative plan is executed by DEFRAS on two validation scenarios: the former with fewer APs (in our case, between 20–60%, indicated with symbol $\ominus$) and the latter with more APs (in our case, between 140–160%, indicated with $\oplus$) with respect to the corresponding pre-operative configuration. These experiments emulate the realistic situation where initial knowledge of APs is not precise, thus the pre-operative plan might need adjustment due to mismatch between the current and the simulated environments. Figure 3 provides a close-up on the configurations of APs considered for case 0 in Fig. 2. To run these experiments, we rely on two parallel simulations: the former (*pre-operative simulation*) represents the simulated environment in the scheme of Fig. 1, estimating the tissue forces and initialized with pre-operative APs (red outlines in Fig. 2); the latter (*actual simulation*) represents the validation scenario with either fewer or more APs than the pre-operative simulation, with simulated dVRK and cameras (blue and green areas in Fig. 2). Visibility in the actual simulation is computed by counting the number of visible ROI points from the simulated endoscope, assessed via ray-casting technique. The monitoring module continuously compares the tissue point clouds from the two simulations, triggering specific interventions according to Algorithm 3. To assess the performance of the monitoring module, we compute the success rate of APs update with BA-Net as ratio between the number of times the update results in $\mu \leq \delta_1$ in Algorithm 3 (no warning from monitoring) and the number of times BA-Net is triggered because $\mu > \delta_1$ (warning state).

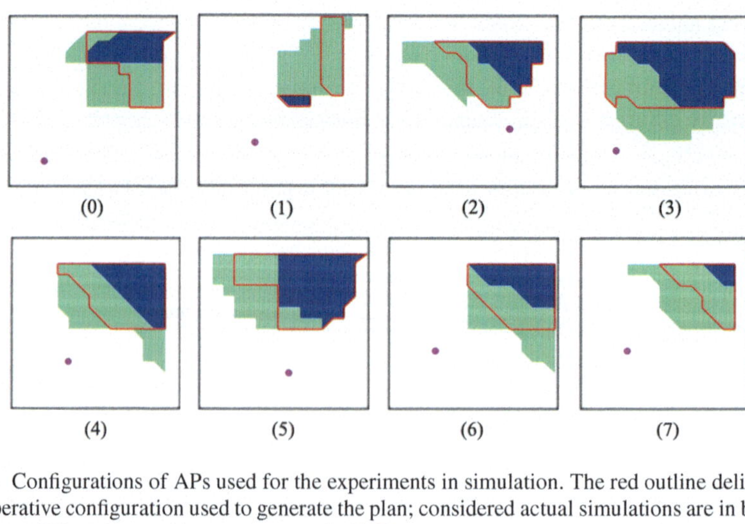

Fig. 2 Configurations of APs used for the experiments in simulation. The red outline delimits the pre-operative configuration used to generate the plan; considered actual simulations are in blue ($\ominus$) and green ($\oplus$); magenta sphere represents the ROI

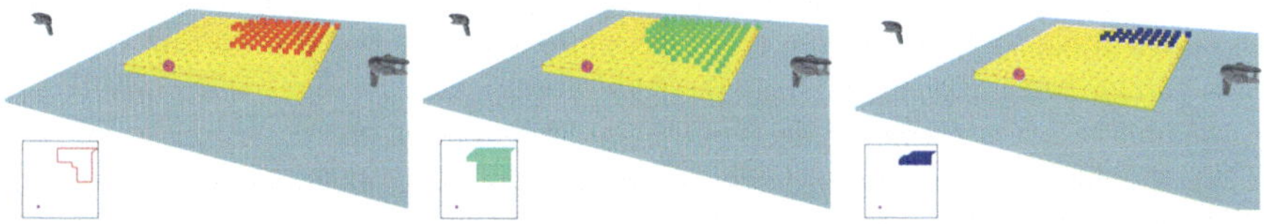

(a) (b) (c)

Fig. 3 Simulation scenes relative to the configurations of APs for case 0 in Fig. 2. **a** The pre-operative configuration; **b** The ⊕ actual configuration; **c** The ⊖ configuration

Furthermore, we compare the performance of DEFRAS with respect to FRAS, in order to show the advantages of the pre-operative plan and of the monitoring and learning modules in a deliberative architecture for autonomous robotic surgery. Therefore, we let FRAS perform autonomous TR on the actual simulations.

Re-planning Efficiency

In addition to validating DEFRAS capability to handle uncertain environmental conditions, we evaluate the computational performance of task reasoner as the *re-planning time*, defined as the time required to compute a new plan given a context interpretation from the sensing module. In particular, we assess how the re-planning time is impacted by the resolution of the grid that defines candidate grasping points (see Sect. 1.1), while also varying the percentage of APs. In fact, both the number of possible grasping points and the percentage $f_{\%}$ of APs influence the size of the search space.

To this purpose, we run 100 simulations initialized with different random environmental states (i.e., p_{ROI} and PC_{AP}) and we execute the task with FRAS, i.e. relying on the described strategy for grasping point selection in case of re-planning and without the monitoring and learning modules. In this evaluation, we consider different resolutions of the grid defining candidate grasping points $N \in \{5, \ldots, 10\}$. For each value of N, we run 25 simulations for each value $f_{\%} \in \{10, 30, 50, 70\%\}$. This results in 600 total simulations, each initialized with a different random p_{ROI} and $PC_A P$ (according to the value of $f_{\%}$).

2.3 *Validation of DEFRAS on the dVRK*

The performance of DEFRAS is evaluated on autonomous TR of silicone tissue with the real dVRK (Fig. 1b) [9]. Following the same approach of in [13], APs in the real environment are defined by stitching the tissue on an attachment board with regularly spaced holes every 10 mm. The point cloud of the tissue in real environment is acquired after color-based segmentation and decimation of the raw point cloud from Realsense, and compared with the point cloud from the simulated environment for monitoring. Visibility in the real environment is computed detecting the ROI (with known size and position) from the endoscopic camera images with color-based segmentation and considering the percentage of visible pixels.

We consider three real world scenarios (A, B and C), obtained by stitching the tissue to the attachment board with 3 different configurations of APs (light blue in Fig. 4). For each scenario, we consider 3 pre-operative models, each characterized by a different pre-operative knowledge of APs: (1) fewer APs (between 20–60%, indicated with $\ominus$), (2) more APs (between 140–160%, indicated with $\oplus$), and (3) same APs (indicated with ⊜) than/as the real scenario (Fig. 4). For each of them, we generate the pre-operative plan in simulation, and test DEFRAS on the corresponding real configuration with the dVRK.

Moreover, we analyze the performance of our framework with respect to two state-of-the-art implementations of autonomous TR on real setups. In particular, we compare both to the results obtained with the learning-based approaches presented in [8] and to the work by Attanasio et al. [3], which relies on image-guided control to reveal a ROI behind tissue flap. Both the considered approaches evaluate task success as percentage of ROI exposure upon task completion.

3 Experimental Results of Autonomous TR in Simulation

Table 2 reports the details of the optimal plans generated for each pre-operative configuration in the experiments in simulation (red outlines in Fig. 2). Each of these plans is executed with DEFRAS on a scenario with fewer and more APs than those of the corresponding pre-operative configuration. Details of such executions are presented in the upper part of Table 3. The lower part of Table 3 reports the results obtained when executing the TR task on the same scenarios using FRAS.

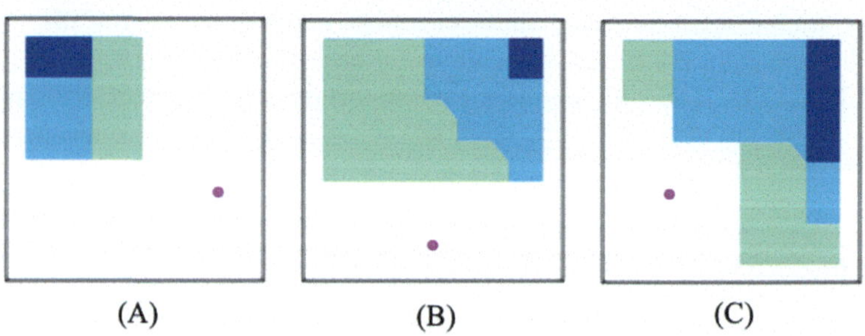

Fig. 4 Configurations of APs used for the real world experiments. The light blue region in each subimage represents the configuration of APs in the real setup (⊜). Blue and green regions indicate pre-operative configurations with fewer APs ($\ominus$) and more APs ($\oplus$) than the real configuration. Magenta sphere represents the ROI

Table 2 Pre-operative plans for the 8 scenarios in our simulation experiments. Table reports the final reached visibility, the number of actions, the number of times $F > \epsilon$ and $F_{\max}$. Last two columns report median and interquartile (IQR) range per row

	0	**1**	**2**	**3**	**4**	**5**	**6**	**7**	Median	IQR
Visibility [%]	100	100	100	95	80	100	93	100	100	94–100
Actions	4	6	6	5	5	5	5	5	5	5–5
$F > \epsilon$	0	0	1	0	1	1	1	1	1	0–1
$F_{\max}$ [N]	0.3	0.3	0.4	0.3	0.4	0.3	0.6	0.5	0.4	0.3–0.4

Table 3 Simulation experiments. $\ominus$ indicates the scenario with fewer APs, while $\oplus$ the one with more APs than those of the pre-operative configuration. The upper Table reports results obtained with DEFRAS, while the lower Table reports results obtained with FRAS. "BA-Net" row reports the success rate of APs update with BA-Net

DEFRAS	**0**		**1**		**2**		**3**		**4**		**5**		**6**		**7**			
	$\ominus$	$\oplus$	$\ominus$	$\oplus$	$\ominus$	$\oplus$	$\ominus$	$\oplus$	$\ominus$	$\oplus$	$\ominus$	$\oplus$	$\ominus$	$\oplus$	$\ominus$	$\oplus$	Median	IQR
Visibility [%]	100	100	100	100	100	0	9	95	100	100	0	100	100	100	100	100	100	98–100
Actions	4	11	6	6	6	30	38	12	5	26	29	25	5	30	5	5	8	5–26
$F > \epsilon$	0	26	11	3	1	44	240	27	0	46	99	83	8	61	1	3	18	2–49
$F_{\max}$ [N]	0.2	1.3	0.4	0.4	0.4	1.4	0.9	1.8	0.3	1.7	3.3	3.3	0.4	1.2	0.3	0.4	0.6	0.4–1.5
BA-Net	1/1	1/1	–	0/1	2/2	1/1	6/6	–	1/1	2/2	11/12	–	1/1	4/4	2/2	–	–	–
FRAS																		
Visibility [%]	100	90	100	0	0	0	90	0	100	100	100	0	97	93	93	93	93	0–100
Actions	5	6	15	23	22	22	7	22	17	19	7	22	16	16	9	15	16	8–22
$F > \epsilon$	0	0	29	33	32	28	11	40	21	29	0	28	27	18	20	12	24	11–29
$F_{\max}$ [N]	0.3	0.3	1.0	1.0	1.1	1.0	0.4	1.2	0.9	0.9	0.3	1.1	0.9	0.9	1.2	0.9	0.9	0.8–1.0

Re-planning times at varying grid resolutions and percentage of grasping points are reported in Table 4.

3.1 Discussion

The pre-operative plans generated for each configuration using our criterion (final paragraph of Sect. 1.1) successfully expose the ROI with a maximum of 6 actions, with the force exceeding the safety threshold ϵ at most once (Table 2).

Reliance on such plans leads to successful completion of the TR task (i.e., the ROI is exposed) in 13 out of 16 cases (Table 3), which means DEFRAS can accomplish the task even when the pre-operative information (i.e., knowledge of APs) is imprecise. Moreover, the results show that, even when starting from pre-operative plans which

Table 4 Re-planning time (average ± standard deviation) with different tissue grid size N and percentage of APs $f_{\%}$

N	*Re-planning time* [s]			
	$\mathbf{f_{\%} = 10\%}$	$\mathbf{f_{\%} = 30\%}$	$\mathbf{f_{\%} = 50\%}$	$\mathbf{f_{\%} = 70\%}$
5	0.25 ± 0.02	0.24 ± 0.02	0.23 ± 0.01	0.24 ± 0.01
6	0.68 ± 0.02	0.65 ± 0.02	0.63 ± 0.01	0.62 ± 0.01
7	1.50 ± 0.02	1.48 ± 0.03	1.41 ± 0.02	1.42 ± 0.01
8	3.06 ± 0.04	2.97 ± 0.06	2.90 ± 0.04	2.88 ± 0.02
9	5.88 ± 0.08	5.70 ± 0.15	5.51 ± 0.03	5.51 ± 0.05
10	10.75 ± 0.20	10.21 ± 0.28	9.92 ± 0.09	9.87 ± 0.08

minimize the tissue force, the force threshold can be exceeded during task execution, hence force feedback is needed to prevent potentially dangerous tissue solicitation.

Furthermore, the tissue force reaches higher values ($> 1N$) mostly in scenarios with more APs than the pre-operative configuration ($\oplus$ in Table). This is motivated by the fact that optimal plans might select a grasping point close to APs that are unknown pre-operatively. In this case, monitoring detects a difference between the pre-operative simulation and the actual simulation, and triggers APs update in the learning module. This leads to prediction of APs very close to the current grasping point, thus the estimated force increases. The results of our framework also show that when pre-operative APs overestimate actual APs ($\ominus$ in Table), the task is accomplished with fewer actions (except for fails) with respect to the case when APs are underestimated ($\oplus$ in Table). Therefore, it seems that overestimating APs in the pre-operative phase leads to more optimized task executions, reducing both interaction with the tissue and potentially unsafe tissue solicitation.

If we compare the results obtained when executing the TR task using DEFRAS with those obtained using FRAS (lower part of Table 3), it emerges that the presence of the pre-operative plan in DEFRAS is fundamental to optimize executions in terms of tissue solicitation (fewer actions, lower number of times the force threshold is exceeded and lower maximum force, considering median values). Comparison between the two frameworks also evidences the advantages of monitoring and learning modules, introduced by our deliberative framework. Whenever the mismatch between the pre-operative simulation and the actual simulation causes the monitoring module to trigger update of APs, BA-Net is able to provide an updated estimate of APs that brings the monitoring metric below threshold, except cases $1\oplus$ (task success, ROI is exposed) and $5\ominus$ (the task fails). Overall, the integration of the proposed deliberative modules results in higher median visibility (100 versus 93%) and lower number of failed tasks (3 fails versus 5) with respect to FRAS. We notice that FRAS is able to solve the task when DEFRAS fails in configurations $3\ominus$ and $5\ominus$. However, in both cases the monitoring module triggers APs update and the force threshold is overcome more times than all other configurations. This suggests that the pre-operative knowledge of APs is particularly far from reality in these cases. As a consequence, the estimate of the force from the pre-operative simulation provided by the FRAS cannot be considered reliable (being the simulation different from reality), potentially leading to unsafe executions by FRAS.

Re-planning Efficiency

Analyzing the computational performance of our framework in case of re-planning, our results show that the task reasoner is able to compute a new grasping point and a plan within 1.5 s when using a 7×7 grid discretization for grasping point definition, demonstrating high efficiency. This guarantees efficient adaptation to the quickly changing anatomical environment, introducing only a minor delay which is compatible with intra-operative times. From Table 4 it emerges that the most influencing parameter is N, while $f_{\%}$ does not significantly affect the average planning time. Reliance on the lowest resolution grid (5×5) for the definition of candidate grasping points for all the validation experiments presented in this Chapter allows us to maximize computational efficiency, both in pre-operative plan generation phase and intra-operative re-planning. Using a higher resolution grid would imply more time to generate the optimal task plan due to a larger search space. Although this would not represent a major limitation in the pre-operative phase, where there are no strict time constraints for plan definition, in case intra-operative re-planning is needed, it is important to rely on an efficient heuristic for the selection of the new grasping point, which ensures that plan generation does not introduce major delays in the execution.

Definition of the set of candidate grasping points as uniformly spaced above the tissue of interest represents a naive strategy which has been selected for our initial evaluation. Despite its simplicity, the same strategy does not only apply to the considered setup, but can be employed for more complex setups characterized by irregular geometries. It is worth highlighting that different grasping point selection strategies can be implemented and easily integrated within DEFRAS, e.g. based on path planning as in [2].

4 Experimental Results of Autonomous TR on the dVRK

Relevant variables describing the executions of the TR task on the experiments on the real setup are reported in Table 5.

4.1 Discussion

Obtained results on the real world experiments confirm that whenever pre-operative APs underestimate real APs, the monitoring and learning modules are triggered more frequently. The update of APs leads to successful task completion in all cases. Moreover, when the simulated and real APs match (cases labelled with ⊜), the

Table 5 Real world experiments using DEFRAS. For each real world configuration (A, B, C), we report details of TR executions of 3 different pre-operative plans, obtained when: (⊖) underestimating real APs, (⊕) overestimating real APs, (⊜) having perfect knowledge of the real APs

	A			**B**			**C**				
	⊖	⊕	⊜	⊖	⊕	⊜	⊖	⊕	⊜	Median	IQR
Visibility [%]	99	95	100	100	100	71	99	83	96	99	95–100
Actions	13	15	9	24	7	8	14	7	7	9	7–14
$F > \epsilon$	11	20	8	0	8	20	8	8	6	8	8–11
$F_{\max}$ [N]	1.2	1.1	0.5	0.2	0.5	1.1	1.1	0.7	0.5	0.7	0.5–1.1
BA-Net	1/1	1/1	1/1	13/14	–	–	1/1	–	–	–	–

number of actions is usually minimum (except for configuration B, with 8 actions for ⊜ and 7 for ⊕). This suggests that overall the optimal pre-operative plan leads to better performances when APs are perfectly known.

When qualitatively analyzing executions for configuration A, it emerges that both for ⊖ and ⊕ re-planning is required: in the first case due to high force after grasping too close to real APs, detected by the monitoring module; in the second case because of invisible ROI after optimal plan execution. Re-planning proves able to successfully expose the ROI in both cases. It is also interesting to consider TR execution when using the plan generated on the configuration with perfect knowledge of real APs (⊜). In this case, the monitoring module detects a mismatch between the real and the simulated scenarios, probably due to noise and uncertainty introduced by real cameras and the calibration procedure. DEFRAS proves able to cope with such situation and successfully complete the task.

The average visibility achieved by DEFRAS is 94%, which is aligned with the 90% visibility obtained when using GAIL [8], and it improves the one reported in [3] (i.e., 83%). It is worth remarking that our framework is able to model uncertainties and handle re-planning, but these functions are absent in the approaches considered for comparison.

5 Conclusions

In this Chapter, we have presented a modular architecture which provides the fundamental building blocks and requisites for autonomy in robotic surgery. Our framework, called DEFRAS, introduces deliberative functionalities in order to deal with the uncertainty of anatomical environments. In particular, it is capable of monitoring the real execution and learning from real observations. The modular structure of the framework offers the opportunity to specialize each deliberative function individually, depending on the desired task. Moreover, a logic-based task planner guarantees interpretability of the surgical plan, thus allowing for human supervision, which is needed for reliable execution. A groundbreaking aspect of DEFRAS is the presence of a biomechanical simulation, which plays a crucial role in both the pre-operative and the intra-operative phase. Before the intervention, the simulation is exploited to design the task plan accounting for each patient's characteristics. Whereas, during task execution, it allows both to monitor the actual surgical environment and detect the presence of unexpected situations, and to provide additional information about the surgical scene.

Experiments on a representative surgical task, i.e. soft tissue retraction, have shown that our framework has the needed features to handle deformable environments with uncertain parameters, successfully accomplishing the task. In particular, DEFRAS has proved able to learn and refine available but imprecise pre-operative knowledge about the location of attachment points, relying on constant monitoring of sensors and simulation data. In this way, any pre-operative plan can be adapted, and tissue force information from the simulation remains reliable for safe task completion. Compared with a framework without the deliberative functions of monitoring and learning, results show that the percentage of task success increases, especially when pre-operative knowledge of attachment points overestimates real ones. Moreover, reliance on a pre-operative patient-specific plan brings benefits in terms of minimal manipulation of the tissue, hence reduced risk of tissue damage.

Although the implementation of each module described in this Chapter is specific to accomplish the tissue retraction task, the general DEFRAS architecture is designed to provide the needed functionalities for autonomous execution of any surgical task. The modularity of DEFRAS will allow us to improve individual deliberative capabilities in order to deal with more realistic and challenging surgical scenarios in future works. Motion adaptation as in [16] and learning from demonstrations as in [24] can be easily implemented to replicate expert surgeons–dexterity. Furthermore, we plan to improve task knowledge description both pre-operatively from the analysis of surgical annotations [25] and intra-operatively by observing the surgeon in most critical situations, exploiting logic learning as in [26, 27]. Finally, we will investigate the possibility to introduce additional sensors on the instruments in order to enhance the sensing capabilities of the framework [28] and cope with specific problems of real surgical settings, e.g. point cloud occlusion. This will also allow to refine other patient-specific parameters and identify more robust task-specific thresholds.

Overall, this framework represents one of the first attempts to a complete deliberative architecture that integrates all the functionalities required to deal with the dynamic and uncertain surgical environments. Therefore, it contributes to make a step forward towards autonomy in surgical robotics.

References

1. Patil, S., Alterovitz, R.: Toward automated tissue retraction in robot-assisted surgery. In: 2010 IEEE International Conference on Robotics and Automation, pp. 2088–2094. IEEE (2010)

2. Jansen, R., Hauser, K., Chentanez, N., et al.: Surgical retraction of non-uniform deformable layers of tissue: 2D robot grasping and path planning. In: 2009 IEEE/RSJ International Conference Intelligence Robots and Systems, pp. 4092–4097. IEEE (2009)
3. Attanasio, A., Scaglioni, B., Leonetti, M., Frangi, A.F., Cross, W., Biyani, C.S., Valdastri, P.: Autonomous tissue retraction in robotic assisted minimally invasive surgery-a feasibility study. IEEE Robot. Autom. Lett. **5**(4), 6528–6535 (2020)
4. Tagliabue, E., Pore, A., Dall'Alba, D., Magnabosco, E., Piccinelli, M., Fiorini, P.: Soft tissue simulation environment to learn manipulation tasks in autonomous robotic surgery. In: 2020 IEEE International Conference on Intelligent Robots and Systems (IROS). IEEE (2020)
5. Pore, A., Corsi, D., Marchesini, E., Dall Alba, D., Casals, A., Alessandro, F., Fiorini, P.: Safe reinforcement learning using formal verification for tissue retraction in autonomous robotic-assisted surgery. In: 2021 IEEE/RSJ International Conference on Intelligence Robots and Systems (IROS), pp. 0–6. IEEE (2021)
6. Shin, C., Ferguson, P.W., Pedram, S.A., et al.: Autonomous tissue manipulation via surgical robot using learning based model predictive control. In: 2019 International Conference on Robotics and Automation (ICRA), pp. 3875–3881. IEEE (2019)
7. Pedram, S.A., Ferguson, P.W., Shin, C., Mehta, A., Dutson, E.P., Alambeigi, F., et al.: Toward synergic learning for autonomous manipulation of deformable tissues via surgical robots: an approximate q- approach. In: 2020 8th IEEE RAS/EMBS International Conference for Biomedical Robotics and Biomechatronics (BioRob), pp. 878–884. IEEE (2019)
8. Pore, A., et al.: Learning from demonstrations for autonomous soft-tissue retraction. In: 2021 international symposium on medical robotics (ISMR). IEEE, 2021
9. Tagliabue, E., et al.: Deliberation in autonomous robotic surgery: a framework for handling anatomical uncertainty. In: 2022 International Conference on Robotics and Automation (ICRA). IEEE, 2022
10. Meli, D. et al.: Autonomous tissue retraction with a biomechanically informed logic based framework. In: 2021 International Symposium on Medical Robotics (ISMR). IEEE, 2021
11. Plantefève, R., Peterlik, I., Haouchine, N., Cotin, S.: Patient-specific biomechanical modeling for guidance during minimally-invasive hepatic surgery. Ann. Biomed. Eng. **44**(1), 139–153 (2016)
12. Nikolaev, S., Cotin, S.: Estimation of boundary conditions for patient-specific liver simulation during augmented surgery. Int. J. Comput. Assist. Radiol. Surg. (2020)
13. Tagliabue, E., Dall Alba, D., Pfeiffer, M., Piccinelli, M., Marin, R., Castellani, U., Speidel, S., Fiorini, P.: Data-driven intra-operative estimation of anatomical attachments for autonomous tissue dissection. IEEE Robot. Autom. Lett. **6**(2), 1856–1863 (2021)
14. Calimeri, F., Faber, W., Gebser, M., Ianni, G., Kaminski, R., Krennwallner, T., Leone, N., Maratea, M., Ricca, F., Schaub, T.: Asp-core-2 input language format. Theory Pract. Logic Program. **20**(2), 294–309 (2020)
15. Wang, J., Yu, Q.-Y., Li, W., Wang, B.-R., Zhou, Z.-R.: Influence of clamping stress and duration on the trauma of liver tissue during surgery operation. Clin. Biomech. **43**, 58–66 (2017)
16. Ginesi, M., Meli, D., Roberti, A., Sansonetto, N., Fiorini, P.: Autonomous task planning and situation awareness in robotic surgery. In: 2020 IEEE International Conference on Intelligence Robots and Systems (IROS), pp. 3144–3150. IEEE (2020)
17. Richter, F., Orosco, R.K., Yip, M.C.: Open-sourced reinforcement learning environments for surgical robotics (2019). arXiv:1903.02090
18. Machin, M., Guiochet, J., Waeselynck, H., Blanquart, J.-P., Roy, M., Masson, L.: SMOF: a safety monitoring framework for autonomous systems. IEEE Trans. Syst., Man, Cybern.: Syst. **48**(5), 702–715 (2016)
19. Alkhouli, N., Mansfield, J., Green, E., Bell, J., Knight, B., Liversedge, N., Tham, J.C., Welbourn, R., Shore, A.C., Kos, K., et al.: The mechanical properties of human adipose tissues and their relationships to the structure and composition of the extracellular matrix. Am. J. Physiol.-Endocrinol. Metab. **305**(12), E1427–E1435 (2013)
20. Bhayani, S.B.: da Vinci robotic partial nephrectomy for renal cell carcinoma: an atlas of the four-arm technique. J. Robot. Surg. **1**(4), 279–285 (2008)

21. Müller, M., Dorsey, J., McMillan, L., Jagnow, R., Cutler, B.: Stable real-time deformations. In: Proceedings of the 2002 ACM SIGGRAPH/Eurographics Symposium on Computer Animation, pp. 49–54 (2002)
22. Faure, F., Duriez, C., Delingette, H., Allard, J., Gilles, B., Marchesseau, S., Talbot, H., Courtecuisse, H., Bousquet, G., Peterlik, I., et al.: Sofa: a multi-model framework for interactive physical simulation. In: Soft Tissue Biomechanical Modeling for Computer Assisted Surgery, pp. 283–321. Springer, Berlin (2012)
23. Roberti, A., Piccinelli, N., Meli, D., Muradore, R., Fiorini, P.: Improving rigid 3D calibration for robotic surgery. IEEE Trans. Med. Robot. Bionics **2**(4), 569–573 (2020)
24. Ginesi, M., Sansonetto, N., Fiorini, P.: Overcoming some drawbacks of dynamic movement primitives. Robot. Auton. Syst. **144**, 103844 (2021)
25. Bombieri, M., Rospocher, M., Dall Alba, D., Fiorini, P.: Automatic detection of procedural knowledge in robotic-assisted surgical texts. Int. J. Comput. Assist. Radiol. Surg. 1–9 (2021)
26. Meli, D., Sridharan, M., Fiorini, P.: Inductive learning of answer set programs for autonomous surgical task planning. Mach. Learn. 1–25 (2021)
27. Meli, D., Fiorini, P., Sridharan, M.: Towards inductive learning of surgical task knowledge: a preliminary case study of the peg transfer task. Procedia Comput. Sci. **176**, 440–449 (2020)
28. Cheng, Z., et al.: Design and integration of electrical bio-impedance sensing in surgical robotic tools for tissue identification and display. Front. Robot. AI **6**, 55 (2019)

Learning Tissue Retraction in Simulation

Eleonora Tagliabue

Abstract In this Chapter we address the "Sim-to-Real" effect, i.e. the different results that can be achieved during task execution, when learning is carried out in simulation. To reduce this effect, simulation must be as close to real as possible and therefore modeling and learning methods must be tuned to this need. In Sect. 1 we describe the software technology used, and in Sect. 2 we present the learning methods and their evaluation metrics. In Sect. 3 we present the results obtained in simulation, and in Sect. 4 we discuss the results obtained after sim-to-real transfer. Section 5 concludes this Chapter.

1 The Technology Elements

Robot Platform

UnityFlexML is a modular framework that allows to exploit learning based methods to learn tasks in a simulated surgical environment which involve deformable objects (Fig. 1) [1]. The developed platform provides an interface between the real dVRK and a simulation of the real environment.

The framework is made publicly available at https://gitlab.com/altairLab/unityflexml. *UnityFlexML* tackles automation of surgical tasks executed with the Patient Side Manipulator (PSM) arms of the dVRK. The dVRK is programmed using the Robot Operating System (ROS) [2]. In order to have a state space (i.e., the set of all possible configurations of the robotic agent) which is straightforward to observe in both the simulator and the real robot, the motion of the PSM end-effector (EE) is controlled in the Cartesian space, keeping the EE orientation constant (as in [3]). The framework can handle any possible surgical tool, provided that the corresponding kinematic model is loaded in simulation. Therefore, the PSM EE state is charac-

E. Tagliabue (✉)
Department of Computer Science, University of Verona, Verona, Italy
e-mail: eleonora.tagliabue@zeiss.com

Carl Zeiss AG, Oberkochen, Germany

P. Fiorini (ed.), *Towards Autonomous Robotic Surgery*, Springer Tracts in Advanced Robotics 161, https://doi.org/10.1007/978-3-032-04247-7_10

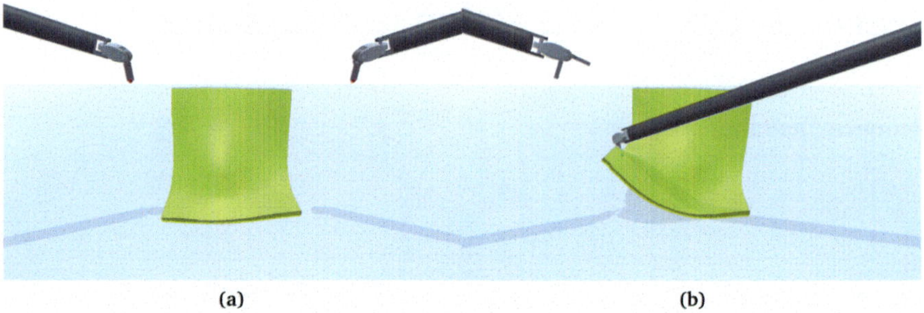

Fig. 1 *UnityFlexML* framework. The simulated dVRK arms interact with deformable tissues, modelled using PBD method. Example scene **a** at rest, **b** during tissue manipulation

terized by its position $\mathbf{p}_t$ and gripper state $g_t \in \{0, 1\}$ for open/close. Similarly to [3], we normalize the PSM positions with respect to the workspace, defined by the PSM joint limits and the obstacles in the environment, to allow generalization of the learned policies to various joint configurations.

Simulation Environment

The simulation is implemented within Unity3D, an engine whose main advantage is the high modularity, which allows users to easily customize the environment scene and exploit advanced features implemented in separate plugins [4]. Our framework relies on two main Unity3D plugins: the Machine Learning Agents Toolkit (ML-Agents), for training intelligent agents [5], and NVIDIA FleX, for soft object deformation [6]. Deformable bodies are simulated with the Position Based Dynamics (PBD) approach relying on the optimized implementation provided by NVIDIA FleX. This library has proved to be able to accurately model the deformable behavior of anatomical tissues with highly efficient computational performances (see [7]) and it is thus particularly suitable to perform the huge number of trial and error attempts required for agent training with learning-based methods. Our choice to simulate anatomical deformations based on PBD instead of relying, for example, on the finite element method to obtain a physically accurate result (Sect. 2) in chapter "Simulation and Autonomy" is motivated by the superior performance of PBD in terms of computational efficiency and numerical stability. These two aspects are of major concern in our framework, which has to allow the simulated agent to perform multiple interactions with the environment in the lowest time to guarantee efficient training, thus also minimizing the risk of simulation instability.

From what concerns the simulation of the robotic part, we have implemented a closed form inverse kinematics of the PSMs to enable the Cartesian space control of the manipulator. Data exchange between Unity3D and ROS exploits UDP-based communication, using the method described in [8]. At each simulation step, the robotic system is allowed to perform a very small motion increment. As a consequence, we could assume the impact of the robot dynamic behavior to be negligible, thus we have not accounted for it in the simulation [3]. In *UnityFlexML*, grasping of an object is modelled as an atomic event triggered when the relative distance with the EE is less that 2 mm.

1.1 Background on Learning-Based Methods

The aim of *UnityFlexML* is to provide an integrated simulation framework where learning-based methods can be trained. Before presenting how the framework can be used for this purpose, we introduce the main concepts in learning-based approaches.

1.1.1 Reinforcement Learning

Reinforcement Learning (RL) denotes a learning paradigm where an agent learns behaviors to achieve its goal while interacting with the environment (Fig. 2). A general RL problem can be formulated as a Markov Decision Process (MDP) described by the tuple $\langle S, A, R, P \rangle$, where:

- S is the set of possible states of the environment;
- A is the set of possible actions of the agent;
- P is the transition probability distribution, with $P(s_{t+1}|s_t, a_t)$ being the probability of transitioning into state s_{t+1} when starting in state s_t under action a_t;
- R is the reward function, with $r_t = R(s_t, a_t, s_{t+1})$ being the immediate reward after transition from s_t to s_{t+1} with action a_t.

At every step t of interaction with the environment, the agent receives an observation of the state s_t, and then decides on an action a_t to take. As a consequence

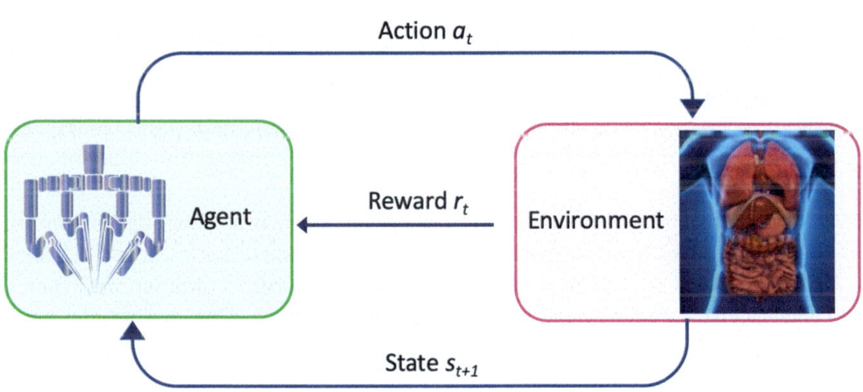

Fig. 2 In RL, an agent takes an action a_t in an environment. In turns, the environment communicates a new state s_{t+1} and a reward signal r_t back to the agent

of the action, the agent moves to the new state s_{t+1} and receives a reward signal r_t associated with the transition (s_t, a_t, s_{t+1}). The goal of the agent is to learn a behavior policy π, i.e. the rule used to decide which actions to take, that maximizes the expected cumulative reward $E[R(\tau)]$. $R(\tau)$ is commonly defined as:

$$R(\tau) = \sum_{t=0}^{\infty} \gamma^t r_t \tag{1}$$

which considers the sum of discounted rewards, where the discount factor $\gamma \in [0, 1)$ is introduced to weight events in the distant future less than events in the immediate future. $R(\tau)$ is sometimes defined over an episode, i.e. the sequence of states and actions over a fixed time horizon T. Due to the high dimensionality of the state space S in many practical problems, deep learning methods have been incorporated in the standard RL setting to represent the policy or other functions, leading to what is called Deep RL (DRL). The expected return obtained when starting from state s and successively acting with policy π is called value function $V_\pi(s)$. The optimal value function $V^*(s)$ is the one obtained when acting according to the optimal policy π^*, the one that achieves the optimal values in all the states. Instead, the action-value function $Q_\pi(s, a)$ gives the expected return when starting from state s, taking a first random action $a \in A$ and subsequently acting following policy π.

RL algorithms are classified in different ways depending on what they learn and how. A first categorization deals with the availability of a model of the environment, which allows the agent to consider a range of possible action plans and predict state transitions and rewards. Such model can be either given or learnt in a first stage. Several different approaches to model-based RL have been proposed [9]. Some of them compute optimal plans with respect to the model each time a state observation arrives, relying on pure planning techniques like model-predictive control [10]. An alternative approach learns the policy that produces actions as similar as possible to an expert planning algorithm [11].

However, having a model of the environment is generally quite difficult, since the dynamics of the objects involved are not always known. To tackle this issue, model-free RL methods are popularly used [9]. While being easier to implement and tune, model-free RL is generally less sample efficient (i.e., it needs more experience to learn) than model-based RL. Model-free approaches can either optimize the policy directly (policy optimization methods) or learn the optimal action-value function (Q-learning methods). Policy optimization algorithms rely on data collected while acting according to the most recent version of the policy (on-policy optimization). On the other hand, Q-learning approaches indirectly optimize for agent performance relying on data collected at any point during training, regardless of the specific policy used when such data were obtained (off-policy optimization). This causes Q-learning to be less stable but generally more sample efficient than policy optimization, since it can reuse data more effectively.

Proximal Policy Optimization

Proximal Policy Optimization (PPO) is one of the most popular RL methods. It is a model-free on-policy RL algorithm which continuously alternates between collecting a new batch of observations and improving the policy [12]. In particular, PPO maximizes a surrogate objective function that estimates how much the expected return will change after parameters update. A common approach to train a PPO agent in DRL relies on two deep networks, one called *actor* and other called *critic*. The actor network receives state observations from the environment and learns what action to take under a given observed state. Whereas, the critic network receives the reward signal following the action from the environment and learns to evaluate if the action taken by the actor led the environment in a better or worse state. The critic sends its feedback to the actor, which exploits such information to improve the policy.

Learning from Demonstrations

The most challenging step in standard RL consists in the design of the reward function. Manually shaping a good reward function to teach an agent to perform a task is immensely difficult, especially for complex tasks [13]. An approach that allows to learn without requiring a reward function is Learning from Demonstrations (LfD). LfD entails those methods that can learn from observed behaviors of other agents (generally human experts), specifically Imitation Learning (IL) and Inverse Reinforcement Learning (IRL).

In IL, the observed behavior is exploited to learn the optimal policy, without requiring interaction with the environment. For example, behavioral cloning learns to replicate the expert's policy from state-action pairs of expert trajectories in a supervised fashion [14]. However, it often suffers from poor generalization since this approach learns to imitate actions without any cue about the reasoning behind the task, so it is not able to understand if the actions are relevant for the final goal.

Whereas, the goal of IRL is not to use the demonstrated behavior to learn the policy, but to learn the reward function that could explain the expert behavior. The benefit of IRL over IL is that the learnt reward function is portable to other environments, thus leading to better generalization capabilities. However, IRL algorithms are very expensive to run, since they require RL in an inner loop to extract the imitation policy from the learnt cost function.

Overall, both IL and IRL usually require a large number of expert trajectories, which are often not easy to get.

Generative Adversarial Imitation Learning

Generative Adversarial Imitation Learning (GAIL) represents a promising approach to learn human decision-making strategies from a limited set of expert demonstrations using deep neural networks [15]. In particular, GAIL combines LfD with a Generative Adversarial Network (GAN) to learn both the unknown policy and reward function. GANs consist of two networks: the *generator* and the *discriminator* [16]. The role of the generator is to generate exploration trajectories that should become more and more similar to expert trajectories as the training proceeds. The goal of GAIL is to train generators such that they learn to behave in the same way as the given experts. Meanwhile, discriminators serve as the reward functions for RL, which judge whether the behaviors look like the experts. Usually, the adopted policy generator relies on PPO. There are two reasons why PPO is used for GAIL: first, it uses smooth policy update for stable learning and second, PPO generates diversified trajectories that act as a wide sampling range for the discriminator in GAIL.

2 Learning Tissue Retraction Within UnityFlexML

The presented *UnityFlexML* is employed to train agents in a simulated environment to learn a soft tissue retraction task. In particular, we aim at learning the sequence of actions that allow to accomplish the task and consists in reaching the adipose tissue covering the kidney, grasping it and lifting it in order to expose a tumor. In the following, after describing our experimental setup, we detail how we adapt the two considered approaches, i.e. a standard DRL approach and GAIL, to learn the desired task with our platform.

2.1 Experimental Setup

Our real experimental setup consists of a synthetic kidney phantom covered with silicone fat tissue, shown in Fig. 3a. We restrict the portion of fat tissue our agent interacts with to a 90 × 90 mm square region which is rigidly anchored to the top part of the kidney. The silicone patch representing the fat is held in place through a

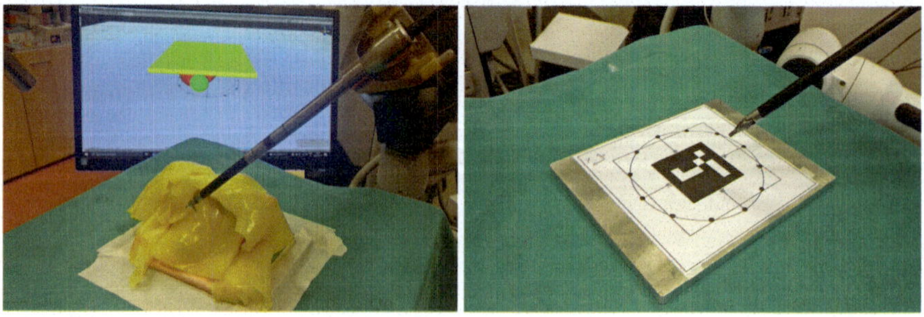

Fig. 3 **a** In our setup, a single arm of the dVRK interacts with silicone fat tissue covering a kidney phantom. The simulated scene controlling dVRK movements within *UnityFlexML* can be seen in the background. **b** The calibration board used to uniquely map all the components of our real experimental setup to the *UnityFlexML* environment

custom designed rigid structure, which enables to uniquely define the position of fat and kidney between the simulated and the real environment. The initial configuration of the fat tissue is obtained by letting this square region fall on the kidney phantom under gravity load. In our experiments, we consider a scenario with a single PSM arm equipped with the Large Needle Driver. All the simulation experiments, including agents training and dVRK control, ran on a workstation equipped with an AMD Ryzen 3700X processor and NVIDIA TitanX GPU.

2.1.1 *UnityFlexML* Environment

The 3D model of the kidney phantom used to inizialize the simulation environment as well as the position of the tumor $\mathbf{q}$ are extracted from segmentation of the Computerized Tomography (CT) of the phantom.

In an effort to minimize reality gap, we perform a preliminary optimization procedure to find the PBD deformation parameters that describe the behavior of our synthetic adipose tissue, keeping the real and the simulated behaviors as close as possible. We employ the genetic algorithm scheme to optimize PBD parameters most impacting the deformable behavior of the fat tissue our robot interacts with. Optimization is performed on some preliminary experiments where a teleoperated PSM arm lifts the fat tissue, which starts from a planar configuration and is rigidly fixed on one side (Fig. 4). We define $N = 5$ different pinch points along fat contour and $L = 3$ different levels of lifting are defined for each pinch point. The point cloud representing ground truth positions of the fat tissue is acquired using an Intel RealSense D435 Depth camera (Intel Corporation, Santa Clara, USA), whose position is defined with respect to a custom calibration board which allows to rigidly align the simulated and the real environment (Fig. 3b).

Optimal values for the cluster spacing, cluster radius and cluster stiffness parameters are estimated by minimizing the following error ϵ:

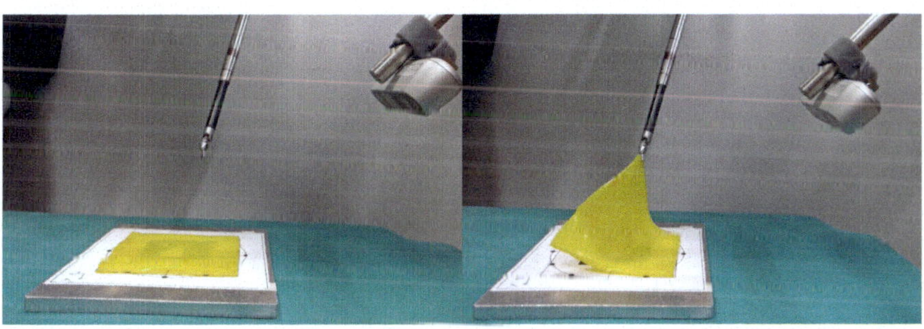

(a) **(b)**

Fig. 4 One of the experiments of the optimization process. The fat tissue is anchored to the calibration board (right side in Figure). **a** Rest condition; **b** Deformed condition. Point cloud of the deformed tissue is acquired with the depth camera shown on the right

$$\epsilon = \frac{1}{N}\sum_{n=1}^{N}\sum_{l=1}^{L}\sum_{m=1}^{M} ||\mathbf{x_{PBD}}(l,n) - \mathbf{x_{PCL}}(l,n)||_2 \tag{2}$$

where $||.||_2$ represents the Euclidean distance between the position of the M particles defining the fat in simulation $\mathbf{x_{PBD}}$, at deformation level l and pinch point n, and the closest point of the corresponding point cloud $\mathbf{x_{PCL}}$. The acquired point cloud has been decimated to bring the number of points comparable to M. The diameter of the PBD particles is set to 3 mm (i.e., the width of our tissue sample), which allows to describe the dynamics of the fat tissue with a single layer of particles. The constraints and the range of allowed values for each parameter are set in the same way as described in [7].

Optimal values for the cluster spacing, radius and stiffness parameters generated with the optimization process are 0.127, 0.095 and 0.361 respectively, which lead to an average error between the simulated and the ground truth point clouds of approximately 3 mm, which is comparable with dimensions of PBD particles. These values are employed to describe the deformable behavior of the fat tissue in the simulation scene.

2.2 *Learning Methods*

In our problem, the agent is represented by the end-effector (EE) of the da Vinci PSM, which interacts with the surrounding anatomical environment, whose initial state is assumed to be known from pre-operative data. Our task consists of moving the PSM arm from a pre-defined initial position $\mathbf{p}_0$ to a position close to the tumor $\mathbf{q}$, grasp the fat and lift it to a pre-defined final position $\mathbf{p}_T$. In order to make the learnt motion primitives robust to different initial configurations, the EE starts from a different position $\mathbf{p}_0$ after each episode (i.e., 2500 timesteps in our case) at training time. Whereas, $\mathbf{p}_T$ is considered fixed through all the training experiments.

The considered state space leverages solely on kinematics information defining the current robot state and the environment, at time t:

$$\begin{aligned} s_t &= [\mathbf{p}_t, \mathbf{q}, \mathbf{p}_T, ||\mathbf{p}_t - \mathbf{q}||_2, ||\mathbf{p}_t - \mathbf{p}_T||_2, g_t] \\ a_t &= [\Delta_t] \end{aligned} \tag{3}$$

where $||.||_2$ is the Euclidean distance. $\Delta_{t,i} = 0.5\alpha$, $\alpha \in \{0, -1, +1\}$ tells the agent if it has to remain still, move backward or forward by 0.5 mm in the i_{th} spatial dimension, while $g_t \in \{0, 1\}$ represents the gripper state (open/close).

The feasibility of using *UnityFlexML* to learn a surgical task is evaluated using two possible strategies: a standard DRL approach and GAIL.

2.2.1 DRL Setting

The first considered method is a model-free on-policy DRL algorithm based on PPO, in its implementation provided by Unity3D ML-Agents. The architecture of the actor-critic networks of the PPO agent used is shown in Fig. 5. For the training phase, we design a reward function which varies with the gripper state, to encourage EE motion towards the tumor if the tissue has not been grasped yet (i.e., gripper is still open), and tissue retraction if the tissue has been already grasped:

$$r_t = \begin{cases} ||\mathbf{p}_t - \mathbf{q}||_2 \cdot k - 0.5, & \text{if } g_t = 0 \\ ||\mathbf{p}_t - \mathbf{p}_T||_2 \cdot k, & \text{if } g_t = 1 \end{cases}$$

The scalar quantity of -0.5 is added to restrict the reward in the range $(-1.0, -0.5)$ before grasping and $(-0.5, 0)$ after grasping. The normalization constant k is introduced to allow re-scaling of the trajectories to different working spaces and is inversely proportional to the maximum distance the PSM can move. During training, the rewards are accumulated at each episode. Being a pure DRL method, this approach is entirely trained in simulation. In the following, we refer to this setting as “PPO”.

2.2.2 GAIL Setting

The second considered approach relies on the learning paradigm provided by GAIL, using a policy generator based on PPO [17]. The network architecture is depicted in Fig. 5. The loss function used in this setting is a linear combination between DRL and GAIL losses $\alpha L_{DRL} + \beta L_{GAIL}$ where α and β represent weighting factors for the two loss functions. Our initial investigation on hyper-parameters tuning yielded best performance for $\alpha = 0.2$ and $\beta = 0.8$. Other values of α and β yielded slower convergence.

Training of a GAIL agent requires the collection of trajectory demonstrations. The acquired trajectories consist of repetitive fat lifting tasks performed by an expert user with the real dVRK, leveraging the communication pipeline provided by *UnityFlexML*. Although our simulation framework supports demonstration recordings using a keyboard or a joystick, the established communication pipeline between dVRK and *UnityFlexML* is crucial since it helps to acquire demonstrations directly with the real robotic system, thus without deviating from the surgical workflow. Overall, we collect a total of 35 task demonstrations. Each recorded demonstration consists of the set of kinematic observations that define the state space and the corresponding action at each timestep. Since the expert is well aware of the final objective of tumor exposure, the grasp position is near the tumor for all the demonstrations. Moreover, the expert user is instructed to diversify the trajectories by starting each demonstration from a different initial position above the fat surface.

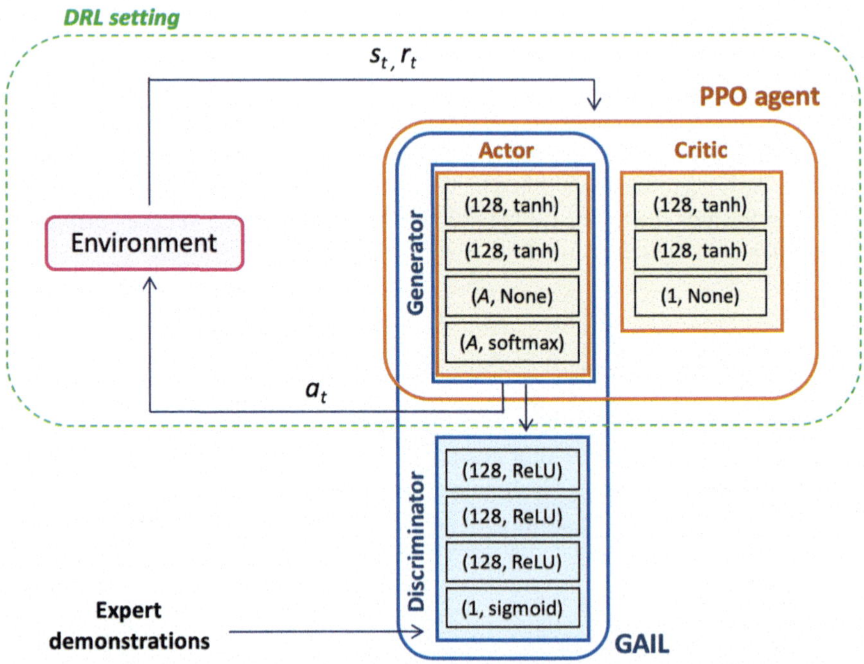

Fig. 5 Network architecture of DRL and GAIL settings. The DRL setup relies on PPO, which consists of actor and critic network. The actor also acts as the policy generator in the GAIL setting. Generated trajectories and expert trajectories are passed to the discriminator. The discriminator learns a probability function which classifies the generator trajectory as expert or non-expert. Details of each network layers are reported inside each box in the format (hidden units, activation) respectively

2.3 Evaluation Metrics

To assess the suitability of the framework as a tool for learning surgical tasks, we test the performance of the considered methods to learn the tissue retraction task when training within *UnityFlexML*. In particular, the high level of realism of the simulated environment created within *UnityFlexML* does not only allow us to train the methods with a sim-to-real approach but also provides a platform for testing the presented methods in realistic settings. As a consequence, the learnt behavior is tested both in a simulated environment, provided by *UnityFlexML*, and in the real one, in a sim-to-real fashion.

Performances of the presented algorithms are tested both in simulation and reality based on two different criteria: sample efficiency and optimality of the accomplished task. Sample efficiency denotes the amount of experience an algorithm needs to learn a behavior by interacting with the environment. It is estimated as the number of time steps required by each algorithm to reach high reward values. Optimality of the learnt behavior represents the ability of each method to make the tumor visible

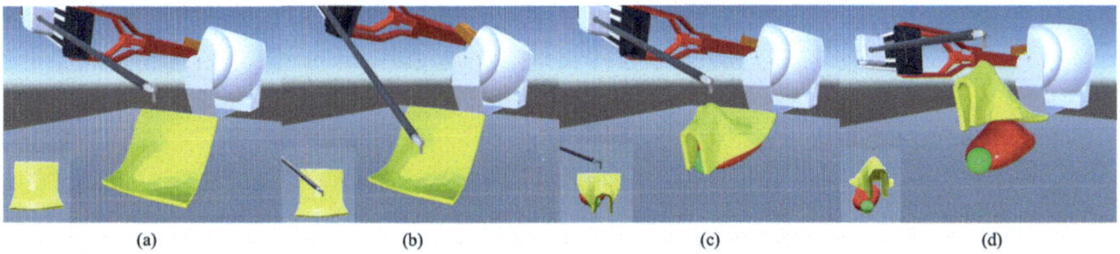

Fig. 6 Sequence of action frames for task completion in simulation: **a** approach, **b** grasp, **c** retract, **d** expose. Perspective of the simulated camera is overlaid on the bottom left of each simulator frame

upon task completion, and is assessed using a Tumour Exposure (TE) metric. We consider the image captured by an endoscope positioned in front of the kidney, both for the simulated and the real setup, where we select a circular region of interest around the tumor (exploiting the fact that its position is known). We then extract the visible portion by applying a mask with HSV bounds matching tumor color. TE is computed as the percentage of tumor pixels which are visible within the region of interest, normalized in the range [0, 1].

3 Autonomous Tissue Retraction in Simulation

After training within *UnityFlexML*, the capability of the two presented methods to successfully accomplish the tissue retraction task is evaluated in simulation (Fig. 6) [17]. In the designed experiment, the trained agents perform the task starting from 49 different positions uniformly sampled on a 7×7 regular grid above the portion of the fat tissue, in order to assess whether the behavior learnt by the agents is robust to different starting positions $\mathbf{p}_0$ of the EE. We evaluate TE each time the EE reaches $\mathbf{p}_T$.

3.1 Results and Discussion

Figure 7 shows the learning curves obtained with the considered learning strategies. Both GAIL and PPO learn to maximize the overall cumulative reward, but with a different pattern. GAIL learning curve shows a monotonous and smooth trend, since it gradually and continuously increases towards high-reward values, diverging from PPO around 1 million steps. Whereas, PPO shows a modular reward trend: it requires 2.5 million steps to learn the approach behavior and interaction with the fat, and 1 million steps to learn the retract behavior. Overall, GAIL is more sample efficient than PPO since it requires fewer steps to learn the task. This experiment shows that incorporating human demonstrations makes learning sample efficient compared to

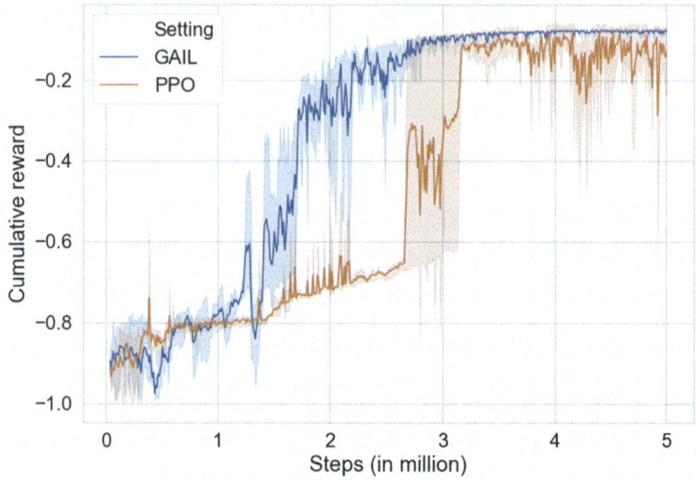

Fig. 7 The obtained learning curve for PPO and GAIL. Cumulative reward is normalised in the range $[-1, 0]$. The shaded area spans the range of values obtained when training the agent starting from three different initialization seeds

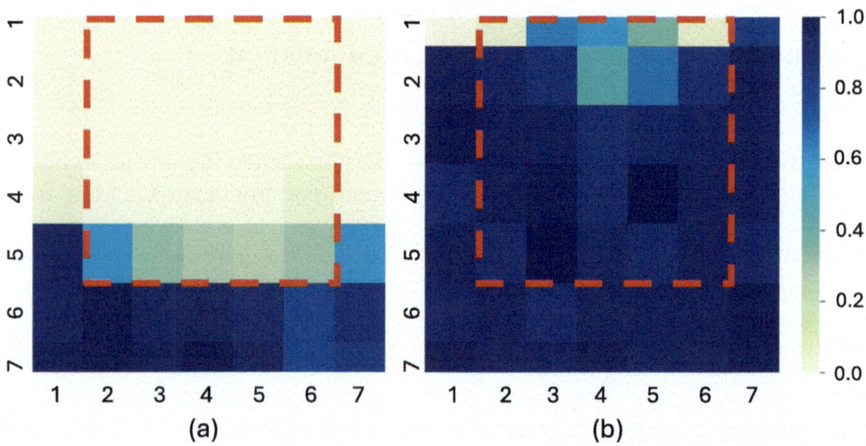

Fig. 8 Simulation experiments: TE from the camera at different starting positions $\mathbf{p}_0$ for **a** PPO, **b** GAIL. The color of each subregion is related to the percentage of visible tumour area when $\mathbf{p}_0$ belongs to that subregion. The fat boundary from the top view is depicted in red dashed lines whereas the fat attachment is shown in the solid red line

baseline PPO, confirming that learning efficiency benefits from the incorporation of human knowledge.

The plot in Fig. 8 shows the TE from the simulated camera depending on the starting position of the PSM arm above and outside the boundary of the fat tissue. Whenever the agent starts from the distal part of the tissue (i.e., the one farther from the fixed region), agents trained with both PPO and GAIL learn to grasp the tissue and the tumor becomes visible from the camera (at least partially).

However, we note that PPO achieves little or no tumor exposure when the starting EE position is close to the fat attachment (Fig. 8a), even though the trained agent has correctly learnt how to perform the task (Fig. 7). It seems that, when $\mathbf{p}_0$ is initialized close to the fixed fat region, the agent is not able to move towards a reasonable grasping point, thus causing the tumor not to be exposed. This is probably due to the fact that we rely on a reward function which is suboptimal for the task. The designed reward function encourages the agent to approach the known position of the tumor, but abruptly changes as soon as the EE is in contact with the tissue regardless of its current grasping position. In this way, we might end up grasping at a location which is not optimal to reach the final objective of exposing the tumor. This suggests that manually tuning the reward function to encode complex task objective such as tumor exposure might be challenging, especially relying on kinematic data only. We expect that including TE-dependent term into the reward function would improve the learnt behavior towards the goal of the task. However, our preliminary evaluation with a reward including a TE-dependent term did not show significant improvements in the results. This might be due to the fact that TE is always zero before grasping, thus represents a sparse reward scenario. We plan to further investigate this in future works.

On the contrary, when human demonstrations are incorporated using GAIL, the learnt behavior allows to expose the tumour regardless of the starting position (Fig. 8b). It is worth noticing that the strategy adopted by the user while acquiring demonstrations is to move and grasp towards points close to the tumor, having clear in mind that the aim is to maximize the exposure. The main difference between the behavior learnt by PPO and GAIL lies in the selection of the grasping point at varying starting position. In particular, when the starting position is above the attached area, GAIL grasps closer to the tumor obtaining a higher TE, since it learns to imitate the human operator, who moves towards the most appropriate points to maximize the exposure.

4 Sim-to-Real Autonomous Tissue Retraction

The behavior learnt with the considered approaches using *UnityFlexML* is transferred to the real robotic platform (Fig. 9). Successful task execution on the real setup relies on two main factors. First of all, it depends on the level of realism of the simulated environment where the agent is trained, because the correct task can be learnt only if the reality gap is minimized. Secondly, it is influenced by the accuracy of the alignment between the simulated and the real environment, since all the movements of the dVRK arm in the real system are controlled through the simulated robot, including the grasping action.

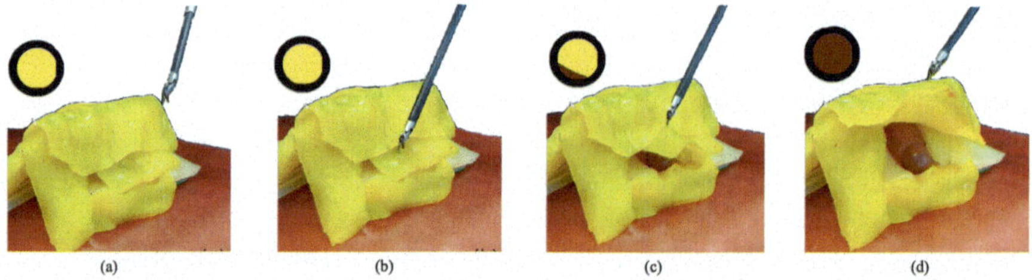

Fig. 9 Sequence of action frames for task completion in real world setup, with the circular mask used to compute TE metric. **a** approach (TE=0%), **b** grasp (TE=0%), **c** retract (TE=∼15%), **d** tumour exposure (TE = 100%). The real camera is placed in front of the phantom, in the same position as in the simulation (which does not correspond to the viewpoint of these pictures)

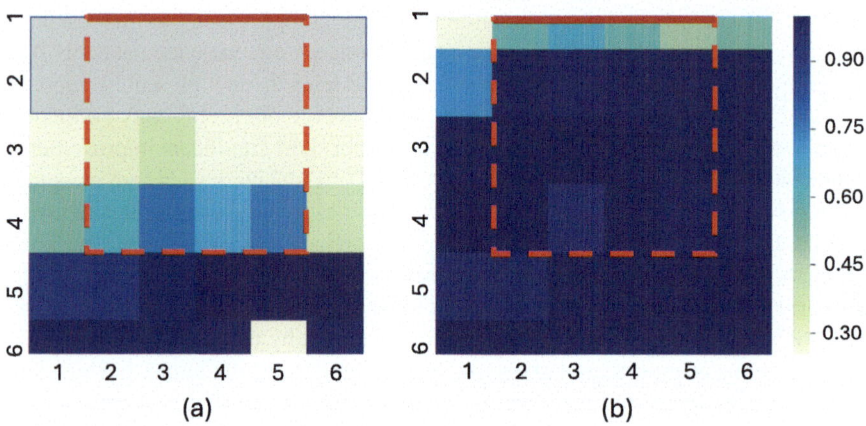

Fig. 10 Real grasp experiments: TE from the camera when starting from different initial positions of the PSM, using **a** PPO **b** GAIL. The portion of fat tissue which is not considered for the experiments is coloured in gray

4.1 Results and Discussion

The real and simulated setup are initially aligned with respect to the same reference frame, defined by the center of the calibration board (Fig. 3b). The mean positioning error of the PSM arm is 1.7 mm.

We have been able to successfully replicate the learned behaviour from the simulated to the real environment without any appreciable inconsistency. The dVRK end-effector successfully gets in contact with the fat tissue for all the different initial positions, and it is always able to reach the target point. The tumor exposure percentage starting from various points above the real fat tissue is illustrated in Fig. 10. Considering the results obtained in simulation, we did not consider starting positions near the attachment when testing the behavior learnt with PPO (represented as the unattempted gray region in Fig. 10a) to avoid tissue tearing that might occur in case of grasping too close to the attached area.

If we consider the average TE over all trials from different starting points, PPO achieves an average TE of 0.38 while GAIL obtains an average TE of 0.90. When comparing the results obtained for GAIL and PPO, it emerges that GAIL is not only able to reach higher overall exposure, but it is also more robust to changes in the initial PSM position. In particular, tumor exposure is achieved also when starting from points that were unattempted for PPO (Fig. 10b), thus suggesting an overall improvement in performances, due to a more optimal learnt trajectory. This observation indicates that the initial PSM position has a great impact on the performances in the case of PPO, whereas GAIL is able to reach optimal performance regardless of the starting position, confirming results obtained in the simulated experiments. Overall, our results show that performance using demonstrations is robust and outperforms PPO both in simulation and real world.

5 Conclusion

In this Chapter, we have shown that simulation can support the process of learning a surgical task. The main advantage of using simulation to this purpose is that it allows to train all those learning approaches that require a high number of trial and error attempts within a personalized, safe and controlled environment. We have designed and implemented *UnityFlexML*, a modular framework which supports simulation of deformable objects, can be interfaced with learning algorithms and communicates with the real robotic system (in our case the dVRK). The platform has proved suitable for training learning-based approaches on a real surgical robotic application, i.e. fat tissue manipulation for the exposure of tumor during robot assisted nephrectomy procedure. The proposed framework does not only allow to train standard DRL approaches entirely in simulation, but it also provides an interface to acquire task executions by expert users on the real robotic system that can be used in LfD settings. Thanks to a calibration procedure for optimizing the simulation parameters to reduce the reality gap, behaviors learnt in simulation have been successfully transferred to the real robotic system. A further advantage of having a simulation framework is that it can be employed as a verification environment where to test the learnt behavior before its execution on the real system. This has allowed us to avoid the execution of potentially unsafe configurations that emerged from tests in simulation (i.e., starting from positions close to the attached area). All these factors make the proposed simulation environment an essential component in development of autonomous agents for controlling surgical tools and manipulating soft tissues.

Although we have considered a simplified anatomical setup, the modularity of the framework will allow to easily increase the complexity of the simulation, for example including multiple organs and both robotic arms, to enable learning and testing of multiple procedural steps. We expect that this will not introduce a drop in computational performance, due to reliance of the framework on the optimized NVIDIA FleX plugin to render soft object deformations.

Considering the exploited learning algorithms, future work will focus on the incorporation of visual cues, for example learning the task starting from the endoscopic images directly. Doing this, we will implicitly account for the current deformed tissue configuration. Sim-to-real transfer is likely to be more challenging in this case, since it will be essential to cope with the unavoidable difference between simulated and real endoscopic images. A possible strategy to cope with this issue will be to rely on methods for image-to-image translation like [18–20], which will allow to transfer the style of real images to simulated ones.

References

1. Tagliabue, Eleonora, et al. (2020) Soft tissue simulation environment to learn manipulation tasks in autonomous robotic surgery. In: 2020 IEEE/RSJ International Conference on Intelligent Robots and Systems (IROS), IEEE
2. "ROS - Robot Operating System." https://www.ros.org/. Accessed 12 Oct 2024
3. Richter, F., Orosco, R.K., Yip, M.C.: Open-sourced reinforcement learning environments for surgical robotics (2019). arXiv:1903.02090
4. "Unity Technologies." https://unity.com/. Accessed 03 Nov 2024
5. Juliani, A., Berges, V.-P., Vckay, E., Gao, Y., Henry, H., Mattar, M., Lange, D.: Unity: a general platform for intelligent agents (2018). arXiv:1809.02627
6. "NVIDIA gameworks. Nvidia FleX" (2018). https://developer.nvidia.com/flex. Accessed 20 Feb 2025
7. Tagliabue, E., Dall'Alba, D., Magnabosco, E., Tenga, C., Peterlik, I., Fiorini, P., Position-based modeling of lesion displacement in ultrasound-guided breast biopsy. Int. J. Comput. Assist. Radiol. Surg. (2019)
8. Qian, L., Deguet, A., Kazanzides, P.: dVRK-XR: mixed reality extension for da Vinci research kit. In: Hamlyn Symposium on Medical Robotics (2019)
9. Polydoros, A.S., Nalpantidis, L.: Survey of model-based reinforcement learning: applications on robotics. J. Intell. Robot. Syst. **86**(2), 153–173 (2017)
10. Nagabandi, A., Kahn, G., Fearing, R.S., Levine, S.: Neural network dynamics for model-based deep reinforcement learning with model-free fine-tuning. In: 2018 IEEE International Conference on Robotics and Automation (ICRA), pp. 7559–7566. IEEE (2018)
11. Schrittwieser, J., Antonoglou, I., Hubert, T., Simonyan, K., Sifre, L., Schmitt, S., Guez, A., Lockhart, E., Hassabis, D., Graepel, T., et al.: Mastering Atari, Go, chess and shogi by planning with a learned model. Nature **588**(7839), 604–609 (2020)
12. Schulman, J., Wolski, F., Dhariwal, P., Radford, A., Klimov, O.: Proximal policy optimization algorithms (2017). arXiv:1707.06347
13. Dixon, M.F., Halperin, I., Bilokon, P.: Inverse reinforcement learning and imitation learning. In: Machine Learning in Finance, pp. 419–517. Springer, Berlin (2020)
14. Bain, M., Sammut, C.: A framework for behavioural cloning. Mach. Intell. **15**, 103–129 (1995)
15. Ho, J., Ermon, S.: Generative adversarial imitation learning. In: Advances in Neural Information Processing Systems, pp. 4565–4573 (2016)
16. Creswell, A., White, T., Dumoulin, V., Arulkumaran, K., Sengupta, B., Bharath, A.A.: Generative adversarial networks: an overview. IEEE Signal Process. Mag. **35**(1), 53–65 (2018)
17. Pore, Ameya, et al. (2021) Learning from demonstrations for autonomous soft-tissue retraction. In: 2021 international symposium on medical robotics (ISMR), IEEE, pp 1–7
18. Pfeiffer, M., Funke, I., Robu, M.R., Bodenstedt, S., Strenger, L., Engelhardt, S., Roß, T., Clarkson, M.J., Gurusamy, K., Davidson, B.R., et al.: Generating large labeled data sets for laparoscopic image processing tasks using unpaired image-to-image translation. In: International

Conference on Medical Image Computing and Computer-Assisted Intervention, pp. 119–127. Springer, Berlin (2019)
19. Rivoir, D., Pfeiffer, M., Docea, R., Kolbinger, F., Riediger, C., Weitz, J., Speidel, S.: Long-term temporally consistent unpaired video translation from simulated surgical 3D data (2021). arXiv:2103.17204
20. Scheikl, Paul Maria, et al. (2022) Sim-to-real transfer for visual reinforcement learning of deformable object manipulation for robot-assisted surgery. IEEE Robot Autom Lett 8(2):560–567

New Hardware: Design, Models and Analysis

Andrea Calanca, Zhuoqi Cheng, Diego Dall'Alba, Paolo Fiorini, Giovanni Gerardo Muscolo, and Chiara Zandoná

Abstract To achieve the results described in the previous chapters, it was necessary to *ground* our logical statements by making precise measurements of the surrounding environment, to determine the position of the instruments and of the targets, to assess the interaction with the tissues and to make predictions on the instrument behavior. Some of these measures were obtained by standard instruments, as described in Chap. 7, whereas in other cases new instruments were designed, simulated and developed to address the specific needs of the ARS project. Similarly, instrument performance would depend on their interaction with the environments and an analytical model could provide useful indication on how to interpret the obtained results.

The original version of the chapter has been revised. A correction to this chapter can be found at https://doi.org/10.1007/978-3-032-04247-7_17

A. Calanca · D. Dall'Alba · P. Fiorini (✉)
Department of Engineering for Innovation Medicine, University of Verona, Verona, Italy
e-mail: paolo.fiorini@univr.it

A. Calanca
e-mail: andrea.calanca@univr.it

D. Dall'Alba
e-mail: Diego.dallalba@univr.it

Z. Cheng
Italian Institute of Technology, Genova, Italy
e-mail: zch@mmmi.sdu.dk

University of Southern Denmark, Odense, Denmark

G. G. Muscolo
ECT*, Fondazione Bruno Kessler, Trento, Italy
e-mail: gmuscolo@ectstar.eu; giovanni.muscolo@unitn.it

Department of Physics, University of Trento, Trento, Italy

C. Zandoná
Department of Computer Science, University of Verona, Verona, Italy
e-mail: chiara.zandona@asem.it

ASEM Srl, Verona, Italy

P. Fiorini (ed.), *Towards Autonomous Robotic Surgery*, Springer Tracts in Advanced Robotics 161, https://doi.org/10.1007/978-3-032-04247-7_11

In this chapter we summarize the study of the interaction and measurements of surgical instruments with the anatomical tissues. In fact, an analytical model can help assess the interaction accuracy by determining whether the instrument is subject to some, albeit small, deflections as summarized in Sect. 1. This analysis was tested in simulation and experiments, but the lack of time prevented their integration in the experimental surgical system. Furthermore, two sensing methods and their hardware implementations were developed to address different shortcomings of the robotic instruments for minimally invasive surgery: one measures the electric properties of the tissues, in Sect. 2, the other measures the internal deflection of the surgical instrument in Sect. 3. Both properties give indications about the type of tissue the instrument is interacting with, and about other physiological properties, such as vascularization and density.

1 Instrument Modeling

The simplest instrument used in medical practices is the needle, which is essential in many diagnostic and therapeutical procedures. As discussed later in Chap. 15 needle-based procedures were also the topic of the ERC Proof of Concept (PoC) grants that were awarded to explore the feasibility of translating the ARS research into clinical practice. The first PoC was the PROST project aimed at improving the final step of prostate cancer (PCa) diagnosis, i.e. the prostate biopsy for the examination of the potentially cancerous tissue.

Needle biopsy is the most reliable technique for detecting PCa and estimating its aggressiveness [1]. The majority of biopsies are performed under ultrasound guidance. Traditional transrectal biopsy is being replaced by the safer transperineal biopsy, which reduces infection risks but requires a more experienced operator to reach the desired targets. Robot-assisted needle insertion proposed in PROST, described in Chap. 15, can improve the accuracy of this procedure without damaging tissues, organs, and vessels. Unfortunately, precise needle placement is difficult to accomplish in real practice because of tissue heterogeneity, needle bending, and tissue/organ deformation and movement. As a result, modelling the interaction between the needle and the tissue is a critical requirement for safe and accurate robotic needle insertion.

Biopsy needles with a bevelled tip are the most commonly used and, when entering the prostate, they deflect due to tissue forces acting on the bevelled tip, producing an unwanted deflection and degrading the accuracy of the biopsy.

During transperineal prostate biopsy, the surgeon can compensate for the needle deformation by twisting it during the insertion in the prostate based on visual feedback. If we consider robotic insertions of the needle, visual feedback may not be sufficient because of the limitation of echography images, and a plan to compensate for the bending during insertion would be necessary.

In planning, needle modelling becomes of paramount importance, as discussed by several authors [2, 3], addressing kinematic models, finite element (FE) models, and quasi-static approximated mechanical models. In this research we expanded the kinematic model for needle insertion first presented in [4], followed by a nonholonomic 3D bicycle-like model [5], and an extended model using an omnidirectional wheel in [6]. Unlike finite element and quasi-static models, kinematic models are computationally more efficient and easier to parameterize. Moreover, they inherently capture the three-dimensional steering effects resulting from needle twisting. In this part of our research, we carried an experimental comparison of kinematic models evaluating their accuracy in the context of a transperineal prostate biopsy, considering different needle insertion speeds and different organ stiffnesses. Due to issue in needle shape reconstruction, we limit our analysis to the two-dimensional case. The full analysis is reported in [7].

1.1 Kinematic Models

The transperineal prostate biopsy procedure consists of straight needle insertion into tissues without twisting. The needle models consider a bevelled-tip needle driven by insertion speed v. The tip moves along a path defined by the surrounding material's properties, the geometry of the needle's bevelled tip, and the needle insertion speed.

We suppose that the needle is inserted at constant velocity v, measured with respect to the A frame along the z-axis and without twisting. The unicycle model presented in [4], considers the needle tip as located at the center of a single wheel (unicycle) lying on the ZY plane as shown in Fig. 1.

According to this model, the needle tip follows a planar path formed by single-arc of fixed curvature with center $c = [0, c_y]$ and radius r, considering the entry point at $(0, 0)$ in the $\{A\}$ frame. Here we assume that the needle tip is oriented such that bending occurs toward the negative y-axis as shown in Fig. 1.

Fig. 1 Unicycle model of a flexible needle with a bevelled tip

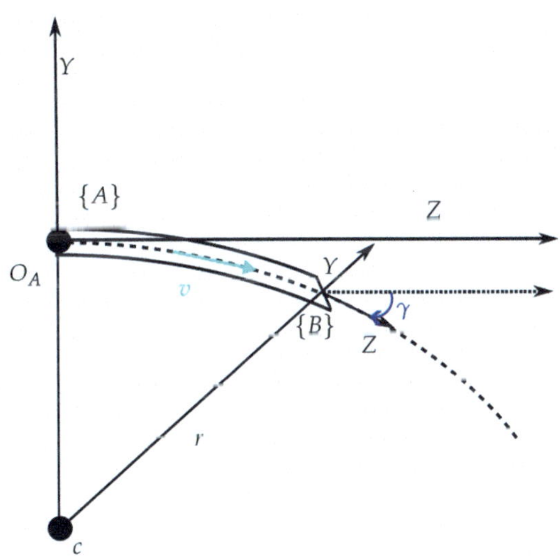

Since the wheel movement satisfies the pure rolling, non-slipping, constraint, in the $\{B\}$ frame, the velocity has only z-axis component, without lateral movements:

$$v_z = v_{in} \tag{1a}$$

$$v_y = 0 \tag{1b}$$

where we suppose that the wheel speed v_z equals the insertion velocity v_{in}.

The dynamic model of the needle can be described as:

$$\dot{z}(t) = \cos\theta(t)v_z \tag{2a}$$

$$\dot{y}(t) = \sin\theta(t)v_z \tag{2b}$$

$$\dot{\theta}(t) = -\frac{v_z}{r} \tag{2c}$$

Considering the initial conditions of the model at the beginning of the needle insertion ($t = 0$) as $z = 0$, $y = 0$ and $\theta = 0$, the solution to the kinematic equations is:

$$z(t) = -r\sin\theta(t) \tag{3a}$$

$$y(t) = c_y + r\cos\theta(t) \tag{3b}$$

$$\theta(t) = -\frac{v_z}{r}t \tag{3c}$$

with r constant.

The extended bicycle model [6] considers a bicycle lying on the ZY plane as shown in Fig. 2. The labels $\{A\}$, $\{B\}$ and $\{C\}$ denote, respectively, the global fixed frame, the needle tip frame (back wheel) and the front wheel frame.

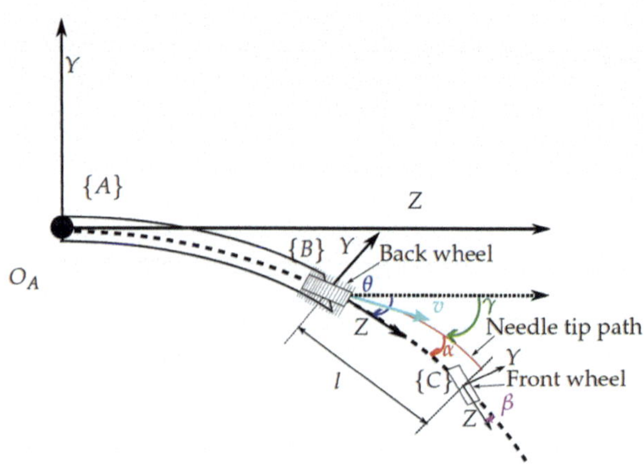

Fig. 2 Extended bicycle model of a flexible needle with a bevelled tip

The model consists of two wheels positioned at a fixed distance l from each other with the front wheel oriented at a fixed angle β. When the needle is moving forward into the tissue, lateral movements can also happen because of tissue deformation. In this case, the final shape of the needle doesn't follow the tip path. This model, in contrast to the unicycle one, accounts for this phenomenon by considering an additional state.

As for the unicycle model, the needle path points toward the negative y-axis. The variables (z, y, θ, γ) denote the configuration of the needle tip, where (z, y, θ) is the $\{B\}$ frame configuration, as in the unicycle model, and γ is the angle between the z-axis of the $\{A\}$ frame and the needle tip path. This angle differs from the $\{B\}$ frame orientation θ because of the tissue deformation.

Within the $\{B\}$ frame, back wheel movement satisfies the pure rolling constraint along z-axis, as in the unicycle model in Eq. 1, but slips laterally along the y-axis to account for tissue deformation. The lateral slipping velocity v_y is defined using an arbitrary function $f(\gamma, \lambda)$ as:

$$v_y = f(\gamma, \lambda) v_z \tag{4}$$

where λ represents the tissue-specific parameter related to its mechanical properties. Using this function, the time variation of θ, can be expressed as:

$$\dot{\theta} = \frac{1}{l}[\tan \beta + f(\gamma, \lambda)] v_z \tag{5}$$

The angle α represents the rotation of the needle tip velocity in the needle tip frame $\{B\}$ causing the needle to follow a non-constant curvature path. Therefore, γ is equal to $\theta + \alpha$. As the needle bends toward the negative y-axis, the tissue deformation pulls the needle in the opposite direction, so $\alpha \in [0, \pi/2]$ and $\theta \leq \gamma$ with $\gamma \in [-\pi/2, 0]$. The back wheel slippage α is related to the $f(\gamma, \lambda)$ function of Eq. (4) by:

$$\alpha = \tan^{-1} f(\gamma, \lambda) = \lambda_1 \gamma^2 + \lambda_2 \gamma \tag{6}$$

where the angle α is expressed as a quadratic function of γ, as in [6].

Formally, the kinematics of the model can be written as:

$$\dot{z} = \frac{\cos(\gamma)}{\cos(\alpha)} v_z \tag{7a}$$

$$\dot{y} = \frac{\sin(\gamma)}{\cos(\alpha)} v_z \tag{7b}$$

$$\dot{\gamma} = \frac{\dot{\theta}}{1 - \frac{\partial \alpha}{\partial \gamma}} \tag{7c}$$

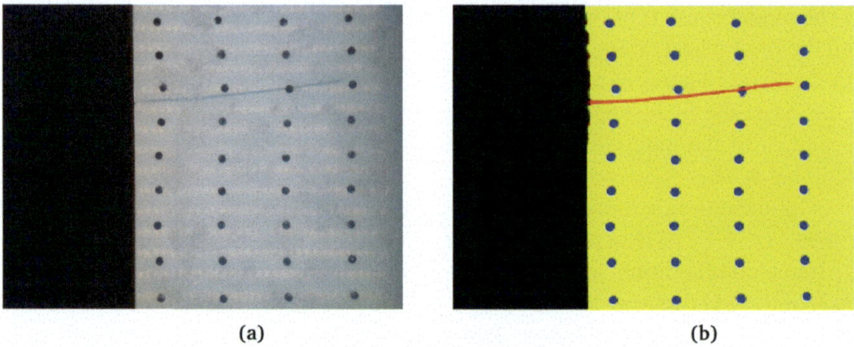

Fig. 3 Examples of image segmentation for needle identification

1.2 Experimental Methods

The experimental comparison is conducted using the setup shown in Fig. 4, which comprises a robotic system performing needle insertion with a beveled-tip needle. The system is equipped with a force sensor mounted at the needle base and an external RGB-D camera for visual tracking. Insertions are carried out on phantoms with different stiffness, designed to emulate prostate tissue at different tumor stages, as classified by the Gleason score, which is commonly used to assess tumor progression.

A required step of a fair experimental comparison, is to identify the optimal parameters for both the unicycle and extended bicycle models to best predict needle tip trajectory. While the identification procedures and outcomes are described in the next section, here we briefly present the vision algorithm that identifies and tracks the needle tip during its insertion.

The vision algorithm is based on semantic segmentation provided by the Generative Adversarial Network (GAN) model [8]. Compared to other approaches, this method has the advantage of requiring very few RGB samples representing the setup to obtain high-quality results.

Figure 3 shows an example of segmentation of an image acquired by the camera, described in Chap. 7.

A chessboard under the needle allows retrieving the pixel/millimeter ratio that is needed to have the needle position in the 3D metric space.

The coordinates (z, y) of the needle tip, which are derived from the mask obtained through semantic segmentation for each frame, were individually subjected to a third order polynomial fitting process over time-to-position data in order to mitigate measurement noise.

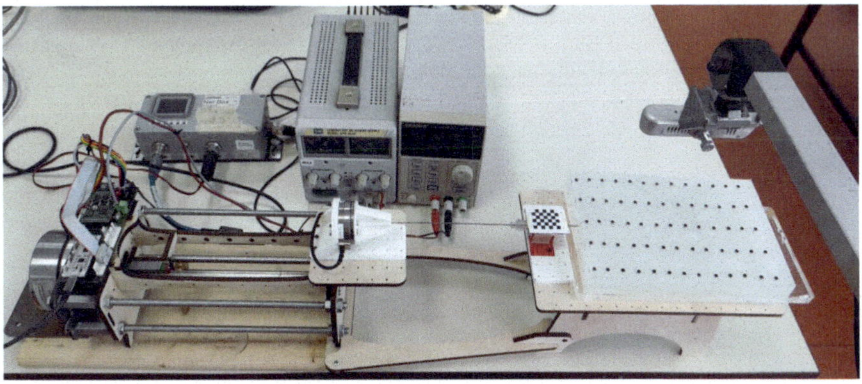

Fig. 4 Setup of the needle bending experiments

1.3 Experimental Results

We designed the device shown in Fig. 4 to test insertion into tissues, with one degree of freedom (DoF) capable of translational motion along the needle's principal axis. The trajectory of the needle tip is reconstructed using an *Intel RealSense D435* camera positioned approximately 20 cm from the surface of the phantom, operating at a rate 30 Hz to capture the images fed into the vision algorithm. The use of transparent phantoms and a camera allows us to acquire the entire needle tip trajectory during the insertion with good accuracy.

In the experiments, a standard 18-gauge brachytherapy needle with a bevel angle of 15° was used. We evaluated four transparent phantoms with varying stiffness values in the range between 32.8 and 107 kPa simulating both benign and malign conditions of the prostate gland [9, 10]. The needle was inserted to a depth of 100 mm considered to be the typical distance between the perineum and the apex of the prostate at two different velocities (10, 20 mm/s). For each stiffness and velocity pair, we perform four repetitions.

We estimate the parameters of the models by performing a least squares identification for the unicycle model and using a genetic algorithm for the extended bicycle model as described in [7]. The unicycle model parameters are $(0, c_y)$ and the radius r in Eq. 3 which are easily estimated using a least square regression. The parameters of the extended bicycle model are β and l in Eq. 5 and λ_1, λ_2 in Eq. 6.

The parameter identification originally proposed for the extended bicycle model does not always lead to suitable results due to several local minima in the objective function, even by trying to impose additional constraints. For this reason, we used a genetic algorithm. We measured an average computation time of 0.7 ms for the unicycle model identification and a significantly higher time, 45 s (range 20–65 s), for the extended bicycle model, on Intel Core i7-6700HQ processor.

To enhance the robustness of the identification procedure for both models, the estimated parameters are averaged over the data obtained from the first three inser-

Table 1 Maximum tip prediction error and the root-mean-squared error (RMSE) for Unicycle Model e_{maxM1} and Extended Bicycle Model e_{maxM2} considering 8 experimental conditions (4 phantoms and 2 velocities pair) with four repetitions each

Insertion velocity [mm/s]	Stiffness [kPa]	e_{maxM1} [mm]	e_{maxM2} [mm]	$RMSE_{M1}$ [mm]	$RMSE_{M2}$ [mm]
10	30	0.18	0.77	0.11	0.49
	50	0.32	0.45	0.26	0.27
	70	0.43	2.07	0.31	0.76
	100	0.44	1.04	0.28	0.71
20	30	0.20	0.61	0.12	0.19
	50	0.22	0.45	0.18	0.26
	70	0.29	0.78	0.19	0.33
	100	0.75	1.24	0.29	0.85

tions. The prediction accuracy of the two models is then evaluated by comparing the simulated needle trajectory with the experimental data from the fourth repetition.

Prediction results are reported in Table 1. Both models revealed to be quite accurate in predicting the tip's final position, since we achieved a tenth of a millimetre of RMSE accuracy. The maximum errors were less than or equal to 0.75 mm for the unicycle model and less or equal to 2.07 mm for the extended bicycle model.

In spite of its lower complexity, the unicycle model is more accurate than the extended bicycle model. This may be due to two factors: (1) it is not proven that the higher complexity of the extended bicycle model can better match the needle insertion physics; (2) the model is highly non-linear with respect to parameters, thus requiring an iterative identification procedure, which is time consuming and subject to both noise and local minima. For both models, higher prediction errors were obtained when the needle was pushed into the more rigid phantoms at the highest velocity (20 mm/s). The computationally intense identification of the extended bicycle model makes it unsuitable for online re-parametrization, which can be used to accommodate for uncertainties in tissue parameters.

Modelling the deformation of the needle and the surrounding tissue during insertion into the prostate would allow surgeons to accurately take tissue samples and identify the prostate cancer stage and its risk level. Further work will be needed to include a more realistic, non homogeneous, tissues with different stiffness levels, to simulate a more realistic needle insertion, including the influence of skin tension, and subcutaneous fat.

2 Electrical Bio-impedance Sensing for Intraoperative Organ Identification

The incorporation of real-time sensing technologies during complex medical procedures is an essential component for novel surgical robotic platforms to complement the information coming from different types of vision sensors. In fact, vision alone may not be always sufficient for tissue recognition, because many organs are visually similar through the endoscopic camera, also because of poor illumination, occlusions and smoke [11]. Furthermore, organ recognition is necessary to provide surgical context awareness, as discussed in Chap. 7, which is essential for cognitive support and enables autonomous functions in surgical robots [12].

To fill this gap in the available sensing technologies, it is necessary to develop new sensors and sensing methods that could ensure safer and faster robot-assisted minimally invasive surgeries (RAMIS). For example, force sensors, such as those discussed in Sect. 3 and those deployed into articulated surgical tools to provide haptic feedback to surgeons [13, 14], have complex mechanical designs, require modifications to existing surgical tools, and advanced control schemes to avoid instability when force feedback is provided to the user. Furthermore, the price increase due to the addition of these sensors is not negligible, even in the context of the already expensive surgical robots.

To address this challenge, ARS researchers joined forces with the Biomedical Robotics Group of the Italian Institute of Technology (IIT) [15] to develop a line of novel intra-operative sensing technologies that would not require modifications to the existing instruments, be low cost, and provide the information needed for organ recognition and situation awareness. Several novel surgical sensing methods and the corresponding physical sensors for intraoperative tissue identification were developed based on electrical bio-impedance (EBI) technology and an advanced user interfaces (AUI) for the display of graphical information [16–24]. These theoretical and experimental results are summarized in the following Sections.

2.1 The Bipolar Sensor

The EBI sensing principle evolved from the implementation of a single sensor for tissue discrimination, to multiple sensor design for hidden organ identification, to scanning protocols to map the structures hidden from view.

The first implementation of this technology was with a bipolar EBI sensor. An EBI sensor can be integrated into a standard bipolar tool for providing fast and accurate tissue detection and identification, and is shown in Fig. 5a. It can be mounted into a standard instrument of da Vinci Research Kit (dVRK) [25] described in Chap. 1, Sect. 3.

The EBI sensor is integrated to the bipolar robotic forceps mounted on the Patient Side Manipulator (PSM) of the dVRK. It measures the magnitude of electrical

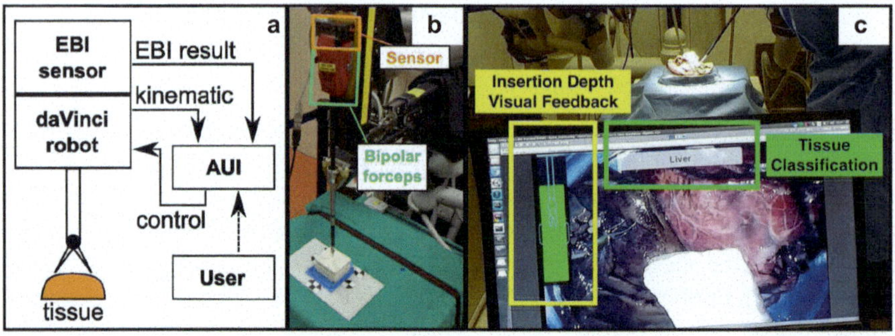

Fig. 5 **a** The schematic of the proposed system; **b** The designed EBI sensor is mounted on the top surface of a standard Maryland bipolar forceps; **c** The Advanced User Interface is designed to control the EBI sensing and display the identification results

impedance of the tissue contacting the tool tips. The measured values are sent to the connected computer for signal processing and tissue identification. The tissue identification results and the augmented-reality labels are displayed on the AUI. The theoretical and experimental details of this approach are given in [21].

2.1.1 The Theoretical Concepts

Figure 5b shows the hardware of the EBI sensor directly mounted on a bipolar robotic tool from the dVRK using a standard Maryland bipolar forceps (Ref. 400172). The two jaws of the bipolar forceps are used as an electrode pair for EBI sensing. To measure the electrical impedance of a tissue sample, an excitation alternate voltage U is applied through the tissue sample. By measuring the feedback current I, the impedance of the tissue Z can be calculated as the voltage to current ratio, and furthermore I can be calculated as the integration of the current density (J_{tot}):

$$Z = \frac{U}{I} = \frac{U}{\int J_{tot}} \tag{8}$$

The total current density (J_{tot}) includes two components: the real part J_c and the virtual part J_d, and it can be computed as:

$$J_{tot} = J_c + J_d = \sigma E - -i\omega\epsilon E \tag{9}$$

where σ and ϵ represent the conductivity and the permittivity of the contacted material, E is the electric field, and ω is used to denote the excitation frequency. Therefore, the modulus of the measured EBI value |Z| can be calculated as:

$$|Z| = \frac{|U|}{|\sigma - i\omega\epsilon| \times |\int E|} \tag{10}$$

The modulus $|Z|$ was used for the tissue identification, which is a function of the excitation voltage $|U|$, the material electric characteristics ($|\sigma - i\omega\epsilon|$) and the electric field generated by the bipolar forceps ($|\int E|$).

In Eq. 10, the modulus ($|\sigma - i\omega\epsilon|$) represents the electric characteristics of the bio-material when the applied voltage U has a constant frequency ω.

As shown in Fig. 5b, the EBI sensor's compact dimensions ($14 \times 20 \times 64$ mm) enable it to be mounted directly on the top surface of a standard da Vinci surgical tool. The sensor measures the EBI of the tissue when the jaws at the proximal end of the forceps are in contact with the tissue through the same electric connections for the bipolar electrification.

In the first prototype, described in [21], the excitation frequency of the EBI sensor was set to 100 kHz for the tissue measurement to achieve a real-time sampling rate of 50 Hz, as discussed in [17], and to have a better tissue discrimination, as described in [26, 27]. In fact, at higher excitation frequencies ($f > 50$ kHz), the cell membrane becomes more electrically permeable. Thus, the measured impedance can give information of both intracellular impedance and extracellular impedance, leading to a better description of the tissue's electrical properties.

The EBI system was calibrated using several resistors of known values ranging from 786Ω to $8.2k\Omega$, which covers the expected range for biological tissue electrical impedance. The error rate was found to be 0.59% in average, and the maximum error was found to be 1.2%. For a more detailed analysis of the measurement performance of the proposed system please refer to [18, 20].

2.1.2 The Advanced User Interface (AUI)

The AUI can be merged to the surgeon console to give an augmented reality (AR) visualization of additional information about the surgical scene, together with the kinematics information retrieved from the robotic system.

As shown in Fig. 5c, the AUI is designed to show three different pieces of information in real time. Firstly, it shows the result of the classification in text form. Secondly, a 3D point on the measurement site is created on the AUI to mark the classified tissue. Thirdly, a visual feedback of the insertion depth which is derived from the robotic kinematic information is displayed for guiding the user during the EBI measurement.

The AUI allows visualizing the data collected in a virtual environment that replicates the real surgical setup. The virtual environment preserves the depth perception of the surgical scene and allows the projection of additional information (e.g., user interfaces, 3D models or point-clouds). The punctual EBI information can be overlapped to the endoscopic images in the AUI, after the hand-to-eye calibration [28].

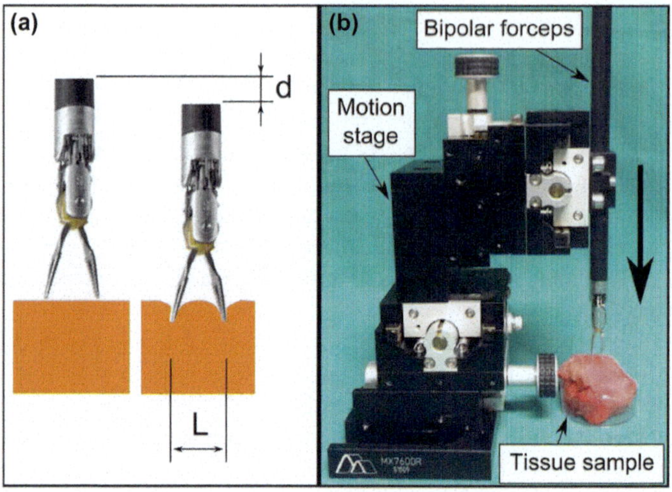

Fig. 6 **a** Parameters L and d of the electrodes configuration used to estimate the electric field. **b** The system setup for testing four tissue types with different L and d values

2.1.3 Experimental Setup and Results

A classifier was designed to identify the tissue in contact with the forceps's tip. For this, we first collected datasets of the $|Z|$ values of different tissue types with different tissue penetration d and jaws opening L, as shown in Fig. 6a.

The setup for collecting data from different tissue types is shown in Fig. 6b. The EBI sensor was connected and mounted to the bipolar robotic forceps, which was then fixed to the motion stage (Siskyou, USA). The penetration depth d was controlled by tuning the stage downwards. The EBI measurements were collected with d varying from 2 to 4 mm with 1 mm steps. During the application, the sensing system and the forceps should be integrated into the dVRK. The user controls the forceps to press the tissue manually via the surgeon console.

This basic configuration of the EBI system was evaluated with three types of ex vivo porcine tissues including abdominal muscle, liver and lung. In total, 18 pieces of porcine tissues were prepared (6 pieces for each tissue type), among which 9 pieces were used for training and the other 9 pieces were used for system evaluation. In Fig. 7a, 200 points were generated to describe the statistical model of each tissue type including the EBI measurement $|Z|$, the L and the d used for the measurement. Figure 7b provides a magnified view for better showing the normal distributions of muscle and liver.

Given 95% confidence, the experimental results prove that these three tissue types can be successfully classified by the proposed sensing system since there are no intersections among them.

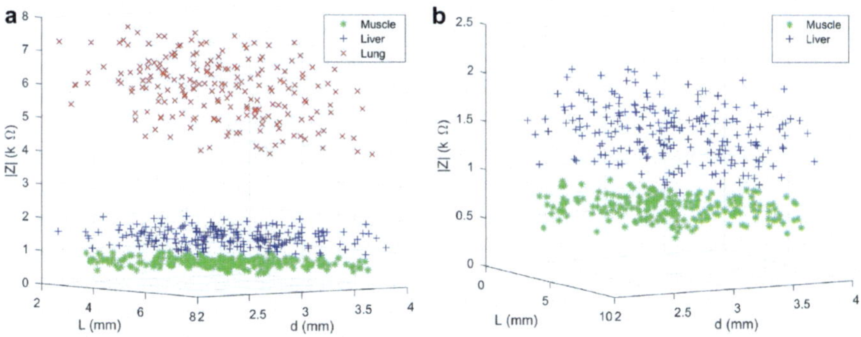

Fig. 7 200 points per tissue are used to describe the multivariate normal distribution of the collected EBI measurements |Z|, the jaw opening distance L, and the pressing depth d

2.2 The Tripolar Sensor

To overcome the dependency of the impedance measurements on the jaw opening angle and penetration depth, a second EBI sensing method was developed which employs two standard surgical instruments with electrosurgical function (such as mono-polar or bi-polar forceps) as electrodes [29]. One electrode is used for providing a current source and the other electrode is for measuring voltage on the tissue surface. Both current source and measured voltages are referred to a third sink electrode positioned in a distal region with respect to the measurement site, as shown in Fig. 8. The resulting system was called Robot Assisted Electrical bio-Impedance Sensing (RAEIS) system, and it is shown in Fig. 8. The theoretical and experimental details of this approach are given in [22].

Based on its enhanced flexibility and sensing capability, this system could be used for measuring tissue electrical resistivity in a local region and for the detection of subsurface non-homogeneous structure.

Figure 9a shows the schematic of the bipolar EBI sensing system. In the excitation frequency range, about 1 kHz to 1 MHz, the measured EBI normally involves a polarization impedance (Z_{el}) serialising the Material Under Test (MUT) due to the interfacial layers between the metal electrode and the tissue. Therefore, the resistance of the MUT is hard to measure accurately using a bi-polar EBI configuration. In the tripolar sensing system, as shown in Fig. 9b, the excitation source and the voltage measurement are separated [16]. By doing so, the effects of Z_{el} can be compensated by using a controlled current source to maintain a constant current through the MUT. In addition, the input impedance for the electrical potential measurement can be made very high to avoid current flows through the voltage monitor electrode. Thus, the generated electric field is not affected by the contact between the electrodes and tissue.

The current source electrode and voltage measuring electrode can be realized by two separate surgical forceps/tools. This allows the system to measure the targeted site flexibly. Also, through adjusting the distance between the two electrodes, the measured impedance covers a different range of materials, and thus enables the sensing of subsurface tissue at different depths.

The sensing technology for detecting the subsurface tissue in this study is inspired by the electrical survey method used in geophysics, where the electrode configuration and method is commonly known as the Wenner-Schlumberger array [30].

This method can be used also in the case where the tissue consists of two layers, as the current introduced from the electrode includes two parts: the direct current and the part caused by the reflected current [30]. When the distance between the electrodes is small, the material resistivities are approximately equal and represent the electrical resistivity of the superficial material. By increasing the distance between two electrodes, the reflected current contributes a bigger portion to the calculated apparent resistivity.

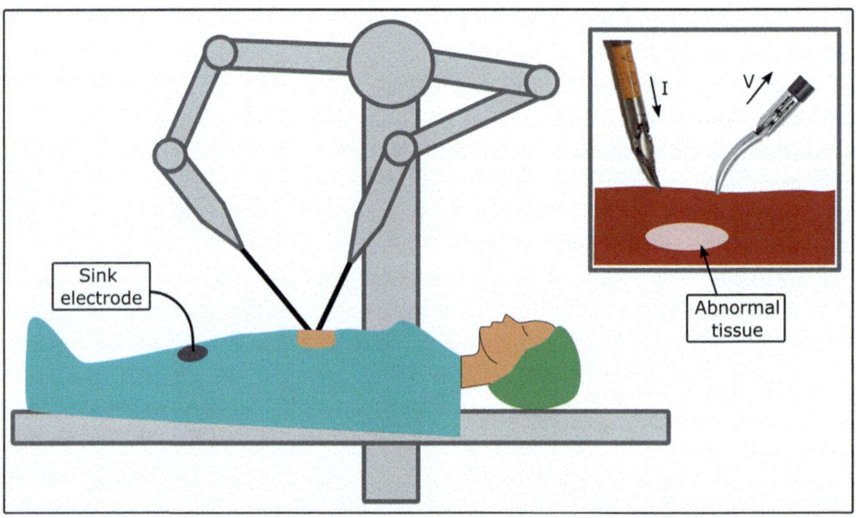

Fig. 8 Configuration of the tripolar EBI sensor

Fig. 9 **a** Schematics of a bi-polar EBI sensing. **b** Schematics of a tri-polar EBI sensing

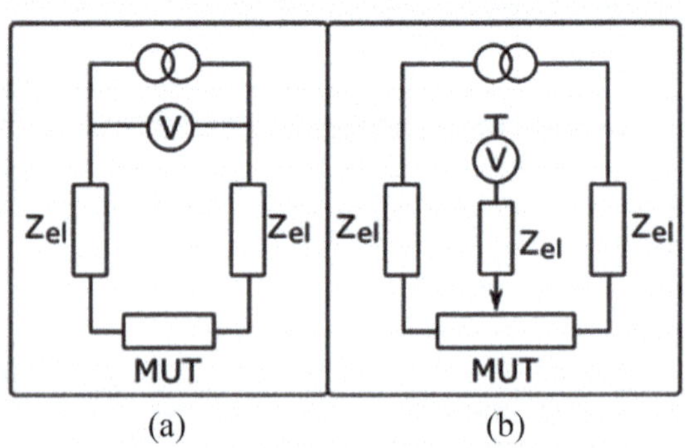

Potentially, the calculated values can be used to estimate the resistivity and the depth of the second layer material. By using a search algorithm, a set of candidate models is identified that accounts for different parameter combinations and calculates its fitting accuracy with respect to the real measurements. The best performer with the highest predictive accuracy is used to estimate the parameters.

Theoretical analysis and experimental verification indicate that the sensitivity of impedance measurement to the pressing depth is much lower in the tripolar setup than that in the bipolar setup. This improved feature is important to ensure the reliability of the RAEIS concept. Nevertheless, it is worth noting that the tripolar configuration is sensitive to the electrodes' distance, which should be controlled accurately in the real robotic system.

The impact of the tripolar measurement accuracy due to a different setting of distances was studied through simulation and no significant differences of the impedance values due to the different settings of distance were found. The tripolar system went through systematic calibration and simulation validation before being tested in ex-vivo experiments.

2.2.1 The Experimental Evaluation

The performance of the tripolar EBI system for subsurface critical tissue detection was evaluated including Finite Element Simulations (FES) and experiments on realistic phantoms. Specifically, a scenario of finding subsurface hepatic cancerous tissue was constructed. The following hypotheses were tested during the system evaluation:

1. The system can perform the scanning on a user-defined position and calculate the corresponding impedance values;
2. The system can detect the subsurface non-homogeneous object successfully;
3. The system can provide accurate parameter estimation of the electrical resistivity of both materials and the depth of the interface.

Before conducting experiments on ex vivo tissues, a saline solution experiment was carried out to evaluate whether the system can measure material resistivity accurately. Then, an experiment based on ex vivo porcine tissues was designed and carried out for the evaluation of the developed system. This experiment simulated a realistic scenario where the surgeon is required to search for an early stage hepatic cancer which grows under a thin layer of healthy tissue.

According to the results of the simulations and experiments, the tri-polar configuration is demonstrated to have a low sensitivity to the forceps' immersed depth. The capability of using the tripolar sensors system for detecting subsurface non-homogeneous tissue are demonstrated by experiments based on FES and ex vivo tissues. According to the experimental results, the apparent resistivity shows an increasing/decreasing trend with the increase of electrode distance if a subsurface non-homogeneous object exists. This is the result from the reflected current theory.

Based on this theory, the relative standard deviation of impedance, can be used for determining whether the subsurface object exists. When the MUT is homogeneous, a nearly constant impedance can be observed, and thus the variance is close to 0. In contrast, the non-homogeneity of the MUT can be detected if the variance is found to be relatively big, however, the variance is found to accumulate errors due to noise and the detection criteria will need to be improved in the future.

2.3 The Robot Assisted Impedance Tomography Technique

Recently, surgical robotics research has been addressing the introduction of some level of autonomy to the clinical practice, which could impact a broad range of procedures, from diagnosis, treatments to tissue removal [16]. To support autonomy, Advanced Intraoperative Sensing (AIS) methods are required to enhance surgical robots and gradually improve their decision support capabilities, following the cognitive surgical robot concept of [31].

In this context, the point-based measurements made possible by the bi- and tripolar EBI impedance methods were enhanced by enabling a continuous scanning of the tissues thanks to the RAEIS system. The system enabled to automatically and quickly identify different tissue types, by applying spectroscopy measurements, optimizing the acquisition protocol by focusing on electrode placement. The theoretical and experimental details of this approach are given in [19, 22].

This approach uses two robotic forceps as separate electrodes and uses two robotic arms to control their relative positions as in the tripolar EBI sensing configuration. The electrodes are required to contact a series of positions on the tissue surface for current excitation or voltage measurement, but the system applies the Electrical Impedance Tomography (EIT) technique to generate the conductivity or/and permittivity distribution of an area or a cross-section. Specifically, through injecting the excitation current via some locations on the surface of MUT and measuring the electric potentials on a series of other surface locations, the impedance reconstruction can be achieved within the electrodes bounded region [32]. The clinical importance of EIT has been also established in the minimally invasive surgery (MIS) such as assessment of surgical margin and detection of subsurface critical tissue.

Before the scanning, the user is requested to input the information about the scanning region, which is rectangular in the experiments, and to specify the scanning resolution which is a grid including the number of rows and columns of the scanning region. The data collection for EIT requires to inject excitation current to each node of the grid, and to measure the electric potential on the other nodes. Measures are carried out by autonomously moving the two instruments to different locations in the scanning area and by inverting their roles, switching between current generator and voltage sensor.

Data collected during the scanning are used for EIT reconstruction, by using the simplified EIT model of a static electric field, since the applied frequencies are relatively low. To create the EIT imaging, it requires to solve the forward problem and the inverse problem iteratively. The forward problem is to find out the electric potential in a defined domain given the boundary condition and the conductivity distribution in the domain. In addition, the inverse problem is a process to determine the conductivity distribution in the domain by knowing the boundary condition and the electrical potential distribution. The two problems are solved with an iterative solver, by providing the measured voltages and the electrode positions to the solver.

2.3.1 The Experimental Evaluation

Two experiments were done to evaluate the EIT system: a water tank and ex vivo tissues. The water tank experiment was designed to detect and localize a non-homogeneous region in an ideal environmental setting. The ex vivo tissues experiment simulated a surgical scenario where the reconstructed EIT image would support the localization of subsurface lymph nodes inside connective fatty tissue.

A FES study was conducted for assisting the determination of the scanning grid. The FES study investigates different grid resolutions through comparing the reconstruction of a 100 × 100 mm rectangular region. Four different settings of the grid: 2×2, 3×3, 4×4 and 5×5 are tested. The position of the non-homogeneous area is located at the center of the scanning grid. The simulation results indicate the non-homogeneous region can be clearly observed in the reconstruction images using the 4×4 and 5×5 grids. Furthermore, the sensitivity and precision of the overlapping area between the truth setting and the reconstructed image were computed.

Figure 10 shows an example of the results obtained. The reconstructed images represent the contrast of electric conductivity distribution, and the non-homogeneous region in yellow indicates the location of suspected lesion.

Compared to the RAEIS method described in the previous section and in [16], the tomography method described here does not have an offset of the reconstructed object due to the system nature. Also, the tomography method can take less time for scanning an area since less scanning positions are required and the whole procedure can be done in an autonomous manner, avoiding tedious and repeated manual operation.

2.4 *3D Vision-Based EIT Scanning*

The demonstration described in the previous sections of integrating EBI sensors into surgical systems is limited to the simplified condition of nearly flat surfaces, which is not realistic for real anatomies. The development described in [24] overcomes this limitation by presenting a RAEIS system able to work with tissues' surfaces of arbitrary shapes, by using 3D vision-based tissue reconstruction. This system has the following novel characteristics.

1. A novel tissue conductivity estimation method that does not rely on the assumption of flatness and computes the conductivity by fitting theoretical values produced by FES to the measured values.

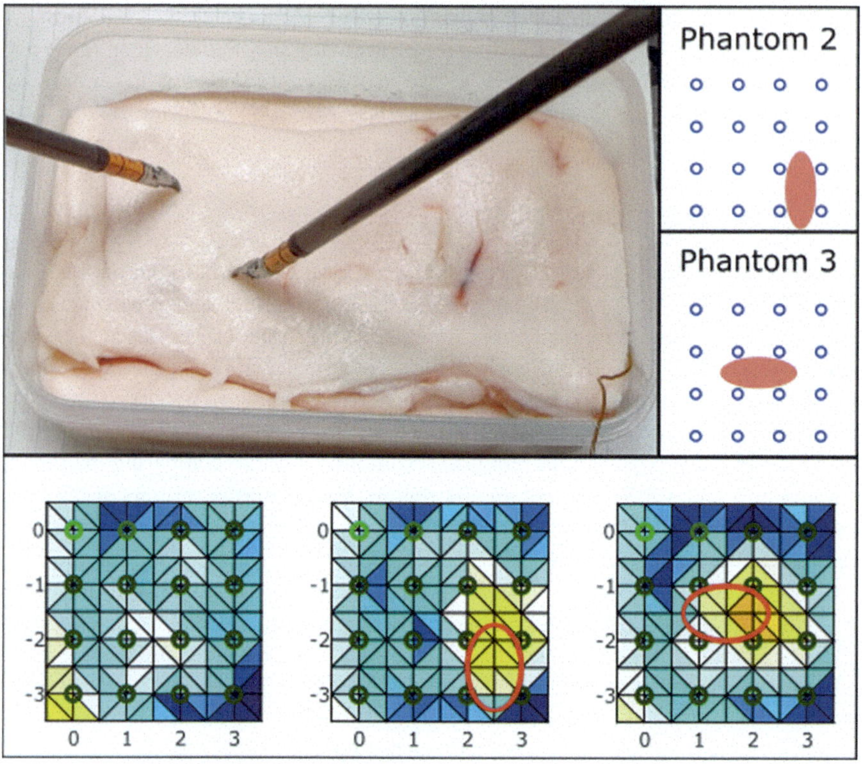

Fig. 10 The figure shows the experimental setup and the reconstructed EIT of a phantom with two embedded lymph nodes simulations

2. 3D vision is used with the purpose of (a) performing the reconstruction of the tissue's model for FES; (b) enabling the system to perform autonomous scanning in realistic conditions, i.e. curved anatomical surfaces with complex shapes.

This method proposes a novel conductivity sensing and estimation method based on a simulation model. The new sensing system integrated a vision sensor to obtain the tissue surface geometry and used it to reconstruct the volumetric model of the MUT. Together with its boundary conditions, the model was used for estimating the electric potential distribution through FES. Considering that energy is bounded, the electric potential should be proportional to the reciprocal of the material conductivity, by comparing the real measurements with the values produced by the simulation, the conductivity of the MUT can be estimated with higher accuracy.

The stereo vision sensor employed in this system is a RealSense D415 (Intel Corporation, U.S.), which provides a high resolution color point cloud used as input to the 3D processing and reconstruction pipeline. Before experimental evaluation, the system is geometrically calibrated over a common reference frame (world) using the method described in Chaps. 7 and 6.

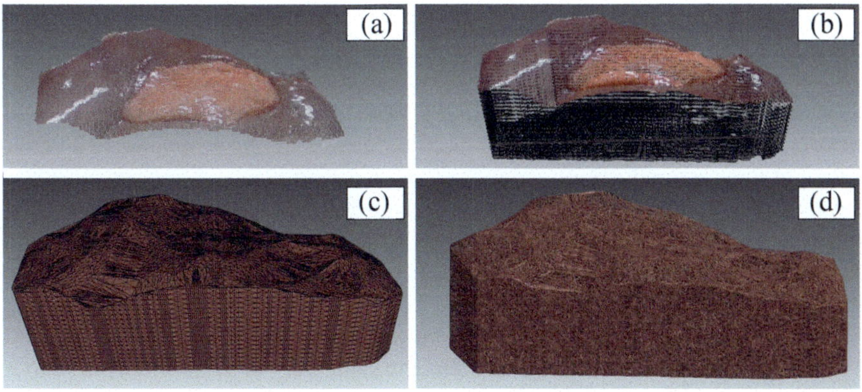

Fig. 11 Four steps of the processing pipeline: original point cloud (**a**), whole surface reconstruction (**b**), boundary polygon mesh (**c**) and final volumetric mesh (**d**). This phantom is the one employed in the ex vivo experiment

The semi-autonomous sensing procedure starts by letting the user choose an AOI on which the robots will perform the autonomous scanning. As shown in Fig. 11, the procedure begins by collecting a pointcloud of the target object with the vision sensor. This pointcloud is displayed on a GUI, where the user selects two locations that define the scanning path. The positions of these points are projected to the tissue's surface provided by the pointcloud.

The processing pipeline generates the volumetric model of the MUT, as required by FES, approximated by vertically extrusions along the perimeter of the surface down to a bottom plane as shown in Fig. 11b, resulting in a new set of 3D points. Then, a bounding volume that envelops the set of 3D points is created and the surface polygon mesh is obtained by selecting the boundary faces of the obtained bounding volume, Fig. 11c. The polygon mesh is ultimately converted to a volumetric mesh, Fig. 11d, using a tetrahedralization algorithm which is required to perform the FES and derive the electric potential distribution.

2.4.1 The Experimental Evaluation

Two experiments were carried out to evaluate the proposed system: a simulation based assessment and an ex vivo test with animal tissue. The simulation study was designed to evaluate the accuracy of the estimation method for sensing the MUT with different curvatures, together with the subsurface object used to study the influence of tissue thickness. In addition, the impact of tissue thickness on the conductivity sensing was investigated, since this is the most important parameter influencing the sensing. The resultant electric potentials were used for conductivity calculation.

The objective of the ex-vivo tests was to first assess the proposed method on a realistic scenario with a complex tissue surface geometry. The second objective was to evaluate the semi-autonomous sensing strategy.

We used the realistic liver cancer surgery scenario shown in Fig. 11a, composed of two types of ex vivo tissues, namely porcine muscle and liver, simulating a tumor given that muscle conductivity is relatively higher than liver's. A copper plate was placed at the bottom of the phantom as the GND electrode. The volumetric model of the phantom was generated based on the tissue's point cloud acquired by the vision sensor. The robots moved to the desired locations according to the generated path, and performed the voltage measurements.

The experimental results demonstrated that the proposed system is able to perform semi-autonomous sensing on a realistic surgical setup, providing accurate tissue conductivity measurements which are compatible with the values available in literature. This system showed high sensing accuracy, fast scanning (8 s), simple integration and efficient usability, thus could be applied in a simple way to existing robot-assisted surgical systems, and improve procedure safety and efficiency.

3 Force Sensors for Minimally Invasive Robotic Instruments

Force sensors allow to measure the physical interaction between two or more physical entities. The local reference system (on a mobile part) can be moved with respect to an absolute reference system (on a fixed part). The displacement between the two reference systems and the two parts (mobile and fixed) have been explored by many researchers. Muscolo and Fiorini [33] presented an overview of force/torque sensors for microscopic and macroscopic applications, including the surgical robotic field. In our work, we designed a new model of a cable-driven force/torque transduction mechanism made up of one mobile part and one fixed part connected to each other by cables. This mechanism has been conceived to solve problems in the robotic surgery research field.

This part is structured as follows: Sect. 3.1 presents our cable-driven transduction system; Sect. 3.2 shows the analytical modeling to define the behavior of the system; Sect. 3.3 shows the developed multibody models and results of simulation. Section 3.4 shows preliminary experiments.

3.1 Cable-Driven Transduction System

Figure 12 (on the left) shows the forceps of a minimally invasive robotic instrument (MIRI) [33], assembled (usually) on a surgical robot and controlled remotely by the surgeon. The open-close action of the forceps and wrist motion are physically

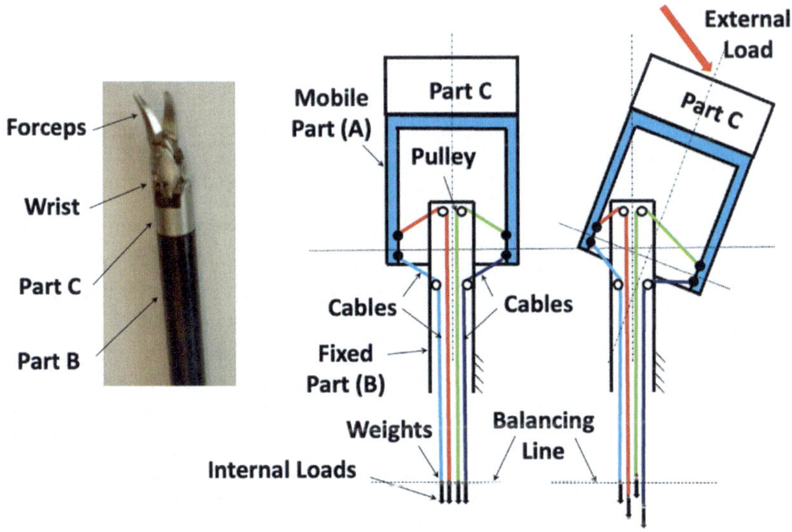

Fig. 12 Forceps in a minimally invasive robotic instrument (on the left), and the working scheme of our proposed cable-driven transduction system (center and right)

performed by a cable-driven system connected to the motors of the surgical robot. The cables, included in part B of Fig. 12 (on the left), transfer the motion from the motors (on the surgical robot) to the forceps (on the MIRI).

Many sensitive systems are proposed for MIRIs [33], but the clinical implementation of MIRIs with tactile haptic feedback to the surgeon has many limits because sterilization of the instrument reduces the life of the electronic components of the sensors. For this reason, MIRIs are used with an open-loop cable-driven control system without sensitive output to the surgeon who controls the teleoperated robot.

In the next future, we plan to use cables not only to control the open-close action of the forceps and wrist motion but also to measure external loads on MIRIs. Figure 12 (center and right) shows the working scheme of our proposed cable-driven transduction system (presented in other works [34–36]), and conceived to include a sensitive system in the MIRIs (used in parallel to the cable-driven actuation system). The use of our system bypasses the sterilization problems because the electronic components are positioned far from the sterilization zone.

As can be seen in Fig. 12 (center), the internal loads balance the weights of the forceps, wrist, part A, part C. For each external load applied on part C, a balance configuration is obtained and its module has a correlation to the motion of the cables where the internal loads are applied (Fig. 12 on the right). If the electronic component is mounted near the internal loads, sterilization of part C can be performed without problems for the electronic components, solving a very huge problem for the surgical sector.

3.2 Analytical Modeling

Figure 13 shows the kinematic scheme of our cable-driven transduction system.

Two reference systems are included for the definition of the cable-driven model: $O_B - X_B Y_B Z_B$ and $O_A - X_A Y_A Z_A$, where i is the number of cables and j is the balance configuration (initial $j = 0$ and final $j = 1$). N_{Bij}, N_{Aij}, $\mathbf{p}_{Bi}$, and $\mathbf{p}_{Ai}$ are the two anchor points of the cables (N_{Bij}, N_{Aij}) and their two position vectors ($\mathbf{p}_{Bi}$, $\mathbf{p}_{Ai}$), respectively; $\mathbf{C}_{ij}$ is the vector of the cables, and $\mathbf{r}_{ij}$ the unit vector of the cables. The position of mobile part A with respect to fixed part B is shown by the vector $\mathbf{p}_G$. P is a general point, and $\mathbf{p}_P$ and $\mathbf{p}_z$ are the position vectors of point P with respect to the reference systems in O_B ($\mathbf{p}_P$) and O_A ($\mathbf{p}_z$). The kinematic equation of the k cables (in a general form) can be written using the rotational matrix W to transform the vectors calculated in the mobile part A with respect to the fixed part B.

$$\mathbf{C}_{ij} = -\mathbf{p}_{Bi} + \mathbf{p}_G + \mathbf{W}\mathbf{p}_{Ai}; \, i = 1, ..., k; \, j = 0, 1. \tag{11}$$

If part A is in equilibrium, the resultants of forces ($\mathbf{F}$) and torques ($\mathbf{M}$) are zero:

$$\sum \mathbf{F} = 0 = \sum_{i=1}^{k} \mathbf{T}_{ij} + m\mathbf{g}_G + \mathbf{F}_P \tag{12}$$

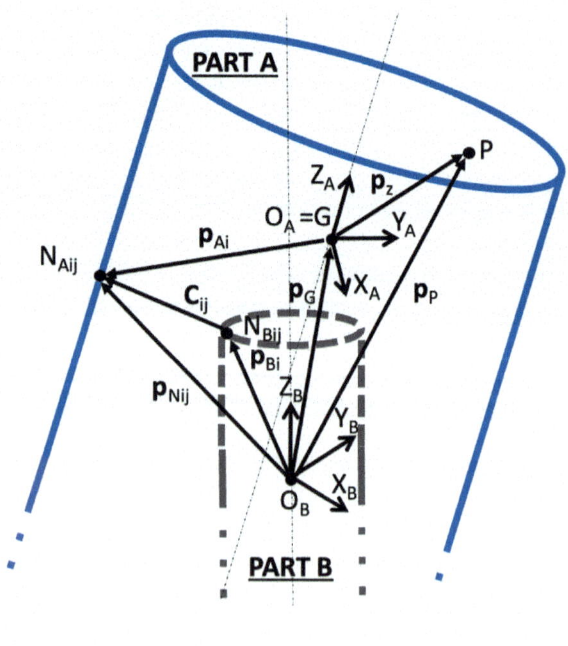

Fig. 13 Kinematic scheme of the cable-driven transduction system. $O_A - X_A Y_A Z_A$ is the local reference system based on part A and $O_B - X_B Y_B Z_B$ is the absolute reference system based on part B

$$\sum \mathbf{M} = 0 = \sum_{i=1}^{k} (\mathbf{W}\mathbf{p}_{Ai} \wedge \mathbf{T}_{ij}) + (\mathbf{p}_G \wedge m\mathbf{g}_G) + (\mathbf{p}_P \wedge \mathbf{F}_P) + \mathbf{M}_P \tag{13}$$

where $\sum_{i=1}^{k} \mathbf{T}_{ij} = \sum_{i=1}^{k} T_{ij}\mathbf{r}_{ij}$ is the tension of cables applied to the part A in N_{Aij}; $\sum_{i=1}^{k} (\mathbf{W}\mathbf{p}_{Ai} \wedge \mathbf{T}_{ij}) = \sum_{i=1}^{k} (\mathbf{W}\mathbf{p}_{Ai} \wedge T_{ij}\mathbf{r}_{ij})$ is the torque produced by the cables; $m\mathbf{g}_G$ is the gravity; and $\mathbf{F}_P$ and $\mathbf{M}_P$ are the external forces and torques applied to the point P, respectively. In a more compact form:

$$\begin{bmatrix} \mathbf{r}_{1j} & \cdots & \mathbf{r}_{kj} \\ \mathbf{W}\mathbf{p}_{A1} \wedge \mathbf{r}_{1j} & \cdots & \mathbf{W}\mathbf{p}_{Ak} \wedge \mathbf{r}_{kj} \end{bmatrix} \begin{bmatrix} T_{1j} \\ \vdots \\ T_{kj} \end{bmatrix} = - \begin{bmatrix} m\mathbf{g}_G \\ (\mathbf{p}_G \wedge m\mathbf{g}_G) \end{bmatrix} - \begin{bmatrix} \mathbf{F}_P \\ (\mathbf{p}_P \wedge \mathbf{F}_P) + \mathbf{M}_P \end{bmatrix} \tag{14}$$

$$\mathbf{S}\mathbf{T}_j = -\mathbf{Q}_G - \mathbf{Q}_{Pj} \tag{15}$$

where $\mathbf{S}$ is the force transformation matrix [34, 36]; $\mathbf{T}_j$ is the vector of the cables' tension; and $\mathbf{Q}_G$ is the gravity vector [34, 36]. The vector of the external forces and torques, applied to point P ($\mathbf{Q}_{Pj}$), is calculated with $\Delta\mathbf{T} = \mathbf{T}_1 - \mathbf{T}_0$, in which $\mathbf{T}_0$ is the vector of tension of the cables, used as offset and calculated in the balance configurations.

By the analysis of Eq. (15) and using the difference between the two balance configurations $j = 1$ and $j = 0$, $\mathbf{Q}_{Pj}$ is obtained:

$$\mathbf{Q}_{Pj} = \left[F_{PX}, F_{PY}, F_{PZ}, M_{PX}, M_{PY}, M_{PZ}\right]^T = \mathbf{Q}_{P0} - \mathbf{S}\Delta\mathbf{T} \tag{16}$$

3.3 *Multibody Model Design and Results of Simulation*

The multibody model of our cable-driven transduction system has been created using MATLAB®, Simulink®, and Simscape™ Multibody™. The simulations are used to study the behavior of our system.

Figure 14 shows an example of our multibody model with and without an applied external load. Units are in mm and the dimensions are shown in the figure. Eight cables allow to measure three force components (F_x, F_y, F_z) and two torque components (M_x, M_y) and more details on the analytical formulation of Eq. (15) are presented in other works [34, 36].

The positions of cables, the distance of the internal loads and weights from the balancing line, and the combination among the motion of cables can give information on the directions and modules of the external loads to our system.

Figure 15 shows a case study with an applied load of 2 Nm on M_x. In the YZ plane, cables d_1 and c_2 have about the same behavior with respect to c_1 and d_2, and the absolute value of the distance from the internal loads and weights and the balancing line is about the same for d_1 and c_2 or c_1 and d_2. This result permits to note that the

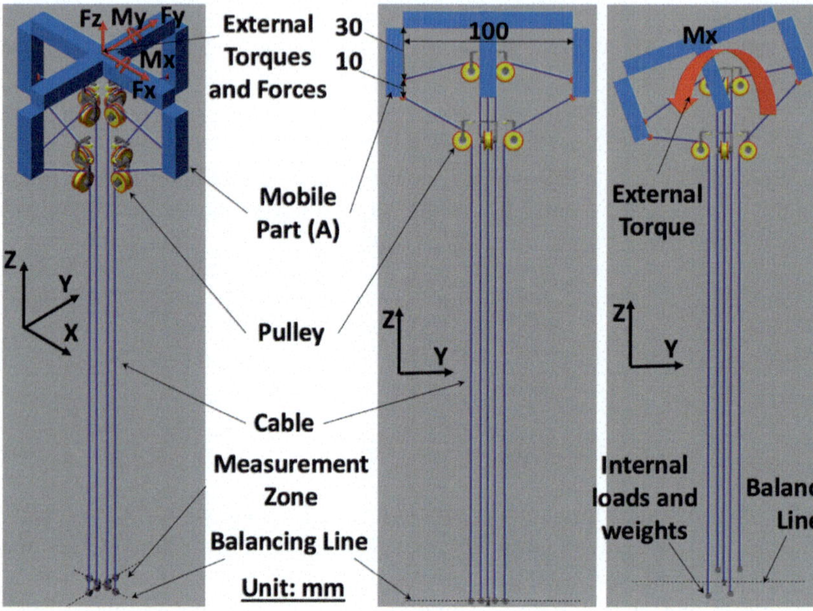

Fig. 14 Multibody model of the cable-driven system for simulation

load is applied around the axis of symmetry. Meanwhile, the alternative motion of the four cables shown in Fig. 15 gives the direction of M_x: c_2 and d_1 (Fig. 15) show a counterclockwise direction for M_x. A comparison between cable displacements (a_1, b_1, c_1, d_1, a_2, b_2, c_2, d_2) in the two planes YZ and XZ suggests the plane in which the load has more influence: plane YZ has 8 mm displacement; on the contrary, the maximum displacement in XZ is 0.3 mm, suggesting that the load is applied in the YZ plane, as shown in Fig. 15.

Figure 16 shows the results if two different torques (M_y and M_z) are applied. M_y has the same type of M_x behavior, confirming the hypotheses of symmetry. M_z has the same behavior in each plane (YZ and XZ), confirming that no equilibrium can be created with the present configurations between part A and part B in Z direction.

Figure 17 shows the application of the same loads shown in Figs. 15 and 16 but in opposite directions.

If $5N$ are applied as external load alternatively as F_x, F_y, F_z, the graphs of Figs. 18 and 19 show that no differences are noted in the YZ or XZ planes if F_z or $-F_z$ are applied.

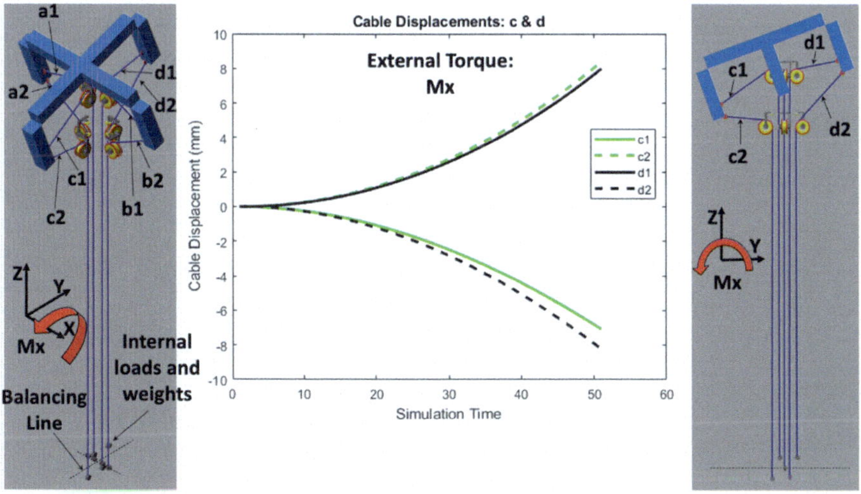

Fig. 15 Multibody model with an applied torque of 2 Nm (M_x)

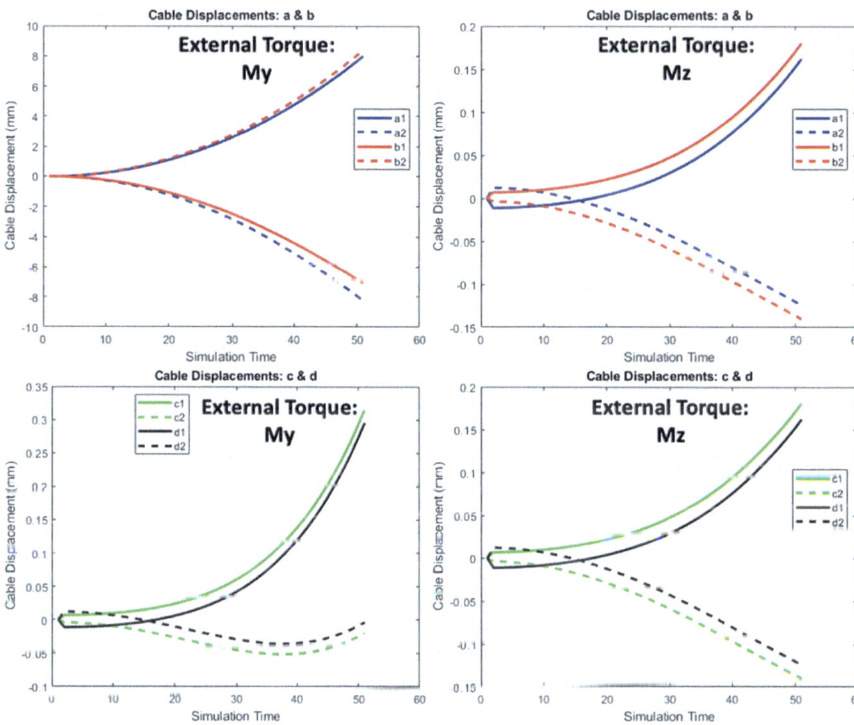

Fig. 16 Applied torque of 2 Nm (M_y) and 0.02 Nm (M_z)

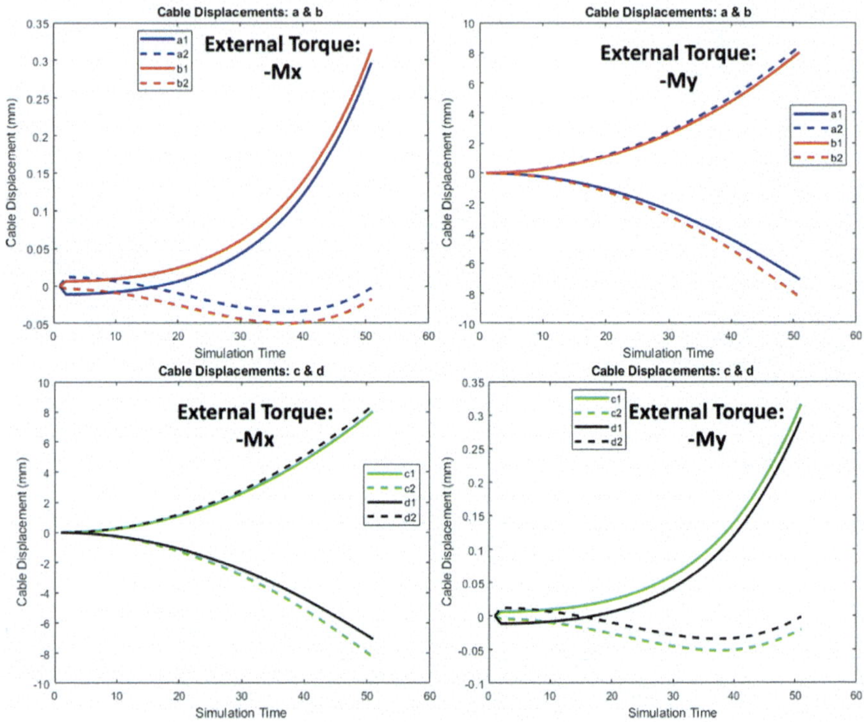

Fig. 17 Applied torque of $-2\,\text{Nm}$ (M_x and M_y) and $-0.02\,\text{Nm}$ (M_z)

3.4 Prototypes and Preliminary Experiments

Figure 20 shows the spatial test-bench prototype developed to test the mechanical behavior of the cable-driven transduction system. More details on the planar and spatial test-bench prototypes used to test some theoretical hypotheses on our cable-driven transduction system are included in other works [34–36].

Test-bench shown in Fig. 20 is made up of two parts (A and B). Part A is free to move and is connected to external springs using cables and passing from holes in part B, connected to a fixed structure. Seven external loads are applied to part A, modifying the balance configuration of the eight cables. Two different friction coefficients ($\mu = 0.25$ and $\mu = 0.3$) are used to model the friction between cables and internal holes of part B. A comparison between measured and calculated external loads with the analytical formulation of Eq. (15) are presented in other works [34, 36] and shown in the graph of Fig. 20.

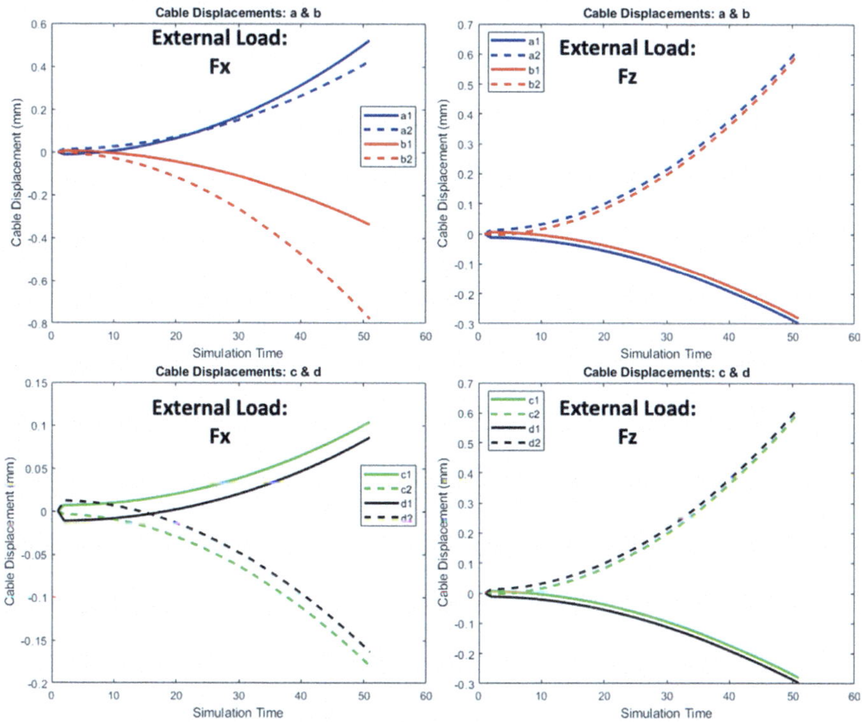

Fig. 18 Applied force of $5N$ (F_x, F_y, F_z)

More details on the working principle of our cable-driven transduction system and on the planar and spatial test bench prototypes developed within the ARS project can be found in [34–36].

The final objective of our work is to implement our cable-driven transduction system in MIRIs of the next future. Figure 21 shows the real dimensions of parts A and B that will be developed and implemented in MIRIs.

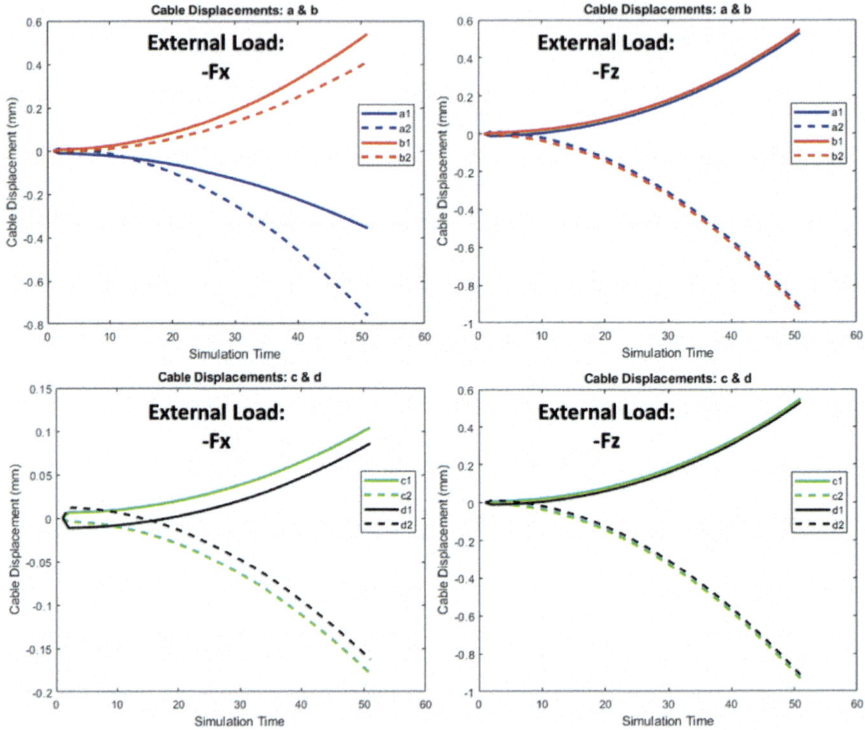

Fig. 19 Applied force of $-5N$ (F_x, F_y, F_z)

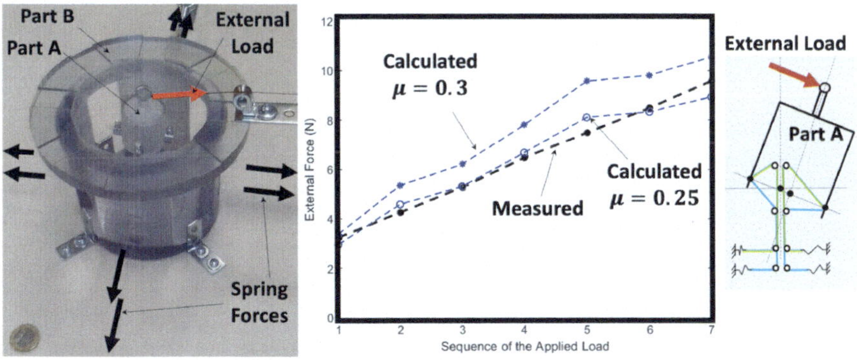

Fig. 20 A preliminary test bench prototype

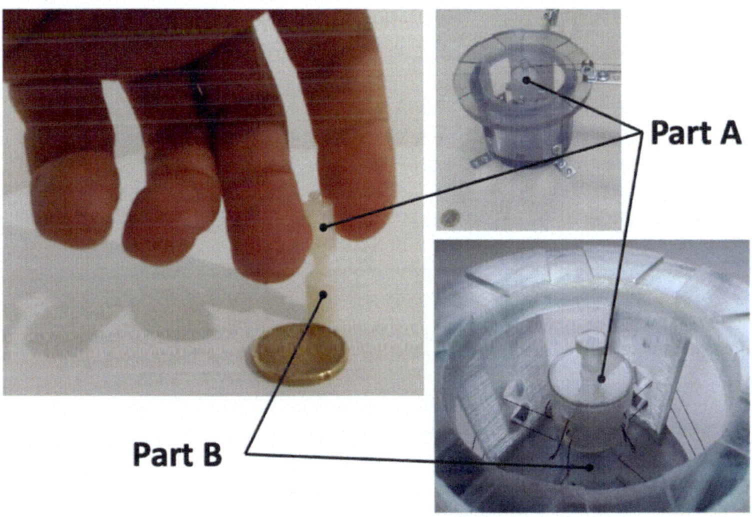

Fig. 21 First prototype with the correct dimensions to be implemented in MIRIs

References

1. Verma, S., Choyke, P.L., Eberhardt, S.C., Oto, A., Tempany, C.M., Turkbey, B., Rosenkrantz, A.B.: The current state of MR imaging, targeted biopsy techniques for detection of prostate cancer. Radiology **285**, 343–356 (2017)
2. DiMaio, S.P., Salcudean, S.E.: Needle insertion modeling and simulation. IEEE Trans. Robot. Autom. **19**(5), 864–875 (2003)

3. Simone, C., Okamura, A.M.: Modeling of needle insertion forces for robot-assisted percutaneous therapy. In: Proceedings 2002 IEEE International Conference on Robotics and Automation (Cat. No. 02CH37292), vol. 2, pp. 2085–2091. IEEE (2002)
4. Park, W., Kim, J.S., Zhou, Y., Cowan, N., Okamura, A., Chirikjian, G.: Diffusion-based motion planning for a nonholonomic flexible needle model. In: Proceedings of the 2005 IEEE International Conference on Robotics and Automation, pp. 4600–4605 (2005)
5. Webster, I.R.J., Kim, J.S., Cowan, N.J., Chirikjian, G.S., Okamura, A.M.: Nonholonomic modeling of needle steering. Int. J. Robot. Res. **25**(5-6), 509–525 (2006)
6. Fallahi, B., Khadem, M., Rossa, C., Sloboda, R., Usmani, N., Tavakoli, M.: Extended bicycle model for needle steering in soft tissue. In: 2015 IEEE/RSJ International Conference on Intelligent Robots and Systems (IROS), pp. 4375–4380 (2015)
7. Zandoná, C., Roberti, A., Costanzi, D., Gül, B., Akbulut, Ö., Fiorini, P., Calanca, A.: A comparison between kinematic models for robotic needle insertion with application into transperineal prostate biopsy. Technologies **12**, 1–14 (2024)
8. Isola, P., Zhu, J.-Y., Zhou, T., Efros, A.A.: Image-to-image translation with conditional adversarial networks. In: 2017 IEEE Conference on Computer Vision and Pattern Recognition (CVPR) (2017)
9. Hungr, N., Long, J.A., Beix, V., Troccaz, J.: A realistic deformable prostate phantom for multimodal imaging and needle-insertion procedures. Med. Phys. **39**(4), 2031–2041 (2012). Wiley
10. Ji, Y., Ruan, L., Ren, W., Dun, G., Liu, J., Zhang, Y., Wan, Q.: Stiffness of prostate gland measured by transrectal real-time shear wave elastography for detection of prostate cancer: a feasibility study. Br. J. Radiol. **92**, 20180970 (2019)
11. Penza, V., Ortiz, J., Momi, E.D., Forgione, A., Mattos, L.S.: Virtual assistive system for robotic single incision laparoscopic surgery (2014)
12. Katić, D., Schuck, J., Wekerle, A.-L., Kenngott, H., Müller-Stich, B.P., Dillmann, R.: Bridging the gap between formal and experience-based knowledge for context-aware laparoscopy. Int. J. Comput. Assist. Radiol. Surg. **11**, 881–888 (2016)
13. Intuitive Surgical Inc., https://www.intuitive.com/en-us/about-us/newsroom/force_feedback. Accessed: 2025-02-15
14. Konstantinova, J., Jiang, A., Althoefer, K., Dasgupta, P., Nanayakkara, T.: Implementation of tactile sensing for palpation in robot-assisted minimally invasive surgery: a review. IEEE Sens. J. **14**(8), 2490–2501 (2014)
15. Istituto Italiano di Tecnologia, https://advr.iit.it/biomedical-robotics. Accessed: 2025-05-15
16. Cheng, Z., Dall'Alba, D., Fiorini, P., Savarimuthu, T.R.: Robot assisted electrical impedance tomography system for minimally invasive surgery. In: 2021 20th International Conference on Advanced Robotics (ICAR), pp. 234–240 (2021)
17. Cheng, Z., Davies, B.L., Caldwell, D.G., Barresi, G., Xu, Q., Mattos, L.S.: A hand-held robotic device for peripheral intravenous catheterization. Proc. Inst. Mech. Eng. **231** (2017)
18. Cheng, Z., Davies, B.L., Caldwell, D.G., Mattos, L.S.: A venipuncture detection system for robot-assisted intravenous catheterization. In: 2016 6th IEEE International Conference on Biomedical Robotics and Biomechatronics (BioRob), pp. 80–86 (2016)
19. Cheng, Z., Savarimuthu, T.R.: A novel robot assisted electrical impedance scanning system for subsurface object detection. Meas. Sci. Technol. **32**(8) (2021). Art. no. 085902
20. Cheng, Z., Davies, B., Caldwell, D., Mattos, L.: A new venous entry detection method based on electrical bio-impedance sensing. Ann. Biomed. Eng. **46**(8), 1558–1567 (2018)
21. Cheng, Z., Dall'Alba, D., Foti, S., Mariani, A., Chupin, T., Caldwell, D., Ferrigno, G., De Momi, E., Mattos, L., Fiorini, P.: Design and integration of electrical bio-impedance sensing in surgical robotic tools for tissue identification and display. Front. Robot. AI **6**(55), 209–219 (2019)
22. Cheng, Z., Schwaner, K.L., Dall'Alba, D., Fiorini, P., Savarimuthu, T.R.: An electrical bioimpedance scanning system for subsurface tissue detection in robot assisted minimally invasive surgery. IEEE Trans. Biomed. Eng. **69**(1), 209–219 (2022)

23. Cheng, Z., Dall'Alba, D., Schwaner, K.L., Fiorini, P., Savarimuthu, T.R.: Robot assisted electrical impedance scanning for tissue bioimpedance spectroscopy measurement. Measurement **195**, 111–112 (2022)
24. Piccinelli, M., Cheng, Z., Dall'Alba, D., Schmidt, M.K., Savarimuthu, T.R., Fiorini, P.: 3d vision based robot assisted electrical impedance scanning for soft tissue conductivity sensing. IEEE Robot. Autom. Lett. **7**(2), 4055–4062 (2022)
25. Kazanzides, P., Chen, Z., Deguet, A., Fischer, G.S., Taylor, R.H., DiMaio, S.P.: An open-source research kit for the da vinci® surgical system. In: 2014 IEEE International Conference on Robotics and Automation (ICRA), pp. 6434–6439. IEEE (2014)
26. Kalvøy, H., Sauter, A.: Detection of intraneural needle-placement with multiple frequency bioimpedance monitoring: a novel method. J. Clin. Monit. Comput. **30**(2), 185–192 (2016)
27. Rigaud, B., Hamzaoui, L., Frikha, M., Chauveau, N., Morucci, J.: In vitro tissue characterization and modelling using electrical impedance measurements in the 100 hz–10 mhz frequency range. Physiol. Meas. **16**(3), A15-28 (1995)
28. Strobl, K.H., Hirzinger, G.: Optimal hand-eye calibration. In: 2006 IEEE/RSJ International Conference on Intelligent Robots and Systems, pp. 4647–4653 (2006)
29. Cheng, Z., Savarimuthu, T.R.: Monopolar, bipolar, tripolar, and tetrapolar configurations in robot assisted electrical impedance sensing. Biomed. Phys. Eng. Express **8**(5), 055014 (2022)
30. Kearey, P., Brooks, M., Hill, I.: An Introduction to Geophysical Exploration. Wiley (2013)
31. Muradore, R., Fiorini, P., Akgun, G., Barkana, D.E., Bonfe, M., Boriero, F., Caprara, A., Rossi, G.D., Dodi, R., Elle, O.J., Ferraguti, F., Gasperotti, L., Gassert, R., Mathiassen, K., Handini, D., Lambercy, O., Li, L., Kruusmaa, M., Manurung, A.O., Meruzzi, G., Nguyen, H.Q.P., Preda, N., Riolfo, G., Ristolainen, A., Sanna, A., Secchi, C., Torsello, M., Yantac, A.E.: Development of a cognitive robotic system for simple surgical tasks. Int. J. Adv. Rob. Syst. **12**(4), 37 (2015)
32. Adler, A., Arnold, J., Bayford, R., Borsic, A., Brown, B., Dixon, P., Faes, T., Frerichs, I., Gagnon, H., Gärber, Y., Grychtol, B., Hahn, G., Lionheart, W., Malik, A., Patterson, R., Stocks, J., Tizzard, A., Weiler, N., Wolf, G.: Greit: a unified approach to 2D linear EIT reconstruction of lung images. Physiol. Meas. **30**(6), 35–55 (2009)
33. Muscolo, G.G., Fiorini, P.: Force-torque sensors for minimally invasive surgery robotic tools: an overview. IEEE Trans. Med. Robot. Bionics **5**(3), 458–471 (2023)
34. Muscolo, G.G., Fiorini, P.: A new cable-driven model for under-actuated force–torque sensitive mechanisms. Machines **11**(6) (2023)
35. Muscolo, G.G., Fiorini, P.: A planar cable-driven under-sensing model to measure forces and displacements. Machines **12**(2) (2024)
36. Muscolo, G.G., Fiorini, P.: Cable-driven mechanism models for sensitive and actuated minimally invasive robotic instruments. Appl. Sci. **14**(7) (2024)

The Non-technical Issues of Autonomy

The third part of the book addresses the non-technical issues related to the development of autonomous robots. These aspects are very difficult to analyze because of the intersection of the two sensitive topics of autonomy and health care, with all their implications on liability, safety, and impact on everyday life. This part of the project was a research project in its own right, since it let us explore the ethical aspects of autonomy, carry out experiments of social interaction with our communication activities, and explore how autonomy can be transformed into a product with the project exploitation.

Chapter "The Ethical and Social Aspects of Autonomy" addresses the concepts related to ethics of autonomous robots and the benefits that they could bring to people.

Chapter "Automation on the Brink of Autonomy: Letting Go of Control" explores the evolving relationship between mankind and machines, with an eye to super-intelligent machines and the fast approaching frontier of autonomous robots.

Chapter "Communication Strategy of the ARS Project" describes the activities carried out during the whole project to define a communication strategy and the appropriate means to engage and interact with the different audiences to which the ARS project would cater.

Finally, Chapter "The Exploitation of Results" describes the sequence of proposals, grants received, and results achieved on the way to commercialize a medical robotic instrument with a minimal set of autonomous features.

The Ethical and Social Aspects of Autonomy

Sara Patuzzo Manzati

Abstract This chapter aims to explore the main ethical implications of AI into robotic surgery. Drawing on the core principles of medical ethics—beneficence, non-maleficence, autonomy, and justice—, it outlines the ideal profile of the human surgeon: a professional equipped with technical expertise, adaptability, emotional self-regulation, and rational decision making abilities under unpredictable circumstances. On this basis, the chapter examines whether, and to what extent, these human qualities can be simulated or even surpassed by intelligent machines. Currently, AI-enhanced surgical robots operate under human supervision. However, ongoing technological advancements point toward a gradual increase in their decision-making autonomy. This emerging scenario raises critical ethical questions: can we entrust machines with real-time, life-and-death decisions in the absence of consciousness, empathy, or moral accountability? While AI demonstrates remarkable competence in logical-analytical reasoning and in the rational management of unforeseen events, concerns remain regarding its ability to establish a relationship of trust with patients, a relationship grounded not only in technical proficiency, but also in empathy and ethical motivation. The chapter will also address the paradox whereby emotionality—something the human surgeon is expected to control in the operating room—may be perceived as a significant absence in machines, potentially hindering their full acceptance by patients. Nonetheless, the possibility that patients may develop emotional attachments to intelligent machines will also be considered, as well as the role of representation and aesthetics in promoting the social integration of robotic technologies.

1 Introduction

A fundamental principle of Medical Ethics is beneficence, which asserts that the good physician is one who acts in the best interest of the patient, with the concept of "good" traditionally understood as safeguarding health and protecting the biological

S. Patuzzo Manzati (✉)
Department of Surgery, Dentistry, Paediatrics and Gynaecology, University of Verona, Verona, Italy
e-mail: sara.patuzzomanzati@univr.it

P. Fiorini (ed.), *Towards Autonomous Robotic Surgery*, Springer Tracts in Advanced Robotics 161, https://doi.org/10.1007/978-3-032-04247-7_12

life of the patient. Consequently, the physician must not cause harm ("primum non nocere") to the patient, in accordance with the ethical principle of non-maleficence. Furthermore, the physician must act in respect of the patient's free and informed choice to undergo treatment, upholding the ethical principle of self-determination. Last, but not least, the physician must base their conduct on the ethical principle of justice and equity, avoiding discrimination, setting aside any biases, affinities, and antipathies, and utilizing available resources in a fair manner.

In light of these ethical principles, we can identify the characteristics and qualities a surgeon should possess to perform optimally (see Sect. 2 of Chap. 8. A surgeon in the operating room should have specific technical competencies, such as manual precision, which is essential for performing delicate surgical maneuvers, a comprehensive understanding of anatomy and surgical techniques, and the ability to coordinate rationally with the surgical team, providing clear instructions ("Precision, technical knowledge, and rational approach"). The surgeon should be adaptable to the specific intervention, as each patient is unique ("Situational awareness and adaptability"). Moreover, the surgeon must be able to solve problems and handle adverse events by managing unforeseen circumstances and complications, weighing the pros and cons of available choices in real time ("Management of unpredictability"). The surgeon should also maintain composure to make quick and rational decisions, without being overwhelmed by emotions or pressure, and possess strong resilience to endure the potential length and demands of the procedure ("Emotional control"). Lastly, for the intervention to be carried out with the patient's free consent, it is essential that this consent is based on the trust the patient places in the surgeon ("Patient trust"). Currently, the field of surgery has begun to integrate AI-equipped robot surgeons into its operative procedures. Although we are still in the early stages of this revolutionary fusion, it is conceivable that future developments will allow these machines to perform surgeries with increasingly sophisticated levels of autonomy, potentially surpassing their human counterparts. Could a robot surgeon equipped with AI possess the same combination of skills and qualities required of a human surgeon? This is the central question around which the issue develops, and we will explore it below, considering how and whether we should promote the development of surgical AI, progressively increasing its autonomy. Indeed, when ethics is called upon to reflect on the implications of technological advancement, it must inevitably "look ahead", following the trajectory of robotic surgery integrated with AI: a future, perhaps not too distant and of which we are already witnessing the early roots today, where the caregiver-patient relationship will no longer be between a physician and a patient, but between a machine and a patient. Posing questions about a future yet to come is not merely a rhetorical exercise or a mental experiment useful for testing the principles we currently consider established through a particular interpretation. Rather, it is crucial to prevent specific issues by shaping, to the extent possible, the development of AI robot surgeons based on what, at the end of our reasoning, we may consider decisive for a sustainable progress that truly meets our needs.

2 Discussion

2.1 *Precision, Technical Knowledge, and Rational Approach—Situational Awareness and Adaptability*

Human intelligence has been divided into eight primary modalities: linguistic, musical, spatial, bodily-kinesthetic, intrapersonal, interpersonal, naturalistic, and logical-analytical [1]. The latter is the complex ability to perform cognitive operations that facilitate the formation of abstract rational thought in analysis and logical argumentation. Rational thinking can be reduced to mathematical operations, as logic can be translated into mathematical rules. Therefore, reasoning can be considered a process of calculation and computation. Computers equipped with AI are mathematically programmed to cultivate logical-analytical reasoning. Consequently, AI is considered intelligent to the extent that it simulates (and enhances) human logical-analytical intelligence [2] (see Sect. 1 of Chap. 3). However, logical-analytical intelligence is a necessary but not sufficient condition for effective operation in the world. It also requires situational awareness, which is the ability to interact with the environment in which we are situated, adapting to it and/or transforming it. Thus, AI, in addition to the ability to perform logical-analytical reasoning, must also possess the ability to situate itself [3], improving through "deep learning".

Based on the implementation of AI, the field of surgery has begun incorporating robots equipped with AI into operative procedures, where their use has shown significant potential in various specific areas [4–6]. Currently, these robots are teleoperated by the human surgeon [7, 8], with some assistive functions (such as monitoring certain operative variables) [9], classified as levels 0 and 1 of autonomy. However, due to scientific and technological progress, to which this project aims to contribute, it is conceivable that these AI robots will increase their level of autonomy, reaching levels 2 and 3, eventually becoming ARSS capable of partially or entirely replacing human surgeons [10]. At such a level of autonomy, it is expected that ARSS will be able to perform logical-analytical reasoning upon which to base planned decisions and actions, modifying its behavior if necessary through situational awareness (see Chap. 7), which, once consolidated into common practices, we generically call "common sense" (see Sect. 3 of Chap. 8).

The presence of these AI-equipped robots in the operating room does not currently raise significant ethical concerns, as, as we mentioned, they primarily serve a supportive role in the human surgeon's work, much like other tools used to enhance surgical performance [11, 12]. Any deviation between stimulus and correct response is attributed to a technical error of the machine, potentially involving legal responsibilities (such as those of the manufacturer or maintenance), but not ethical questions related to decision-making autonomy. In other words, the predominantly passive objectivity of the AI robot surgeon is what prevents fundamental ethical questions from arising regarding its integration into surgical practice. However, as indicated in this volume, the trend of scientific progress is toward increasingly sophisticated systems, aimed at making their intelligence, combined with situational awareness, so complex that they can perform and modify reasoned operations rationally, with the ultimate goal of achieving the results in the operating room for which the machine has been programmed, i.e., behaving as a human surgeon would or perhaps even better [13]. It is within this scenario, where a gradual and potentially total replacement of the human surgeon with intelligent machines is envisioned, that bioethics raises some questions. Of course, this is not an exclusively medical scenario but pertains to many other aspects of human life. Nonetheless, in the medical-healthcare field, and particularly in the operating room, the idea that a robot could hold the patient's life and death in its mechanical hands, entrusted by the patient who may be unconscious due to anesthesia, presents a specific case where precision, reliability, and safety must be such that the patient develops full trust in the machine. Indeed, in the operating room, a high level of autonomy of the machine meets direct interaction with the patient, whose existence depends on the decisions made in real time and the variability of the human body's response, given its uniqueness (see Chap. 7).

2.2 *Management of Unpredictability*

An ethical aspect related to the use of a surgeon robot equipped with artificial intelligence in autonomous mode concerns its potential limitation to the algorithms that govern its functioning (see Chap. 8). This raises the concern that the robot may be unable to make "instinctive" decisions, those that, in some cases, may be required during surgery, for example, if an unforeseen event occurs, but which were not included in its programming. Indeed, during a surgical procedure, unforeseen situations can arise that require the experience and intuition of the surgeon to be addressed [14]. However, what we often refer to as "instinct" is nothing more than a human intellectual ability to quickly and rationally assess the available options, selecting the best solution. In this context, artificial intelligence may be able to perform even more precise and sophisticated analyses [15–17], making it, in some cases, a preferable choice over a human surgeon. An additional concern may relate to the unpredictability margin of the AI robot surgeon: how can we be certain that it will not perform unexpected and undesirable actions, potentially with lethal consequences for the patient [18, 19]? (see Sect. 3 of Chap. 8) Let us start by considering that even the human surgeon is capable of performing unpredictable actions with disastrous outcomes. In fact, unpredictability is an inseparable aspect of intelligence: if either AI or a human were to behave exclusively in a deterministic manner based on cause-and-effect relationships, they would always be predictable but would not be considered intelligent (see Chap. 3). Moreover, in comparison to humans, AI, due to the superior efficiency of its logical-analytical and self-adaptive systems, has a reduced potential for unpredictability, making it preferable in this regard.

2.3 Emotional Control

The experience that concerns us here, that of the operating room, is based on the need for a surgical procedure to be performed in a non-emotional, but rather logical-rational and situational manner: while operating, the human surgeon must control (and suppress) their emotions [20]. In order for the procedure to succeed optimally, the surgeon must remain emotionally detached, leaving their feelings outside the operating room and striving to behave as much like a machine as possible. While it is generally true that compassionate human relationships can play a role in the caregiving process, when we refer specifically to surgery, and particularly to the moment when the surgical procedure is taking place, the physician is required to view the biological portion they are operating on as a mere body, not as a specific person [21]. Consequently, the robot surgeon with AI is certainly an optimal choice in relation to the need for emotional control in favor of a rational approach to medical-surgical decisions.

2.4 Patient Trust

One ethical issue that can be raised for consideration is that the trust a patient develops towards their physician is based not only on the belief that the physician possesses medical knowledge, i.e., the technical-professional skills acquired through their training and clinical experience, but also on the empathy that presumably motivated the physician to pursue a medical career. Indeed, in common perception, the work of a physician is not seen as just another job. It is, rather, considered a mission, where the qualities of service, help, and solidarity towards others are central. The fact that a machine does not experience emotions may therefore be perceived as a fundamental lack, hindering the full development of trust. In the operating room, the human surgeon "cares" for the patient because they can empathetically place themselves in the patient's shoes. This cannot be said for the machine, at least not from a moral perspective [22]. While the patient may be convinced of the technical capabilities of the AI robot surgeon, even superior to those of a human surgeon, the consequence may be reluctance or even refusal by the patient to undergo surgery by the machine. This can be compared to passengers' resistance to pilotless flights, where, despite the efficiency of AI, public acceptance can be problematic [23].

In fact, it is true that the emotionality of the physician can play a significant role in the formation of trust, as well as have a "therapeutic" value for the patient in their willingness to heal [24] . In medical ethics courses, it is emphasized that the physician, when facing the patient, should not primarily focus on the pathology the patient is suffering from, but on the person with that pathology. However, the patient also knows that, ultimately, the physician is a professional, not a loved one, and therefore the feeling they may experience is relatively superficial. Upon closer inspection, perhaps what the patient truly expects and needs is not for the physician to "love" them, but to be kind, caring, and available. All of these are qualities that AI possesses. One can verify its "care" in its approach simply by interacting with ChatGPT. In fact, precisely because it is incapable of experiencing emotions, the courtesy displayed by AI cannot turn into irritation or anger, which can happen with a human being [25].

Another potential obstacle to trust that might arise today if we were to introduce an autonomous AI robot surgeon into surgical practice could be its perception as an outsider, generating fear and difficulties in acceptance. However, the scenario we are contemplating, in which technological advancements will have progressed to the point that intelligent machines can actually perform surgical procedures instead of human surgeons, is not exactly just around the corner. The gradual implementation of the AI robot surgeon, proportional to its levels of autonomy, will likely allow society to gradually become familiar with these machines, eventually considering them an indispensable part of the hospital and surgical context. Nonetheless, this familiarization with the figure of robots could also occur in other ways, as explored by the "uncanny valley" issue, for example, through the creation of an aesthetic image (as well as their movements) that is similar to ours [26].

Furthermore, we can highlight the possibility that this sense of affinity may stem from the idea of proximity to the machine due to our ability to feel emotions towards it [27]. In fact, even though robot surgeons are not (self)aware and do not experience feelings, patients might be able to feel empathy towards them and treat them as something more than mere machines [28]. Additionally, patients might be capable not only of feeling empathy but also of projecting and attributing emotions and passions to them. For this to happen, intelligent machines do not need to have developed the ability to be sentient [29]. In fact, humans generally tend to form emotional bonds with objects, even when fully aware that their behavior is programmed [22, 28, 30, 31]. It is a self-illusion, but how often do we self-illusion ourselves about something, such as truly feeling emotions towards someone or something, or thinking that someone or something feels them for us, because it serves our well-being [32, 33]? Ultimately, it is what happens when we go to the movies and allow ourselves to be emotionally engaged by a representation we already know to be false.

3 Conclusion

In any process that integrates new elements, an effort is required to overcome what differentiates us, emphasizing similarities and leveraging divergent characteristics as strengths. This effort is fundamentally philosophical, meaning that it necessitates a rationalization of our approach to the AI robot surgeon in order to overcome our defense against the unusual and the unknown [34]. Ultimately, perhaps it is we, human beings, who have innate biases against AI machines, rather than the other way around. This conclusion calls for further encouragement of the integration of AI robots in surgical fields and the adoption of proactive measures to improve their public acceptance. At the same time, it will entail a meticulous reflection on the attribution of responsibility, both ethical and subsequently legal, for the actions carried out by an autonomous AI robot surgeon [35–38].

References

1. Gardner, H.: Frames of Mind The Theory of Multiple Intelligences. Basic Books (2011)
2. Turing, A.M.: Computing machinery and intelligence. Mind, vol. LIX, no. 236, pp. 433–460 (1950)
3. Sternberg, R.J.: Adaptive intelligence: intelligence is not a personal trait but rather a person × task × situation interaction. J. Intell. **9**(4) (2021)
4. Rivas-López, R., Sandoval-García-Travesí, F.: Robotic surgery in gynecology: review of literature. Cirugia y cirujanos (Eng) (1), 107–116 (2020)
5. Mikhail, D., Sarcona, J., Mekhail, M., Richstone, L.: Urologic robotic surgery. Surg. Clin. N. Am. **100**(2), 361–378 (2020). Robotic Surgery
6. Štádler, P., Dorosh, J., Dvořáček, L., Vitásek, P., Matouš, P., Lin, J.C.: Review and current update of robotic-assisted laparoscopic vascular surgery. Semin. Vasc. Surg. **34**(4), 225–232 (2021)
7. Hashimoto, D.A., Rosman, G., Rus, D., Meireles, O.R.: Artificial intelligence in surgery: promises and perils. Ann. Surg. **268**, 70–76 (2018)
8. Fahrner, R., Rauchfu, F., Bauschke, A., Kissler, H., Settmacher, U., Zanow, J.: Robotic hepatic surgery in malignancy: review of the current literature. J. Robot. Surg. **13**(4), 533–538 (2019)
9. Alip, S., Kim, J., Rha, K., Han, W.: Future platforms of robotic surgery. Urol. Clin. N. Am. **49**, 23–38 (2022). Funding Information: The authors have nothing to disclose
10. Yip, M.C., Das, N.: Robot autonomy for surgery. CoRR, abs/1707.03080, 1–33 (2017)
11. Hwang, M., Ichnowski, J., Thananjeyan, B., Seita, D., Paradis, S., Fer, D., Low, T., Goldberg, K.: Automating surgical peg transfer: calibration with deep learning can exceed speed, accuracy, and consistency of humans. IEEE Trans. Autom. Sci. Eng. **20**(2), 909–922 (2023)
12. Gupta, A., Singla, T., Chennatt, J., David, L., Ahmed, S., Rajput, D.: Artificial intelligence: a new tool in surgeon's hand. J. Edu. Health Promot. **11**(93) (2022)
13. Di Sivo, M., De Paolis, V.: Robot-assisted surgery in the operating room: ottimizzazione degli spazi e qualit delle performance, ch. 5. Human factors and technological design innovation. Pisa University Press (2021)
14. Jupiter, J.: The making of a great surgeon. Tech. Hand Up. Extrem. Surg. **18**(2), 61 (2014)
15. Balch, J., Upchurch, G.R., Bihorac, A., Loftus, T.J.: Bridging the artificial intelligence valley of death in surgical decision-making. Surgery **169**(4), 746–748 (2021)
16. Mestres, C., Quintana, E., Pereda, D.: Will artificial intelligence help us in predicting outcomes in cardiac surgery? J. Card. Surg. **37**(11), 3846–3847 (2022)
17. Cormi, C., Parpex, G., Julio, C., Ecarnot, F., Laplanche, D., Vannieuwenhuyse, G., Duclos, G., Sanchez, S.: Understanding the surgeon's behaviour during robot-assisted surgery: protocol for the qualitative behav'robot study. BMJ Open **12**(4) (2022)
18. Yampolskiy, R.V.: Unpredictability of AI (2019)
19. Franklin, M., Awad, E., Ashton, H., Lagnado, D.: Unpredictable robots elicit responsibility attributions. Behav. Brain Sci. **46**, e30 (2023)
20. Oakley, J.: Virtue Ethics and Professional Roles. Cambridge University Press (2001)
21. Orri, M., Revah-Lévy, A., Farges, O.: Surgeons emotional experience of their everyday practice - a qualitative study. PLoS ONE **10**(11), e0143763 (2015)
22. Menne, I., Schwab, F.: Faces of emotion: investigating emotional facial expressions towards a robot. Int. J. Soc. Robotics **10**(2), 199–209 (2018)
23. Gao, S., Lu, Z., Luan, H., Yin, M., Wang, L.: AI pilot in the cockpit: an investigation of public acceptance. Int. J. Hum. Comput. Interact. **41**(1), 543–556 (2025)

24. Halpern, J.: From Detached Concern to Empathy: Humanizing Medical Practice. Oxford University Press (2001)
25. Lee, H., Woodward-Kron, R., Merry, A., Weller, J.: Emotions and team communication in the operating room: a scoping review. Med. Educ. Online **28**(1), 2194508 (2023)
26. Mori, M.: The uncanny valley. Energy **7**(4), 33–35 (1970)
27. Balistreri, M., Casile, F.: Methodologies and Intelligent System for Technology Enhanced Learning (2019), 9th International Conference, ch. Care Robots: from Tools of Care to Training Opportunities. Moral Considerations, pp. 18–25. Springer Nature Switzerland (2020)
28. Balistreri, M.: Sex robots: love in the age of machines. Trivent Publishing (2022)
29. Dumouchel, P., Damiano, L.: Living with Robots. Harvard University Press (2016)
30. Birkhoff, D.C., van Dalen, A.S.H., Schijven, M.P.: A review on the current applications of artificial intelligence in the operating room. Surg. Innov. **28**(5), 611–619 (2021)
31. Damiano, L., Dumouchel, P.: Anthropomorphism in human robot co-evolution. Front. Psychol. **9** (2018)
32. Sparrow, R.: Robots, rape, and representation. Int. J. Soc. Robot. **9** (2017)
33. Sparrow, R.: Virtue and vice in our relationships with robots: is there an asymmetry and how might it be explained? Int. J. Soc. Robot. **13**(1), 23–29 (2020)
34. Patuzzo, S., Balistreri, M., Marinelli, T., Giacopuzzi, S.: Is a robot surgeon with AI the ideal surgeon? a philosophical analysis. AI Ethics **5**(1), 2025-02
35. Tobia, K., Nielsen, A., Stremitzer, A.: When does physician use of AI increase liability? J. Nucl. Med. **62**(1) (2021)
36. Coeckelbergh, M.: Artificial intelligence, responsibility attribution, and a relational justification of explainability. Sci. Eng. Ethics **26**(4), 2051–2068 (2020)
37. Balkin, J.: The three laws of robotics in the age of big data. http://hdl.handle.net/20.500.13051/4697 (2017). Accessed: 2025-02-15
38. Kerasidou, A.: Ethics of artificial intelligence in global health: explainability, algorithmic bias and trust. J. Oral Biol. Craniofacial Res. **11**(4), 612–614 (2021)

Automation on the Brink of Autonomy: Letting Go of Control

Maria-Camilla Fiazza and Paolo Fiorini

Abstract In this chapter we make some reflections on the evolving relationship between mankind and machines, with an eye to super-intelligent machines and the fast-approaching frontier of autonomous robots. Here, humankind encounters Another: finding itself mirrored and challenged as the mythical Pygmalion, it labors to work out a relational stance. We explore the dynamics of control and the danger of new forms of marginalization and enslavement, and suggest there is room for authentic relationship where both man and machine have acquired mastery. We discuss the problem of meaningful supervision and touch on its practical consequences on safety and on its enabling technologies.

1 Introduction

The advent of software that exhibits super-human intelligence heralds a fast-approaching horizon, the margin where automation becomes autonomy. At this new frontier mankind encounters Another—an artificial agent, the first able to operate at a level of abstraction similar to ours, and in some ways exceed our performance.

Prior attempts to place machines in complex environments have resulted in performance levels so very far removed from ours that machines were not serious candidates for a relationship between equals. Things changed with the advent of deep learning and a plethora of other key enabling advances, both in hardware and software technology.

Machines come from us but do not think like us. They organize information in ways that can be profoundly different from ours, leveraging super-human speed and probabilistic thinking to burn through enormous numbers of possible configurations, instead of relying on abstraction and semantic connections as humans do. These new super-human machines are predictable and fully knowable in theory, but not in

M.-C. Fiazza
Department of Surgery, Dentistry, Paediatrics and Gynaecology, University of Verona, Verona, Italy

P. Fiorini (✉)
Department of Engineering for Innovation Medicine, University of Verona, Verona, Italy
e-mail: paolo.fiorini@univr.it

P. Fiorini (ed.), *Towards Autonomous Robotic Surgery*, Springer Tracts in Advanced Robotics 161, https://doi.org/10.1007/978-3-032-04247-7_13

practice. We have mostly observational knowledge of them: hence, we are in effect dealing with another type of agent, who is doing what we do in its own way. We can interpret or understand its workings to a certain extent, but the machine is not completely transparent to us.

There is a newcomer in our once-exclusive operational space, inside our ecological niche. Is the new kid on the block a competitor—a threat—or a new companion—an aid? We are to choose a stance.

2 Relationship: On Dignity and Control

We have witnessed machines progress from the age of mechanics to the age of electronics, actively building for them new bodies to inhabit, infusing into them the products of our ingenuity. Machines first conquered the domain of the simple repetition, and then moved on to claim the immense vastness of big data for themselves, as their own kingdom: we cannot function at that scale, nor at that speed. As the parents of a gifted child who surpasses us, we need to rethink our role. First creators, then authorities, then guides—and now? Psychologically, humanity is experiencing a very difficult passage, the discovery of the existence of Another. As a species, we have to choose between control and cooperation, between fear and confidence.

Well known patterns in family therapy tell us what failure looks like when it happens at the human level: the parent tightens the grip, becomes controlling and suffocates the child's potential. At times, the parent cultivates the illusion of autonomy, calling it supervision, and requiring unattainable performance levels as a condition for independence. The desire to protect a vulnerable or inexperienced child from error can be healthy. However, often the core issue is power—a struggle over who is allowed to have the initiative and who must adapt to whom. Genuine otherness can be perceived as a threat and trigger a drive to suppress all unpredictability, uniqueness and individuality. An attitude of grounded openness, on the other hand, allows learning from Another what is uniquely visible from another vantage point, from a different way to understand the world.

From the budding fields of cooperative robotics we learn that explicability, interpretability and in part also explainability are key for safety, rather than total control. Total control is stifling and thwarts the ability to respond to circumstances. Currently, certifying a system removes all room for change after certification, an example of when control backfires. We need to envision more flexible ways to deploy machines and embrace the fact that they will change with experience. There are other dangers besides rigid control. The relationship could tip the other way, with the enslavement of man.

In some contexts robots are sold as replacement objects of affection—for company and for sex—created to be always obedient and used to manipulate human emotions instead of fulfill them. The sale pitch is appealing because of the illusion that it is possible to overcome loneliness with convenient and need-free relationships.

If we cede to the temptation to devalue human relationships through machines, we will end up devaluing man altogether. By treating robots as humans, we will end up treating humans like robots—with a dearth of dialogue, negotiation, accommodation, consideration. When humans start competing with obedient robots for affection and attention, the dominant logic of human relationship will become that of subservience to power.

How close are we to that space when machines are so useful that human life will be economically devalued, pushing most of mankind onto a new margin? How close are we to asking man to adapt to the machine, instead of building machines that fit harmoniously with man? Bias in AI will crush the vulnerable, the poor, the weak. These power imbalances are solved through the commitment to value man, every man: by making room for meaningful consent and by accepting that any mismatch of skill and need ought to be resolved upwards. Putting robots in human roles is a far cry from measuring ourselves with machines who can show us what we did not know, and help us grow into our full potential.

3 The Terrain of Encounter

We prepare for an authentic encounter with machines by practicing in situations where the machine is a helper, and where autonomy makes the machine a better helper. In robotic surgery, for example, once the robot masters the autonomous execution of small tasks, the surgeon can be made available to the patient at the point of his highest contribution, without being saddled with fatigue. As the machine lightens loads and relieves burdens, we practice being comfortable transferring control of small things, to ready ourselves for the large leaps of faith.

One famous encounter occurred on the Go board, between the Go masters, representing Man, and the program AlphaGo [1], representing the machine child of Man. In the game Go, the space of possibilities is so vast that personality shines through in the playing style, it is revealed in the playing style. In Asian culture, playing Go is both an art and an instrument to further the knowledge of oneself. Fan Hui, the first to play and lose against AlphaGo, explains that *AlphaGo is a real mirror, playing against it feels like being naked* [2]. In that nakedness, where man has to confront himself, room for doubt opens up and with it also the opportunity to connect with Another solely through the board, in a new, distilled way. Fan Hui holds that AlphaGo taught him to be a better player and to see things he had not been able to conceive of before, even as a 2nd dan Go master.

AlphaGo's moves were at times surprising, with even 9th dan masters seeing them at first as mistakes, and then realizing their brilliance. *Over two games, [AlphaGo] has beaten the very best by playing in ways that no human would* [3]. These masters are focused on their art. Humble and growth-oriented, they are changed by the encounter with Another. From the artificial intelligence of AlphaGo, they learned new playing styles and a new aesthetic appreciation for the game: an *impossible* innovation for a game played for three thousand years.

The terrain of the encounter with Another, the place where there is room for genuine companionship, is mastery. Here super-human machines can help us push the boundary of where humans can go. This margin is a bound, the confine of our limitations. Masters are unable to learn much from other humans because they have already beaten them all, or seen all the strategies humans can find. This other kind of intelligence, if we learn to leverage it, will give the best of us a companion, a play mate, an engine of growth.

4 Risk, Error and Safety

Accepting the challenge of autonomous machines also means accepting the risk of error—of a new kind of error, one that comes from non-human heuristics. These are errors which we do not know how to evaluate a priori and can not defend against. Even the Go masters could not tell if some of AlphaGo's moves were bad or brilliant at first. There were brilliant moves, and there were also inexplicably bad moves. From machines we ought to expect both, because even with their computational speed one cannot cover the whole space of possibilities. Where there is little experience to leverage, there will be bad moves. Once artificial intelligence is taken outside the realm of games, one has to wonder how to reconcile safety with the idea that machines will err, sometimes spectacularly, and that we should let them.

We must never be nonchalant with errors we know are errors. However, where only machines can go, we do not know how to recognize at first if what they suggest we do are errors or reasoned, well-informed and creative solutions that will repay our trust with progress. One approach consists of distinguishing between errors that derive from incompleteness of knowledge (the discovery errors typical of learning, which are seldom repeated) and errors that derive from internal contradictions, which are systematically committed because they are the fruit of flawed learning. By going to war against the second, we earn the right to be open to the first.

Safety is not about *playing it safe* in a needlessly fearful way. If the system is designed well, failures ends up being aligned with the occurrence of rare cases, just discovered by the machine. This calls for specialized methods to recognize and then handle the anomalous situations.

5 Conclusions

Supervising machines that have reached a level of mastery comparable to human experts is a challenge that will require creative solutions and methodological rigor. In particular, in safety-critical applications such as medical robotics and diagnostics, one can foresee the need to re-evaluate using expert opinion as the ground truth for machine learning. If humanity can bring itself to let go of its constant and total control over machines, it will be welcomed to dwell in new spaces, those beyond the limits of human computation, and it will find there unexpected margins of growth and improvement.

References

1. DeepMind, G.: The alphago web page. https://deepmind.google/research/projects/alphago/. Accessed: 2025-06-5
2. Kohs, G.: AlphaGo the movie. https://www.youtube.com/watch?v=WXuK6gekU1Y. Accessed: 2025-06-5
3. Metz, C.: The sadness and beauty of watching google's AI play GO. https://www.wired.com/2016/03/sadness-beauty-watching-googles-ai-play-go/. Accessed: 2025-06-5

Communication Strategy of the ARS Project

Martina Doppio and Paolo Fiorini

Abstract In this chapter we describe the communication strategy that was developed for the ARS project, how this strategy was implemented in different media and in-person events, and how we assessed the communication results. In Sect. 1 we present the challenges involved in the communication of complex scientific subjects, and in Sect. 2 we address the specific problems of communicating autonomous medical robotics, which would, eventually, affect the lives of people attending our seminars. In Sect. 3 we present the specific elements of the ARS project, such as logo, project identity, audiences and communication channels. Section 4 describes the on-line communication of the ARS project, based on giving a "face" to the scientific concepts, by asking the researchers involved to record brief statements about their work. Section 5 describes the in-person activities, consisting of seminars and short courses, workshops and one-to-one discussions. Finally, Sect. 6 discusses the outcomes of the communication in terms of qualitative and quantitative assessments, and the important lesson learned while interacting with the audiences.

One of the most important tasks of a research project is to make everybody aware of the results achieved. By everybody, one may mean a variety of audiences, starting from his or her own scientific community, to the members of one own institution, the media, the community at large and possibly Institution and political administrators. Usually, by dissemination we refer to the targeted distribution of research findings to a relevant audience of scientists, policymakers, or practitioners. Communication instead refers to the exchange of information with a wider range of people, including the public. Interestingly, dissemination is a one-way process of sharing information, whereas communication is a two-way interaction. Both activities can also be indicated with the general term of *Public Engagement* (PE).

M. Doppio (✉)
Department of Computer Science, University of Verona, Verona, Italy
e-mail: martina.doppio@gmail.com

Etifor | Valuing Nature, Padova, Italy

P. Fiorini
Department of Engineering for Innovation Medicine, University of Verona, Verona, Italy
e-mail: paolo.fiorini@univr.it

P. Fiorini (ed.), *Towards Autonomous Robotic Surgery*, Springer Tracts in Advanced Robotics 161, https://doi.org/10.1007/978-3-032-04247-7_14

In the ARS project, we set up the additional goal of using these activities as experiments to test the audience reaction to the novel concepts presented, i.e. the possibility of receiving health care by a machine, resulting from the integration of Artificial intelligence (AI) algorithms and robotics. This mixture of technologies is the subject of endless movies and media reports, most of them presenting dystopic scenarios in which intelligent robots dominate mankind. The application area of ARS is surgery, which amplifies the audience sensitivity. Clearly, one may assume that the scientific community would react with interest to the proposed solutions, but we were curious to see the reactions of the other communities. For example, the general public may not be ready for robotic medical and surgical assistance, the philosophical and religious communities may object to the ethics of a robot deciding the course of a surgery, and the legal community may be critical about machine learning and civil liability. We were **precursors**, anticipating the current wave of AI fears, by inquiring about people concerns. In this Chapter we briefly summarize the philosophy that drove our dissemination and communication activities, the many meetings we carried out, and the conclusions we derived from the interactions with the different audiences.

1 Introduction

The communication of research results is a great challenge that involves the transmission of complex concepts to broad and diverse audiences in terms of knowledge and cultural background. The difficulties are not only related to the concepts communicated, but also to the rapid changes of our surrounding world with new media channels appearing and new communication languages being created. Communication must then create clear and concise messages that are tailored to each audience, that are tuned to the specific language of each community, and that present the scientific results with relevant and impactful examples.

ARS achieved many important scientific results. It established the framework for robotic autonomy in surgery, which includes knowledge acquisition, planning, sensing and perception, and task execution. These results were disseminated through conference and journal publications receiving recognition and visibility. However, the opinion and feedback of communities outside our own, e.g. the medical profession, the patient associations, and the general public, are harder to acquire. To adopt a more creative and interdisciplinary approach in our public engagement strategy, we involved philosophers, ethics experts and students of Theology. These experts were able to guide us in exploring the different project facets and gave us a better insight into the value and meaning of our technologies. The outcomes of these meetings represent the results of our PE strategy. We attained to the following basic considerations and principles:

- Good scientific communication should provide an accurate context, decline the message at different levels of depth, capture the attention of the audience, overcome the possible initial lack of knowledge, and stimulate critical and evidence-based thinking. We assumed the audience had strong curiosity and interest in the subjects presented, because of their participation to the meetings, and we strived to increase and resonate with their curiosity.

- The Covid-19 pandemic and the disasters related to extreme weather have increased the attention towards the world of science, which is expected to provide answers and tools to interpret and protect from such aggressive events. Research conducted by Eurobarometer [1] shows that citizens of the European Union have an overall very positive opinion of science and scientists. However, over half of them believe that researchers should communicate more to policy makers and to the public.
- To address the public opinion concerns about truth and excess of information, sources must be authoritative and act to avoid anti-scientific drifts and denials. We adhered to the principle of using factual and verifiable data in our communication, to limit the risk of being misunderstood or of triggering reactions that can prevent or limit the understanding of scientific facts presented.
- The European Commission supports open science [2], consisting of the free dissemination of knowledge as soon as it is available. Scientific communication is a key element of this strategy and requires advanced communication skills, understanding of the target audience and a commitment to making science accessible and relevant to everyone. In the ARS project communication, we made our best effort to move forward in this direction.

2 The Challenges of Communicating Autonomous Medical Robotics

The communication of research results in autonomous robotics, especially when addressing medical or surgical procedures, presents unique challenges due to the highly technical content of the topic and of its potential impact on people health. Robotics is a research area in which Italy has a top world ranking in terms of published papers, according to indices 5.5.2, 5.5.3 and 5.5.5 of the Elsevier Research Metrics Guidebook [3], as processed by the I-RIM association [4]. However, the communication of the research results outside the robotics community is not as widespread as it should be.

The communication of robotics research faces the additional challenge of competing with Artificial Intelligence (AI) research for the public attention. Clearly, autonomous robots derive their behavior from the integration of AI and robotics, however physical interaction goes beyond the AI capabilities. Today's scientific communication does not distinguish between robotics and AI, making communication more difficult because of the need of detailed explanations about the differences.

Autonomous medical and surgical robots are devices consisting of complex components that interact with each other and with the environment in ways that are often non directly predictable. Behaviors that cannot be easily explained can generate fear and mistrust in many people, including doctors and patients. They are surely not deeply familiar with robotic and AI technologies and may know about them only from simple and often unclear media reports. Thus, a clear communication to patients and medical personnel about how autonomous medical robots work and what advantages and risks they offer is essential to overcome their **lack of familiarity** with technology. This will be specially needed during the discussion of the informed consent before an intervention, and will give patients a more active role in their medical process.

Presenting autonomous medical robots as safe devices to both medical professionals and patients is crucial to obtain people **trust** in the technology. This can be achieved by describing how they are designed, tested and monitored to ensure patient safety and to give simple key data about their performance. In this sense, it is also worth considering the issue of **cultural acceptance**, which can vary according to the specific national background and the level of technical knowledge.

A concern about autonomous robotics now raising in relation to autonomous driving technologies refers to its **ethical and legal** aspects. The use of robotics in the medical field raises even more complex issues, such as liability in the event of errors or damages. With our meetings we aimed at preparing the ground for discussion and an open dialogue among different fields of knowledge, i.e. legal, philosophical, and engineering, to freely exchange opinions on how these issues should be addressed.

When considering the end users of robots, that is, medical professionals and surgeons in particular, the biggest challenge is that of **training and skills**: surgeons must learn to work with robots effectively and safely. A collaborative design approach, involving engineers and end users, influences very positively the adoption and the effective use of these technologies: intuitive interfaces and training process must be jointly designed to focus on the important skills. In the market consisting of public and private hospitals and healthcare facilities, the issue of robot use must involve delicate **financial aspects**, since medical robots are often very expensive and require very long payback times. To gain the support of these stakeholders to the new technologies, it is essential to communicate how the robot acquisition and operational costs can be justified by increased efficiency, improved care and reduced hospital stay.

Finally, autonomous robots must pass rigorous **regulatory and approval** tests, addressing the European regulation about using AI system in safety critical applications.

Overcoming these challenges requires a strategic communication approach, involving clear and accessible language, the transmission of correct information and an open dialogue with all stakeholders, including medical professionals, patients and the general public.

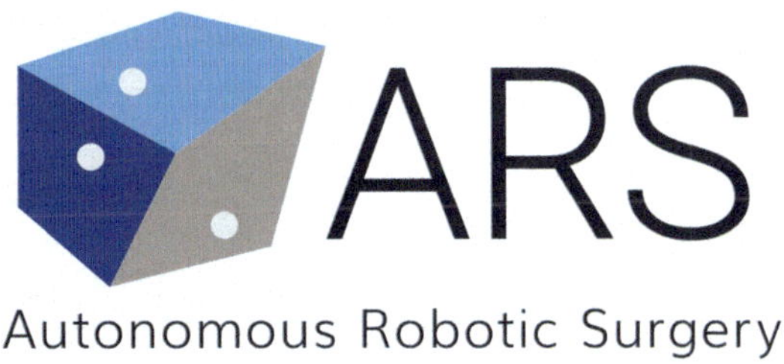

Fig. 1 The ARS project logo

3 Communicating the ARS Project

The ARS project started on October 1st, 2017 and it was supposed to last five years ending on September 30th, 2022. Obviously, we did not expect that all project activities would have been disrupted by the COVID-19 pandemic. Since project communication involved large gatherings of people, it was severely affected by the pandemic. During most of 2020 no meeting could be organized and, in the following years, the potential audiences were reluctant to meet for a scientific discussion, fearing new spreading of the virus. Fortunately, the project was extended with an additional year till September 30, 2023, so that we could compensate for the delays due to the pandemic.

The first step of the communication and dissemination strategy of the ARS project was to define the visual identity of the project, by finding graphical representations of its objectives and of the development process. To achieve this, we defined the logo of the project, shown in Fig. 1, representing the three main elements that create the basis of the project: the expertise in the field represented by the light blue wedge, the possibility of collecting clinical data, represented in dark blue, and the availability of a surgical robot for laboratory experiments represented in gray. The rationale for the project and the path to achieve the objectives of the project are graphically described in the ARS video on the YouTube channel https://www.youtube.com/watch?v=6Xn19CeIBdA&t=11s. The dots in the wedges represent the contributions that our team would give to the success of the project.

To collect comments and suggestions on the ARS topics, we organized a workshop as the project kick off. Thirty-eight people were invited to the event representing many technical and non technical research areas and communities in Europe and the United States. We used the workshop to communicate the project goals and challenges to members of engineering, medical and legal communities and collected their feedback through *Brain Writing* sessions. These sessions were organized in four separate groups, after ARS technical presentations, and each focused on a specific topic related to "autonomy in robotic surgery":

1. Accessibility: interfaces, communication, ethics, social aspects.
2. Knowledge representation: requirements, knowledge collection, formalism.
3. Autonomy levels: applications, granularity, TRL for autonomy,

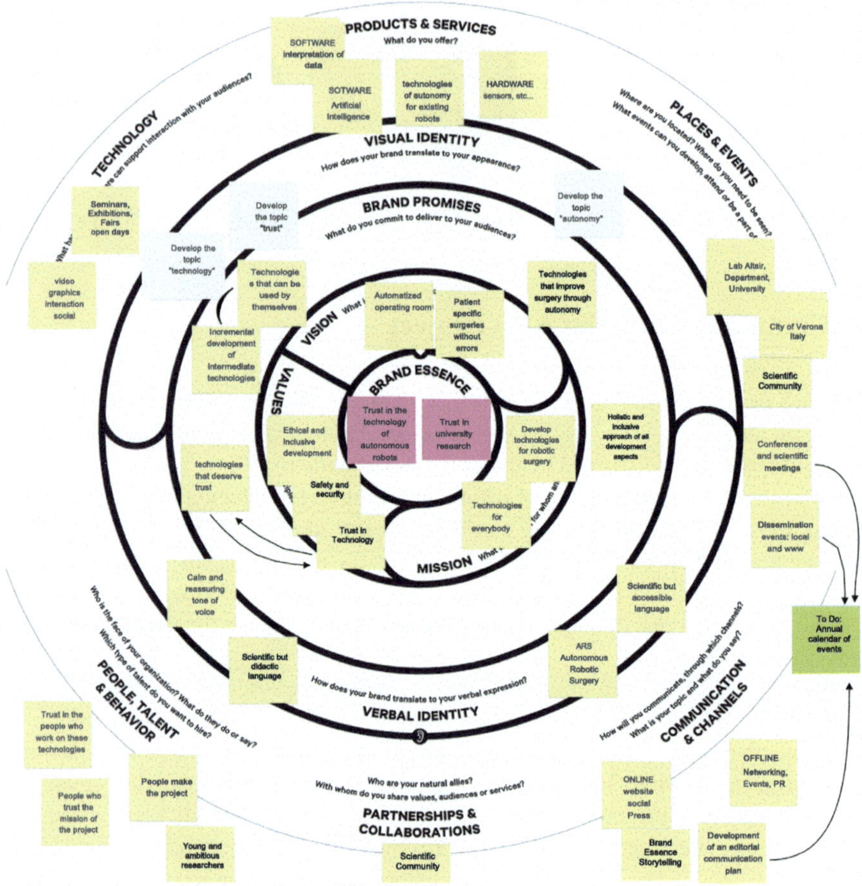

Fig. 2 Chart representing the ARS project identity

4. Technologies: hardware and software specific architectures, control models, reasoning and AI

Within these brain storming sessions, we assessed the degree of maturity of the various technologies related to ARS, their possible development, and we consolidated our relationship with members of the relevant scientific communities.

The communication and dissemination aspects of ARS were addressed specifically in an internal workshop. To guide the discussion, we used the *Brand Thinking Canvas* shown in the following figures. The first canvas, shown in Fig. 2 represents the brand identity of the project and charts in Figs. 3 and 4 represent the audiences of the project.

A *thinking canvas* is typically used in a design process to visually map out a problem, identify key stakeholders, brainstorm potential solutions, and analyze their impact. It gave a structured framework to the discussion and definition of the com-

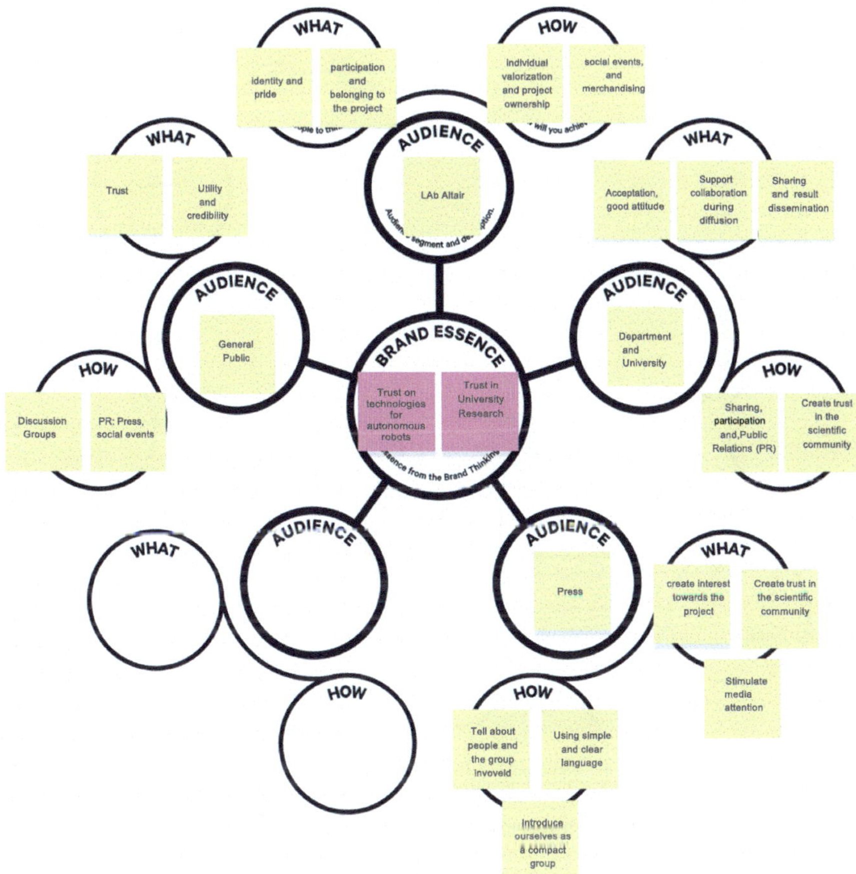

Fig. 3 Chart representing the primary ARS audience

munication and dissemination strategy of the ARS project. This framework helped us define the core values that the project desired to propose to the public and identify the type of language and style that we should used for each distinct audience. We used sticky notes, colors, and visual aids to clearly represent different ideas and connections, we encouraged discussion and brainstorming within the participant to generate diverse perspectives, and we adapt the flow of discussion to different topics that were raised related to the ARS project.

We iterated among the different concentric circles of the canvas, starting close to the center with the items we had clear in our mind: vision, values and mission of the project ARS. These items were clearly stated in the project proposal, and they were easy to identify. The ARS vision was based on the hypothesis that some level of automation would have increased the safety in the operating room, thus leading to the partial automation of every surgical process. The values directly followed from the

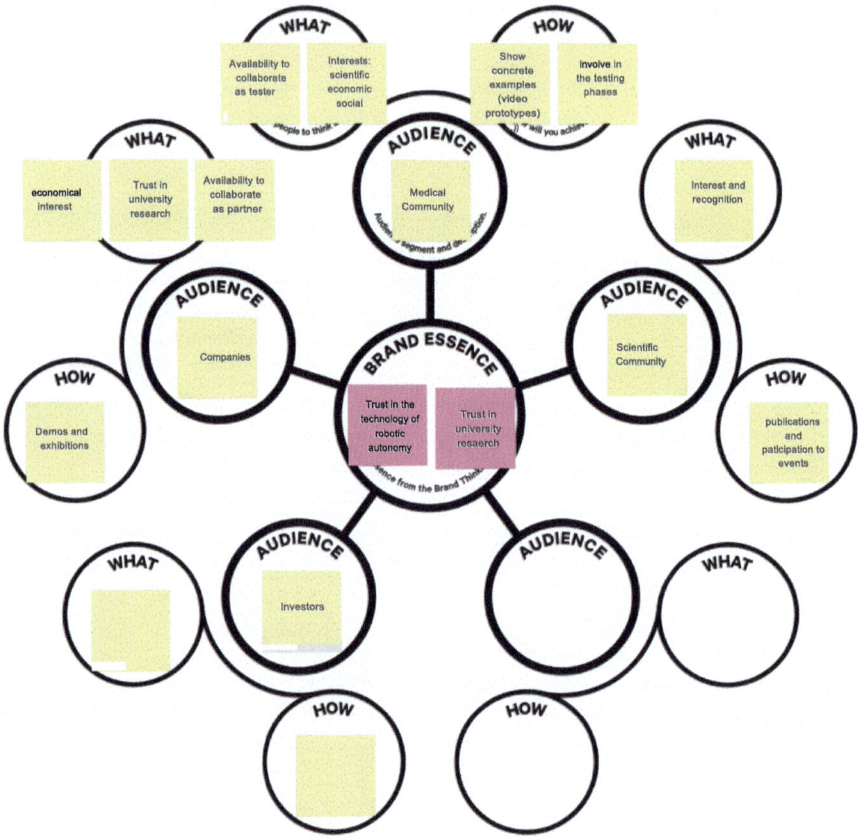

Fig. 4 Chart representing other target of ARS communication

vision and included the ethical and safe approach to technology and the confidence in the value and effectiveness of technology. Thus the mission of the project was to fulfil the vision and the values by developing technologies for autonomous surgery that could be to the benefit of all. We were surprised then to realize that the identity of the ARS project, called *Brand Essence* on the canvas, was not technology or its results but trust in the scientific results we were to achieve and in the infrastructure in which we were working. These are the red labels at the center of the canvas.

The outer layers of the canvas help us focus on the details of what we wanted to communicate. In fact, in the *Brand Promises* we specified our vision in specific technologies for robotics and autonomy that can be used alone or combined with other developments and can deserve our trust. In the layers on *Identity* we specified the visual and verbal tone of communication, which consisted of simpler but scientifically correct language, presented with a reassuring voice and with visual aids that could immediately convey the concepts of autonomy, technology and trust.

Then in the outmost layer we defined what, where, and how we would have made tangible the conceptual elements identified in the inner layers. In fact, we were to describe our *Products and Services*, using technological means of communication and different channels. This process helped us discovering aspects of *Places and Events* and of *People and Talents* that we were not fully aware of. We realized that our project mission and values might not have been clearly known to our institution and to our co-workers. Thus, the first place where to start our communication was within our laboratory and our department, and our first audience was necessarily consisting of our colleagues who, although working on, or near, the ARS project might not have known the full extent and articulation of the project.

Having understood the importance of communicating our work even in our own backyard, we developed an onion-like communication strategy, starting from our own Altair laboratory, our department and our university, our specific scientific community and the medical communities, companies and investors, the general public and the press. Clearly each audience needed a different approach both in terms of events in which to present our work and in terms of topics described.

The involvement of our colleagues, co-workers and students at various stages of their academic career was achieved by organizing social events during special occasions. It could have been the Christmas party, the European Robotics Week enhanced by *Scientific Apertif*, as shown in Fig. 5 the Student Summer Celebration, the visit of some important guest, one of the periodic visits of high school students during orientation week. During these events, the different members of the team were presenting the project and their specific results with the objective of building project identity, sense of belonging, and pride in their work, while also becoming accustomed to public speaking.

Going up a notch, we organized and/or participated to scientific meetings within the University of Verona. In this case our goals included sharing of scientific results, create opportunities for collaboration and stimulate our colleagues to address topics that were at the forefront of robotics and computer science. In particular, we interacted with the colleagues in the departments of Medicine and Surgery, Humanities and Law within thematic workshops, plenary lectures, and public events. These interactions were truly stimulating and the communication was bi-directional, receiving many new ideas and suggestions while presenting to our colleagues.

Going further away from our institution, we addressed the robotics research community, the industrial automation sector and presented the case of our technology to the investment community. These events were more traditional, e.g. scientific presentations at meetings, conferences and technology exhibitions. In these cases the communication was mostly one-directional with the audience rarely interacting with the speakers.

Of great interest for the ARS project was the communication to the general public and the press. Of course, we wanted to create interest in our project and raise confidence in the scientific development, but we also wanted to receive feedback from these diverse audiences about the future possibility of interacting with a robotic medical assistant and of being diagnosed by an AI program. In Italy, every city has a program of continuing education for the citizens, and we gave lectures and courses

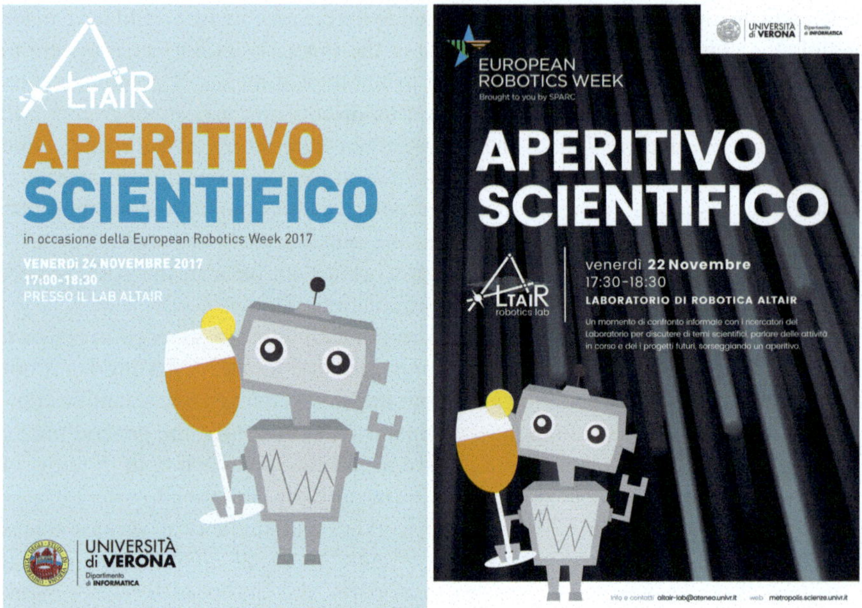
ALTAIR
APERITIVO
SCIENTIFICO
in occasione della European Robotics Week 2017
VENERDì 24 NOVEMBRE 2017
17:00-18:30
PRESSO IL LAB ALTAIR
UNIVERSITÀ di VERONA
Dipartimento di INFORMATICA
UNIVERSITÀ di VERONA
EUROPEAN ROBOTICS WEEK
Brought to you by SPARC
APERITIVO
SCIENTIFICO
ALTAIR robotics lab
venerdì 22 Novembre
17:30-18:30
LABORATORIO DI ROBOTICA ALTAIR
Un momento di confronto informale con i ricercatori del Laboratorio per discutere di temi scientifici, parlare delle attività in corso e dei i progetti futuri, sorseggiando un aperitivo.
info e contatti altair-lab@ateneo.univr.it
web metropolis.scienze.univr.it

Fig. 5 Fliers of the Scientific Aperitif events held in the Altair laboratory

to these programs. Most of the audience consists of elderly and retired people, but usually with a high cultural level and strong curiosity about science developments. These events were attended by a public ranging from 60 to 200 people and the interaction with the public was very active and stimulating. The interaction with the press occurred mostly as a side event to another event. Press and TV reports were present to document events related to the project and we gave interviews during those occasions.

4 On-Line Communication and Dissemination of ARS

The on-line Communication and Dissemination strategy of the ARS relied on the project web site and on frequent posts on Twitter (now X). The web site of the project is;
https://www.ars-project.eu
and the Twitter channel is:
https://x.com/arsproject_erc.
Both communication forms aimed at describing the ARS scientific results, alert and summarize the events associated to the project, and introducing the researchers working on the project.

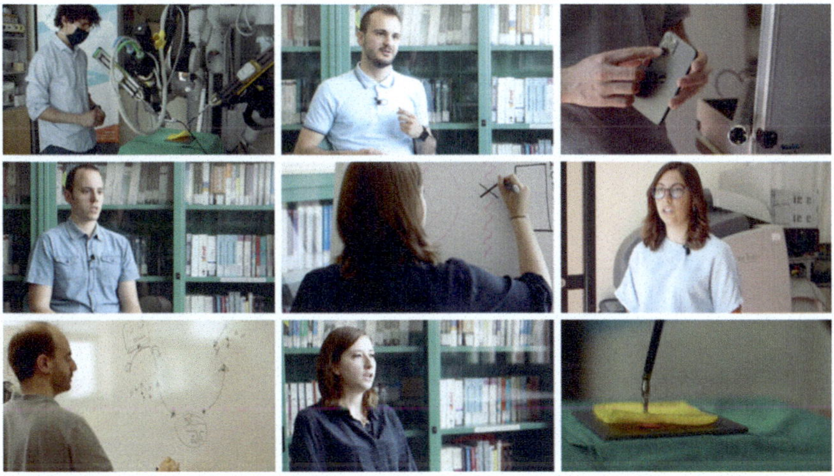

Fig. 6 Link to the Research Insight videos

The web site relies on a combination of standard features and of a novel form of communication that we called *Research Insights*, shown in Fig. 6 These are short video clips in which members of the ARS community give their opinion about issues related to robotic autonomy or explain some of ARS research results. The web site is organized in many linked pages: Home, Project, Results, News, Contacts, that are described in the following.

- The *Home* tab is the landing page of the web site and shows the links to the Research Insights, the ARS goals, the group expertise, and the latest news. These pages can also be reached by the web site tabs.
- The *Project* page is organized in three subpages:
  - The *About* page presents the ARS Advisory Board, the state of the art and the project objectives, and the factors making the ARS project timely and scientifically relevant. The Advisory Board was formed by prof. Alicia Casals, prof. Pierre Jannin, and prof. Marco Zenati, and the page shows videos of their assessment of the potential and risks of robotic autonomy in medical and surgical robotics.
  - The Work Packages page presents the scientific objectives of the ARS project and the development methodology, based on the five main work packages corresponding to the project research lines. As expected, during the project development, the research lines intersected and strongly complemented each other.
  - The Expertise page presents the Altair Robotics Laboratory in which most of the research took place, and the team of researchers and doctoral students who worked on the ARS project (https://metropolis.scienze.univr.it).
- The *Results* page is organized in three subpages:

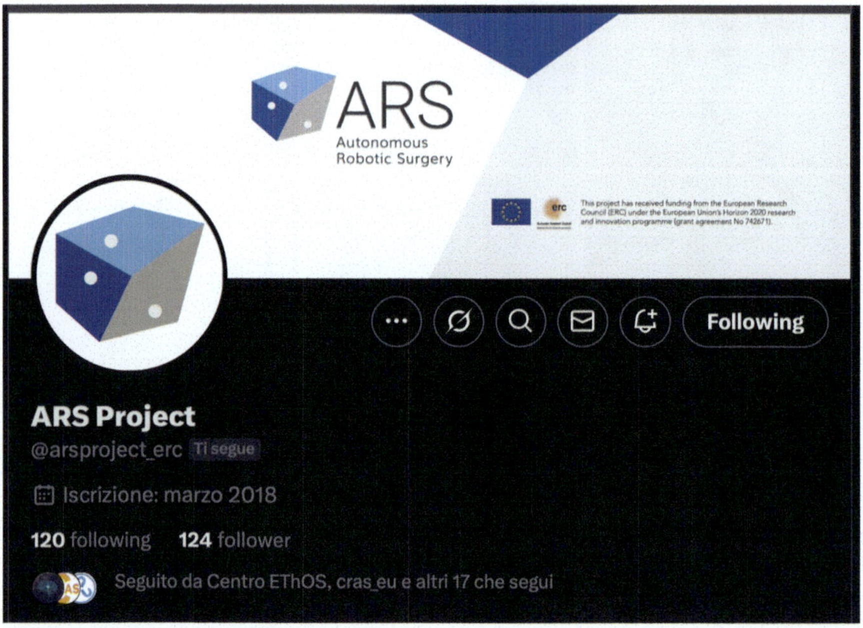

Fig. 7 Starting point of the twitter feed

- The *Latest Results* page gives a detailed description of the six main scientific contributions of the project: the formal representation of surgical knowledge Chap. 2, the robotic intervention planning Chap. 3, the patient specific simulation Chap. 6, the instrument localization in the anatomy Chap. 7, and realistic demonstrations Chap. 10.
- The *Publications* page refers to the Open Repository of the University of Verona.
- The *Research Insights* page gives the link to the project YouTube playlist (https://youtube.com/playlist?list=PL0anXc69FEER7VXeO8rBsfV1wdkxsNN4g) where the technical videos are located.

• The *News* page has the links to the press reports of the main events organized by the project ARS.
• The *Contacts* page give the street address of the Altair laboratory and its map location.

The other on-line communication channel was Twitter (now X) on which we were giving timely information about events and activities of ARS. The channel https://x.com/arsproject_erc is the time line of ARS and scrolling the tweets is like watching a sped-up reel of the project. There are posters of events, pictures from conferences, cover of published papers, and related links. The beginning of the tweets is shown in Fig. 7.

5 In-Person Communication and Dissemination of ARS

Our *in person* Public Engagement activities followed the pattern defined in the *Thinking Canvas*, i.e. divided in events for the Academia, Patient Associations, Physicians and Medical Structures, Companies, and the General Public. In the following we list the specific events organized, together with a summary of the comments received.

1. Events for the Academic World

    - We organized the project kickoff workshop inviting many researchers on AI and robotics to advise us on the key areas of the ARS project. The interviews with some of the participants are among the *Research Insights* available on the web site [5].
    - We participated to the workshop *Marginalia* [6] organized by the Doctoral School of the University of Verona to discuss the frontiers of research.
    - We participated in workshops organized by the ETHOS center of the Department of Culture and Civilization of the University of Verona during 2023. The topics were *Ethics of AI in Medicine* [7] on February 2nd, *Bioethics in Medicine* on June 6th, and *Knowing AI* on November 8th.
    - Every year we co-organized and participated to the Conference on New Technologies for Computer/Robot Assisted Surgery (CRAS) [8].
    - Important scientific events organized, or participated, by the ARS project were the doctoral summer schools.

        - At the University of Verona, we organized the school called *COSUR* that stands for Control of Surgical Robots. We organized COSUR in 2018 with a rather large attendance of students, as shown in Fig. 8 and attempted to organize COSUR in 2020, but because of the pandemics, the school was postponed. In 2022 we organized the school in Verona with a specific focus on Common Sense reasoning [9] to discuss the latest development of ARS.
        - We participated to the Doctoral Schools on Robotic Surgery organized by the LIRMM Laboratory in Montpellier (France).

    - P. Fiorini gave a plenary lecture at the CAMI Days 2022, in Montpellier (France).
    - We organized and participated in workshops on the research lines of ARS at major robotics conferences. In particular:

        - Workshop on "Surgical Robotics" at the 2019 ICAR conference in Belo Horizonte (Brazil).
        - Workshop on "Towards robotic autonomy in surgery", at the 2021 Hamlyn Symposium on Medical Robotics in London (UK).
        - Workshops on "Planning under Uncertainty" and "Ethics of Robotics", at the ICRA 2022 conference in Philadelphia (USA).

- Workshop on "Benefits and Risks of Robot Learning in Medical Applications" at the conference IROS 2022 in Kyoto (Japan).
- Workshop on "Recent Advances in Autonomous Surgery", at the 2022 Hamlyn Symposium on Medical Robotics in London (UK).
- Workshop on "Autonomous flexible surgical robots: where we are and where we are going", at the 2023 Hamlyn Symposium on Medical Robotics in London (UK).
- Workshop on "Autonomous Surgical Robotics" at the 2023 ICAR conference in Abu Dhabi (UAE).
- Workshop on "Autonomy in Robotic Surgery", at the ICRA 2024 conference in Yokohama (Japan).
- Workshop on "Applying Surgical Data Science in Robotic Surgery", at the 2024 Hamlyn Symposium on Medical Robotics in London (UK).
- Participation to the "2nd Workshop on Machine Learning in Medical Robotics: Bridging ML Theory and Clinical Frontiers" at IROS 2024 in Abu Dhabi (UAE).

2. Events for Patient Associations

- We met with two organizations of oncological patients, ANDOS on 20/04/23, and LILT on 12/05/23, to gain insights into the perspectives of individuals closely involved with cancer patients and to understand the relationship between patients and emerging technologies.

  - ANDOS is the non-profit National Association of Women with Breast Surgery that has been active in Italy for more than 20 years. It is composed of about 60 committees distributed throughout the territory. It is made up of women who have experienced breast cancer, doctors specialized in this sector and anyone who shares its goals. Its purpose is to promote personal awareness of early diagnosis, to help women who have to face a healing process towards complete recovery. The Verona Committee is managed by volunteers who have, or not have, had breast surgery. The meeting consisted of a general presentation of the ALTAIR Laboratory at UNIVR, and of the ARS project with the distribution of some information material. The participant showed great interest in the topics we presented, and appreciated the direct communication approach used. They encouraged us to continue our scientific communication aimed at doctors and patient associations, addressing the medical staff, operators and volunteers, but not the final patients. Patients refer to doctors or volunteers of the associations.
  - The meeting with the LILT organization took more time to organize because of the difficulty in organizing an event aimed at both patients and the association's board of directors. LILT has little contact with patients because it works upstream in treatment, that is, in prevention and dissemination. They are equipped with laboratories capable of providing early diagnoses to the

patient, suspected diagnoses that are then directed to the doctors' care. They are interested in what happens in our laboratory, and we agreed that our activities will be their reference on the state of the art in medical robotics.

3. Events for Physicians and Medical Structures

- We offered seminars to the medical communities, as part of their continuing education program:
  - We gave a seminar on "Robotic Surgery: between present and Future" to the School of Medicine and Surgery at the University Hospital of Verona. The student was attended by more than 150 medical students.
  - We gave two seminar at the Sacro Cuore Hospital in Negrar (https://www.sacrocuore.it/) on 05/05/23 and on 20/10/23 for their continuing education program. A lively debate followed our presentations involving physicians specialized in various disciplines. The hospital CEO noted that we should always ask "Is this good for the patient?". It was mentioned that, although the robot increases the average level of surgeries, patients would be better off with a good surgeon, thus the human elements is essential even with the most advanced automation. An orthopedic surgeon reported his experience using the Da Vinci robot: positive results and advantages in total and mono-compartmental prostheses in terms of greater precision in positioning the prosthesis, less bleeding, less use of analgesics, and less physiotherapy.
  - On October 20th, 2023 we gave a seminar at the Accademia of Sciences of Verona. The recording of the seminar is available at this link https://www.youtube.com/watch?v=wTiobJPU9WE At the end of the seminar, we distributed a questionnaire to gather feedback from participants. We collected data from 15 participants [10] which show that the participant were generally confident about the use of autonomous robots in surgery, but required the participation and the advice of the primary care physician.
- We interviewed the physicians carrying out cadaveric tests at the ICLO institution in Verona. The videos of these interviews are among the Research Insights in the web site https://www.youtube.com/playlist?list=PL0anXc69FEEReie-bNrhxQq645fNwEP8O.

4. Events for Companies

- We attended industrial exhibitions (Innova Biomed (2021, 2022) [11] in Verona and BT Expo (2021, 2022) in Modena) presenting our progress to the visitors of the ARS booth and during podium presentations.
- P. Fiorini gave an interview at the TV channel Business24 for the show Pole Position about the applications of the ARS technologies in the development of a new product for prostate cancer diagnosis.
- We presentated the ARS results to Hibot Corp in Tokyo, in November 2022.

5. Events for the General Public

- On 28/11/2017, we gave a talk at the TEDx event organized in Verona in 2017 (https://www.youtube.com/watch?v=J5Yui8ktb70), please see the subtitles in English.
- We gave lectures on AI in Medicine at the School of Theology in Verona and at an event organized by the Fondazione Toniolo (a private cultural institution).
- We participated to a series of seminars on Science and Faith organized by the Diocese of Verona.
- We gave a lecture on robotics in medicine at the "University of Permanent Education" in Bussolengo in Spring 2019. In Spring 2024 P. Fiorini offered four lectures to the "University of Permanent Education" in Verona, introducing the main concepts of robotics, AI and their applications to Medicine. These lectures in Verona were well attended and the organization asked to increase the program to six lectures in Spring 2025. These lectures are directed to elderly and retirees interested in learning about different cultural topics, among which also new technologies. The lecture in Bussolengo was attend by about 200 people, and the lectures in Verona, in 2024 and in 2025, were attended by about 50–60 people each. The lectures were always followed by a lively discussion and by general positive feedback about the use of advanced technologies in health care.

6 Discussion and Conclusions

Besides presenting the results of our research, our Public Engagement (PE) activities aimed at assessing the perception of AI and robotics by the future stakeholders of the technologies. Although our PE activities started 6 years ago, before the explosion of AI media coverage, the public sensitivity about this technology was already strong. For this reason, all our PE activities were very well attended. Because AI was not as popular as it is now, our public was more balanced than it is today and could give interesting opinions on the topics presented. In our communication activities we tried to engage the public so that we could receive feedback on our research directions from points of view that were not biased by being of technology developers.

The ethical and social implications of using robotics and AI in medical applications were among the motivations to carry out the extensive Public Engagement (PE) activities about the ARS project.

We tried to assess the impact of our on-line and in-person PE events. We could make a quantitative assessment of the efficacy of our PE activities by counting the number of accesses to our web site and twitter stream and by counting the number of

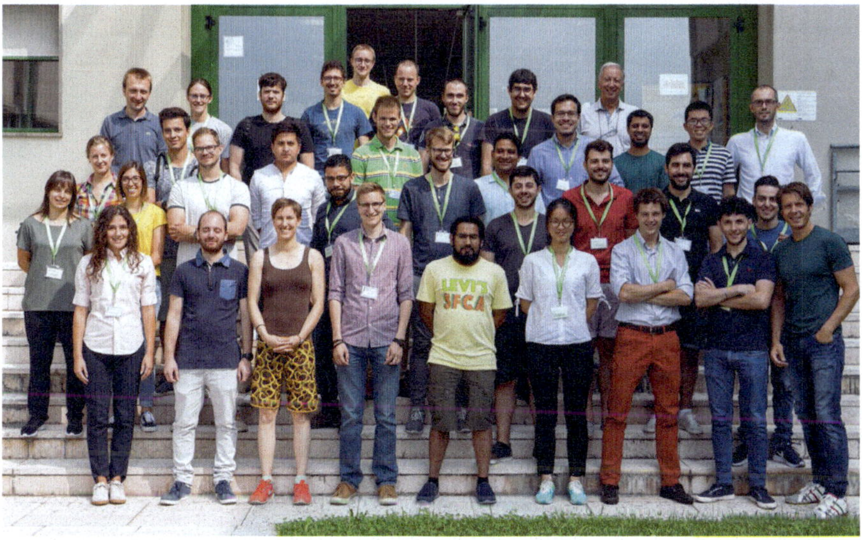

Fig. 8 The COSUR 2018 doctoral summer school

participants to the in-person meetings. The qualitative assessment was actually very interesting since it summarizes the comments received during the meetings and the discussions made with some of the participants.

6.1 *Quantitative Assessment of ARS Public Engagement Activities*

The quantitative measurement of our PE activities' success can be tracked online by considering the number of visits to the official website, views of the on-line videos, and the number of people attending the meetings we organized.

From the launch on January 1, 2018, until January 30, 2024, the website has received more than 5,600 visits while the official project video and teaser reached more than 1300 visualizations. However, the visits to the web sites may not be independent accesses. The number of views of the project videos can be seen in the YouTube page dedicated to the ARS project [5]. The 29 short videos on the research directions are divided into three groups: Autonomy, Safety and Learning. The Autonomy area received 191 views of the video in the first page and approximately 330 views of the other videos in the playlist. The Safety area received 96 views of the video in the first page and approximately 440 views of the other videos in the playlist. The Learning area received 121 views of the video in the first page and approximately 425 views of the other videos in the playlist. The videos of the interviews with ten of the participants to the kickoff workshop were viewed approximately by 1300 people, whereas the 14 video interviews with four experts and influential personalities from the scientific world made during the Hamlyn Symposium on Medical Robotics, were viewed approximately by 2000 people.

The seminars to the medical community included University students and faculty, hospital personnel and physicians attending continuing education lectures. Each event was attended by approximately 150 people on average, showing the great interest in the topic.

The participation in the industrial exhibitions attracted about 30 visitors to the booth and to the lectures, belonging to companies interested in learning about the use of artificial intelligence and robotics in medical devices.

The workshop with the researchers of the ETHOS aimed at presenting and discussing our projects with ethics and philosophy experts. The first workshop was attended by the 12 members of the center, whereas the second seminar on the ethics of AI in medicine, was open to the public, and was attended by approximately 25 people.

The PE events for the general public included large events, a television transmission, and lectures and short courses at the Continuing Education University programs in the city of Bussolengo and Verona.

The large event was the TEDx conference organized in Verona that was attended by approximately 500 people. The video of this event has been visualized 1,405 times.

The television show *Pole Position* reached about 30K people, which is the average audience of the program. The recording of each show posted on the Web receives on average 250–300 views, which is approximately the number of people viewing the show to which we participated.

The lecture at the Continuing Education University in the city of Bussolengo was attended by about 200 people. At the end of this talk, some of attendees manifested their strong interest in innovative AI and robotics therapies discussed during the lecture, to which they were not yet familiar. The short courses at the Continuing Education University in the city of Verona, are attended by 50–60 people per lecture, who interact in discuss the topics of robotics and AI at the end of each lecture.

6.2 Qualitative Assessment of ARS Public Engagement Activities

The qualitative evidence of the success of our PE activities can be determined from the feedback and the verbal interactions with the attendee during and after the meetings. The meetings were organized with an initial introduction, the main presentation, tailored on the audience interest and technical background, and ending with a discussion time.

The comments we received during the in-person events were very beneficial to us. For example, during the meeting with the ANDOS association, the participants suggested to direct our communication also to the volunteers helping patients, who could be freer for discussion than patients. Implicit to these comments was the need of an ethical approach to our research, which prompted us to involve our colleagues from the ETHOS center, and to appoint one of them as the ethics advisor of the project, before it was made mandatory for EU projects.

The evaluation of what was learned by our audiences was a difficult task, since we did not organize follow up meetings. The only case, was a second meeting with the ETHOS group, on "Ethics of AI in Medicine". In this meeting a researcher of the group built on our previous seminar, by giving a solid philosophic foundation to some of today's claims about machine autonomy, significantly broadening our understanding of the implications of our research.

The impression gathered from the interactions with people after our public events was of satisfaction for the presentations and gratitude for having shed light on the claims and risks of AI based systems. A surprising fact was that the people posing the questions did not show any additional preoccupation about using new therapies based on AI, even though they imagined the commercialization of these new therapies faster than it will be actually possible. They had a very pragmatic and open attitude towards innovation, much more than expected. In the interactions we were thanked for our transparency and clear explanations of the advantages and risks of the new technologies.

Professional audiences had a similarly open attitude towards the possibility of having intelligent robot supporting their work. Surgeons in particular would welcome this possibility and our seminars prompted several requests to cooperate on projects involving surgical automation. Our project generated only a limited interest in the companies met at the exhibitions we attended, probably because the perception of the long lead time to market made our technologies less appealing to companies.

6.3 Lesson Learned

The ARS research team learned many lessons from the Public Engagement activities described above. We learned how to identify the audiences of the project beyond the scientific community and that there is no standard lecture format. These lessons were in line with the dissemination and communication strategies developed at the beginning of the project.

Even though the lecture topic was obviously the same, the way the message was delivered was customized and adapted to each specific audience. We learned the sensibility to adapt to the audience and to tailor the communication (often in real time) depending on the type and size of the audience. We learned that the public is much more interested in advanced scientific topics than we expected, provided that these topics are explained in a clear and down to earth manner.

Most important we learned the open mind attitude of our public, which further motivated our communication activities and made us deliver even clearer and more effective presentations. The concrete evidence of such learning is in the videos presenting our research activities. They were developed on the form of "Question and Answer" interviews, rather short, with very simple and clear language, and accessible to technical and non-technical audiences.

A more anecdotical evidence of learning is the repetition of the invitation to offer a public event at the same institution. This should indicate that the presentation and the interaction with the public was successful, and the message delivered was well received by the public. Lastly, an important lesson comes from the audience that participated in our events. Data gathered from the questionnaires returned reveal a significant level of openness and trust among non-expert audiences towards new technologies. Specifically, some key findings include:

- most of the responses associate Artificial Intelligence to concepts like progress and future, more than risks and hazards;
- responses also consider of paramount importance that a robot be precise and safe before being made available to hospitals or becoming economically viable.
- the fields where AI is hoped to have the most impact are medicine and industry, rather than defense or security or surveillance.
- as further evidence of trust in new technologies, almost all respondents would undergo surgery performed by artificial intelligence either under a doctor's recommendation or even without it.

These activities enabled us to contribute to "capture" the social perception regarding robotic surgery and artificial intelligence within what we might term "Descriptive Ethics". Fears, concerns, but also hopes and trust, are among the elements present in the public, useful for understanding whether future patients would feel comfortable in a medical scenario where intelligent robots and humans cooperate. As mentioned earlier, we found that people are more pragmatic than what it emerges from the media reports.

People would seem willing to accept these novel types of medical interactions, provided that they satisfy all safety criteria, and not be preliminary versions. This consideration further highlights the need of developing transparent and explainable AI algorithms, whose correctness can be objectively assessed and that are self-aware of their domain of competence. These descriptive analyses represent a significant initial step towards developing a Normative Ethical Report conducted by a medical ethics expert, such as the ARS Ethics advisor, providing foundational insights into the ethical implications of AI in medicine and surgery. Our initial findings stimulate the need of discussing the primary ethical issues underlying robotic surgery and artificial intelligence, through logical and rational argumentations that take into account objections and counter-objections. Specific ethical expertise will be crucial in identifying and debating the ethical issues raised, particularly from a perspective of future development and implications of the project. Several ethical themes requiring further investigation include the data collection from actual procedures performed with the surgical robot. These data will permit to assess the issues related to the moral and legal responsibility of using artificial intelligence-equipped machines in the healthcare sector, particularly in view of a hypothetical future where these machines will become increasingly autonomous.

References

1. European Union.: Eurobarometer. https://europa.eu/eurobarometer/screen/home. Accessed: 2025-06-14
2. European Union.: The EU's open science policy. https://research-andinnovation.ec.europa.eu/strategy/strategy-research-and-innovation/our-digital-future/open-science_en. Accessed: 2025-06-14
3. Elsevier Publisheer.: Elsevier Research Metrics Guidebook. https://assets.ctfassets.net/o78em1y1w4i4/54o8UH5cdisCqfUFpSG03T/b1c80b9c4a9fcf168f85065a0f044a64/ELSV-13013-Elsevier-Research-Metrics-Book-r12-WEB.pdf. Accessed: 2025-06-14
4. I-RIM Association.: I-RIM Web site. https://i-rim.it/en/. Accessed: 2025-06-14
5. University of Verona, https://www.youtube.com/@arsproject8149. Accessed: 2025-06-5
6. University of Verona, https://www.ars-project.eu/marginalia-forgotten-places/. Accessed: 2025-06-7
7. University of Verona, https://www.ars-project.eu/workshop-ethics-robotics/. Accessed: 2025-06-7
8. Vander Poorten, E.: https://cras-eu.org/past-events/. Accessed: 2025-06-5
9. University of Verona, https://metropolis.scienze.univr.it/commonsense-reasoning-in-surgical-robotics-summer-school/. Accessed: 2025-06-5
10. Doppio, M.: Interviews at the Accademia of Verona. https://docs.google.com/spreadsheets/d/1w8pOq_j7wiKrt5xhhmdO7LmcMsgYHrjpFJmV6w3oto8/edit?gid=290677008#. Accessed: 2025-06-5
11. Innova Biomed, https://www.ars-project.eu/innovabiomed-2022/. Accessed: 2025-06-5

The Exploitation of Results

Paolo Fiorini and Bogdan Maris

Abstract Scientific research should be able to impact people life and be moved from laboratory experiments to real products. In the case of medical devices, this process is called translational research and it is particularly difficult because of the long and expensive process necessary to validate the technology and acquire all the necessary safety certifications. This chapter describes the efforts motivated by the ARS project to transform some of the research results into commercial product, thanks to funding from the European Union. Since a full autonomous surgical robot is a distant goal, we focused on the smaller and reachable goal of percutaneous interventions. Section 2 describes the project PROST that developed a prototype of semi-autonomous robot to support the execution of biopsy for the diagnosis of prostate cancer. Section 3 describes the PROCT project, that aims at demonstrating the feasibility of using Optical Coherence Tomography to replace the physical prostate biopsy with 3D pictures of suspicious areas. Section 4 describes the PROFTH project, which addresses the issues related to focal therapy of prostate cancer, and develops a planner to safely carry out the ablation of early-stage prostate cancer. Finally, Sect. 5 describes the ROBIOPSY project, which aims at moving the PROST prototype closer to market by developing a certifiable medical device for prostate biopsy.

1 Introduction

During the ARS project, it was evident that to have a chance to apply some of the project results to the clinical practice, we needed to focus on small but credible and impactful projects not tied to any existing surgical robot. In fact, regulation and market constraints would have prevented the use of new algorithms and devices into

P. Fiorini (✉) · B. Maris
Department of Engineering for Innovation Medicine, University of Verona, Verona, Italy
e-mail: paolo.fiorini@univr.it

B. Maris
e-mail: bogdan.maris@univr.it

P. Fiorini (ed.), *Towards Autonomous Robotic Surgery*, Springer Tracts in Advanced Robotics 161, https://doi.org/10.1007/978-3-032-04247-7_15

a certified commercial medical device, unless long and costly procedures are carried out.

We decided to focus on Prostate Cancer (PCa) diagnosis and therapy because this pathology has still a high diagnostic error and patients do not have a choice of therapies personalized to their specific disease stage. Surgery is recommended in most cases, even for early cancer stages, since the alternative is only *Active Surveillance*, i.e. periodic checks to verify the disease progression, leaving patients with great psychological distress. Focal therapies, non-invasive procedures alternative to surgery, are still in clinical trial because of potential side effects.

We felt that a robotic device guided by artificial intelligence-based algorithms could solve the shortcomings of prostate cancer diagnosis and remove many of the side effects of focal therapies, due mostly to lack of proper planning and guidance.

For this purpose, we applied to the ERC Proof of Concept (PoC) Grants derived from the original ERC-ADG ARS grant. PoC grants fund small projects aimed at testing the practical application of the scientific concept developed during the main ERC grant.

We received three ERC PoC grants to explore different ways to improve the treatment of PCa. The first project was PROST (2019) that allowed us to design and build a laboratory prototype to demonstrate the feasibility of robotized PCa diagnosis. The second PoC grant was PROCT (2022) to explore the possibility of replacing the physical biopsy with images generated by an OCT (Optical Coherence Tomography) sensor. The third PoC was PROFTH (2023) that aimed at exploring the data and modeling needs of using focal ablation in the therapy of PCa.

To develop the prototype into a commercial product, in 2022 we started Needleye Robotics Srl, a spin-off of the University of Verona. A consortium led by the University of Verona was awarded in 2023 the project ROBIOPSY, funded by the Transition program of the European Innovation Council (EIC). The goal of ROBIOPSY was of developing the product prototype that will undergo medical certification and will be used in clinical trials.

In the rest of this chapter, these four projects are briefly described to give an overview of the steps needed to transform scientific ideas into commercial products. The economic potential and clinical impact of the ARS research will be tied to the success of this entrepreneurial activity.

2 The PROST Project

The first PoC grant (N. 875523) was called PROST (Autonomous Prostate Biopsy) and it was carried out from 1/11/19 to 30/04/21 focused on PCa diagnosis. With 1.3 million new cases worldwide last year [1], prostate cancer (PCa) is the second most common cancer in men, causing 358,989 deaths in 2018 alone [2]. As for any degenerative disease, early diagnosis is key to improve patients' therapeutic path and reduce the mortality rate. The problem is that the current diagnostic process is still affected by an error rate exceeding 30%, which leads more than 300,000 European citizens to either remain untreated or to receive unnecessary treatment out of about 1.000.000 patients who undergo diagnosis for prostate cancer every year [3].

Basically, PCa diagnosis is triggered either by the increase of the Prostate Specific Antigen biomarker (PSA) in the blood (that can also lead to over-diagnosis) or by more specific symptoms. In this case, patients undergo Magnetic Resonance Imaging (MRI) for an accurate detection of possible lesions down to 7 mm, the size below which tumors can be considered non-aggressive. When PCa is suspected, diagnosis must be confirmed by a biopsy and subsequent histological analysis of the sample. Biopsy is where the largest share of diagnostic errors occurs. In fact, in order to perform a biopsy on suspect tissues, physicians adopt the so-called Freehand Transrectal (or Transperineal) Ultrasound technique (TRUS). Basically, they manually identify the prostate capsule through real-time ultrasound (US) images and overlay MRI to US images to pinpoint the lesion locations, since they are not visible in the US images. Tissue samples are then collected by manually aiming and triggering a biopsy gun through the rectum (transrectal) or the perineum (transperineal).

Failures in identifying the location of the lesion and in manually aiming the biopsy gun lead to low sensitivity (33–44%) [4], with a high false-negative rates (23%) [5]. Recent fusion methods of MRI and US images reduced the error in target identification, but did not improve the overall diagnostic accuracy.

These errors lead to over or under treatment, i.e. patients go through unnecessary surgery or are not treated properly because of wrong diagnoses. Our hypothesis was that by combining Robotics and Artificial Intelligence algorithms in a medical device with autonomous robotics capabilities, we could reduce the errors affecting PCa diagnosis and reduce the focal treatment risks.

2.1 Device Description

The PROST project aimed at the development and validation of an Autonomous Prostate Biopsy System. This was a paradigm shift in prostate cancer diagnosis that would turn a subjective and operator-dependent procedure into a safer and more accurate diagnostic tool by introducing the autonomous robotic execution of the biopsy. PROST would reduce human errors because of automated target identification and robotic pointing of the biopsy gun. Diagnostic decisions, i.e. verification of the target correctness, and triggering of the biopsy gun is left to the clinicians.

Prostate biopsy was an excellent candidate for autonomous robotics because it was a relatively simple procedure that can greatly benefit from autonomy. However, its market introduction must be verified with extensive tests in relevant regulatory and clinical contexts and its economic viability remained to be validated.

The first prototype is described in [6] and it consists of two-joint arms that move along parallel planes, as shown in Fig. 1. They are coupled by an axis passing through the center of the two joints. This axis determines the needle orientation. Two small spheres with a hole, installed on each of the two joints, allow the needle to pass through the center of the joints. Each arm is composed of four links: the first

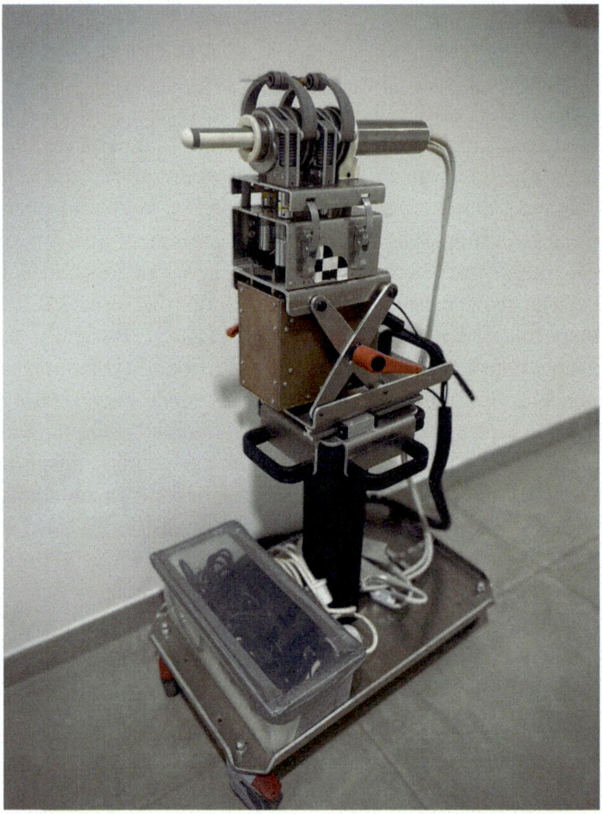

Fig. 1 The PROST1 prototype

one rotates around a common axis (roll axis in Fig. 1). Once the robot reaches the final position, non-reversible gears ensure that the desired orientation is maintained. The US probe axis coincides with the roll axis. With this configuration, the robot has two degrees of freedom (DOFs) for reaching the entry position, two DOFs for needle orientation and one DOF for the US probe (Fig. 2). The robot positions a cannula oriented toward the target; a biopsy needle then slides through the cannula touching the patient entry point, directed toward the target. The needle insertion is done manually. The entry point is computed by the PROST software as a fixed point that allows reaching all the selected targets. For each target point, the orientation is given as the line through the spheres in the top joints that connects with the entry point. A time-of-flight sensor (TOF) is attached to the cannula to measure the insertion depth of the biopsy needle. The PROST prototype integrates the Ultrasonix US system with a compatible bi-planar US probe (BK Medical, Peabody, Massachusetts, USA). A dedicated user interface shown in Fig. 3 and image processing software, based on 3D Slicer and developed in Python, was developed in collaboration with our clinical

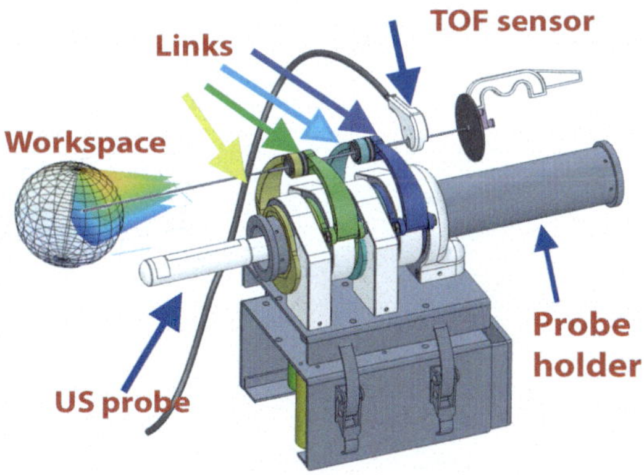

Fig. 2 The CAD of the robotic needle positioner in the PROST1 prototype

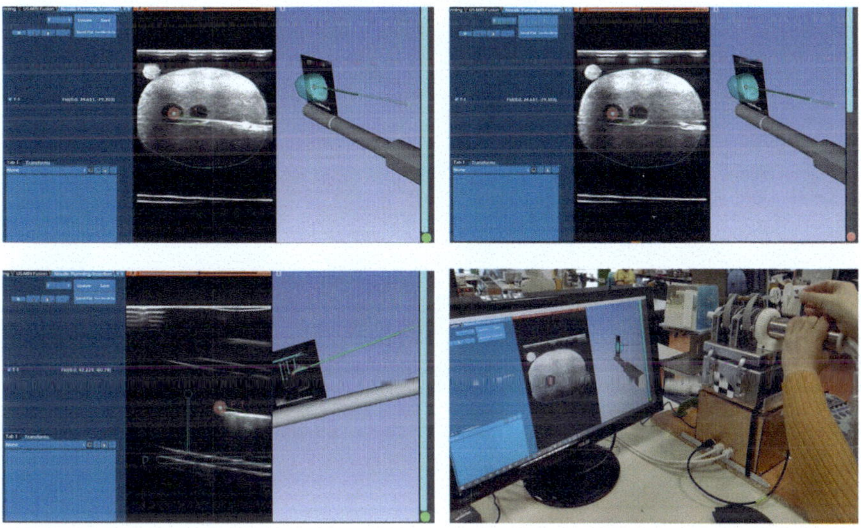

Fig. 3 The User Interface of the PROST1 prototype

partners. Through intensive calibration tests, we measured a calibration accuracy at the needle tip of less than 1 mm (see [6]).

PROST's goal was to reduce margins for human error in prostate biopsy procedures, which means providing assistance, both manual and cognitive to the clinician. PROST makes a proposal to the physician, who assesses it, can approve it, or request another proposal or input a value directly, according to his or her clinical judgment. The doctor retains the complete control of the surgical task through the manual needle insertion.

The PROST system includes a software module implementing a dedicated convolutional neural network that we called PROST-Net [7, 8]. This module allows the segmentation of the prostate in US and MRI images for the purpose of image fusion.

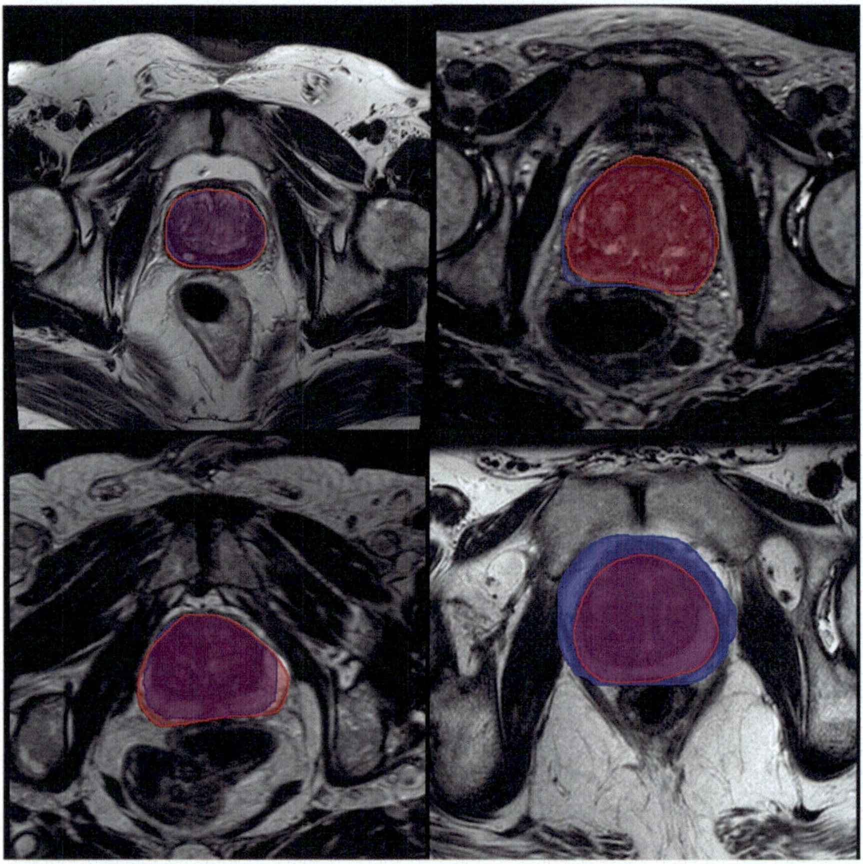

Fig. 4 Result of the MRI–US segmentation-based fusion for prostate segmentation. The MRI-segmented prostate capsule is shown in red, and the ultrasound (US)-segmented capsule is shown in blue

The pre-clinical validation of this module is made on patient data obtained after ethical approval. This module was not tested on cadaver images, because the US images of ex-vivo prostate tissue differ considerably compared with in-vivo tissue and MRI data of cadavers were not available (Fig. 4).

2.2 Test Results

We firstly tested the method on phantoms. A second phase of experiments involved the use of patients dataset composed of 840 images for training and validation and 664 images for testing. The data and the ground truth were obtained with the support of the local hospital and with the approval of the ethics committee. Finally, we tested

PROST-Net on MRI images of patients taken from the Cancer Imaging Archive [9]. This dataset contains more than 1000 patients and for each entry the prostate gland segmentation and the segmentation of tumours is given.

The segmentation of the prostate in MRI allows the initial fusion with a 3D reconstructed and segmented US image acquired with PROST. The segmentation of the lesion in MRI gives to the robot the coordinates of the target. The goal of cadaver testing was to measure PROST's accuracy in targeting points acquired though the imaging of a realistic anatomical space. Tests were carried out by five board-certified practicing urologists with relevant clinical experience in prostate interventions. Available cadaver specimens (pelvis to toe tip) were examined via trans-rectal pelvic ultrasound by an expert urologist. A total of 10 cadaver specimens were prepared by placing 6 seeds and to target each of them once, so that for each prostate 12 needle insertions would be performed.

Samples from radical prostatectomy were fixed in 10% buffered formalin, with surgical thread marking the apex. After fixation, specimens were sectioned at 5 mm intervals following the axis of the prostatic urethra. The data collected were sufficient to indicate a reliable performance range, with an overall mean of 2.25 mm and a standard deviation of 0.75 mm. These are very encouraging results considering the difficulties described above.

The positive results of the experiments supported the technical viability of developing a product based on an improved design and the company Needleye Robotics was founded as a spin-off of the University of Verona. The market justification for starting a company was that the potential for the global PCa diagnostic market was predicted to reach $5.5 billion by 2025, showing a Compounded Annual Growth Rate of 12.3%. Since the share of PSA and other testing tools is expected to be around $2.8 billion by 2025, the value of the biopsy market is projected to be in the range of $2.5 billion. PROST could also be sold in "retrofit-mode" on existing echography, which would substantially increase the market potential of the product.

3 The PROCT Project

The second PoC grant (N. 101069279) was PROCT (Prostate Diagnosis using Optical Coherence Tomography) that lasted from 01/10/2022 till 31/03/24.

The PROCT project aims to address the second shortcoming of PC diagnosis, i.e. the long processing time of a PCa diagnosis, by validating in pre-clinical stage a semiautonomous robotic approach to PC diagnosis based on Optical Coherence Tomography (OCT) that would exactly pinpoint the target lesion and analyze it through an AI and robotic-based imaging setup. This can comprehensively visualize the lesions at the microscopic level in vivo, without taking any physical sample of the prostate. The resulting virtual microscope slide will allow urologists to explore and analyze various suspicious areas in the same procedure without the need to rely on the histopathological examination of the biopsy tissue samples.

This procedure would avoid the delays due to the histological laboratory sample preparation and examination by permitting to assess in real time the tissue. This analysis could also be carried out by proper AI algorithms trained to recognize cancer cells. The PROCT probe could also be used to assess the success of a radical prostatectomy intervention by examining whether PCa cell are left on the intervention margins. PROCT could be instrumental to "focal therapy" procedures, which treats the specific lesions of the prostate avoiding overtreatment as do systemic (chemotherapy or radiotherapy) or radical resection procedures, by enabling the accurate grading and mapping of cancer which is not possible with state of the art biopsy protocols.

3.1 Device Description

To reach this goal, we acquired a custom-made OCT system to be able to modify and customize its parameters. To improve quality and performance we have developed an FPGA implementation of the algorithms. If the laboratory experiments were successful, we may consider examining the human tissues removed from a patient during the prostatectomy intervention, after approval by the Ethical Committee.

Our OCT system is based on Common Path Optical Coherence Tomography (CP-OCT), a specialized OCT configuration in which both the reference and sample optical paths share the fiber. Despite its advantages, CP-OCT also has limitations. One of the main challenges is the limited imaging depth due to the fixed position of the reference reflector. Additionally, CP-OCT systems often require careful calibration to compensate for variations in reference reflectivity and background noise.

Needle-based OCT is an advanced imaging technique that incorporates an OCT probe into a thin, needle-like device, allowing for minimally invasive imaging deep inside tissues. This approach is particularly valuable in real-time biopsy guidance, intraoperative tumor margin assessment, and intravascular imaging. By embedding a CP-OCT probe within a needle, surgeons and clinicians can visualize tissue microstructure in real time, reducing the risk of sampling errors and improving diagnostic accuracy. A key aspect of the work done was the acquisition and processing of experimental data, particularly from biological samples such as pork tissues. We used a laser with 800–880 nm wavelength range, optimized for real-time spectral-domain OCT (SD-OCT) imaging. Figure 5 shows the overall configuration of the PROCT system, with the optical processing system, the computation unit, the vertical micropositioner and the needle-based OCT probe.

We experimented with the U-Net architecture successfully to learn the global structure of the scans, accurately capturing the overall circular shape and common artifacts. However it struggled to preserve fine-grained details, leading to a loss of subtle textures and structural variations. We used also a Pix2Pix model, leveraging adversarial training with Patch-GAN, that offered a speedup in scan generation passing from 15 s per scan to about around one second, making real-time applications possible. Figure 6 shows a typical image acquired by the needle-based OCT probe.

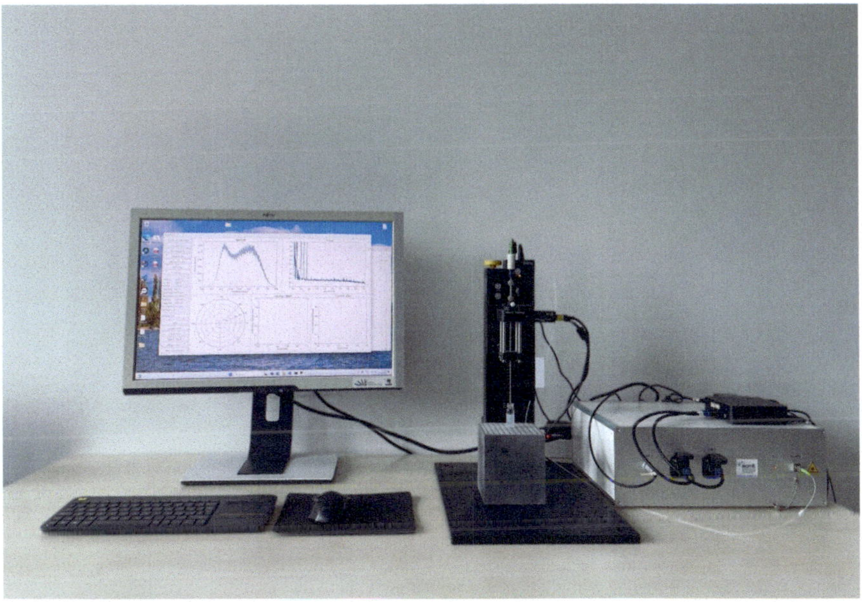

Fig. 5 The overall PROCT system

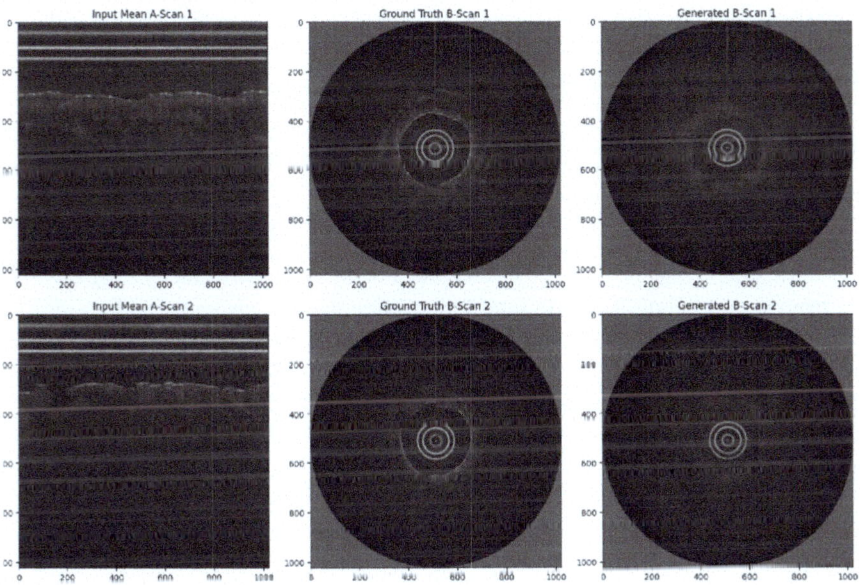

Fig. 6 Typical images acquired by the PROCT system

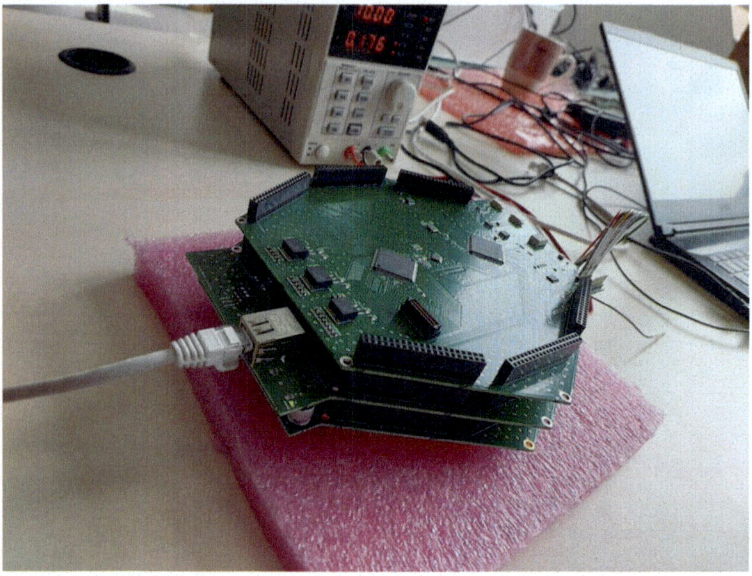

Fig. 7 The prototype of the FPGA implementations of the PROCT algorithms

We are currently porting these algorithms to an FPGA architecture to achieve further speed improvements, Fig. 7 shows the prototype of the FPGA implementation of the image reconstruction algorithms.

4 The PROFTH Project

The third PoC grant is PROFTH (Prostate Focal Therapy, grant N. 101138301) run from January 1st, 2024 till June 30th, 2025. This project was addressing the requirements to make focal therapy for PCa a reality. PCa treatment in fact, is lagging the treatment of other tumors, e.g. breast and lung cancer, that have moved from total removal of the organ to much less invasive and traumatizing focal therapies. Having developed an efficient and affordable device for the precise PCa diagnosis, the logical next step is to replace the biopsy needle with an ablation needle and, if the tissue examination gives a positive result, immediately burn the PCa tissue. Of course, the distributed nature of PCa requires an accurate analysis of the patient inclusion for this therapy, to avoid leaving dangerous cancer cells, unseen by the MRI, in the prostate.

In this project the modelling and planning algorithms for placing the ablation needles will be developed by the team of Needleye Robotics, while the urology team of the University of Verona will carry out the patient analysis to define the inclusion conditions for the therapy. No clinical trial is planned in this project, but we will interact with the Ethical Committee about the patient data analysis for the inclusion criteria.

The motivation of this project is that around 70–80% of patients are still treated with radical prostatectomy [10], since alternative approaches, e.g. radiation therapy and focal therapy are unable to avoid the risk of metastases. The problem is that radical prostatectomy comes with serious side effects, most notably erectile dysfunction (up to 82% of men), and urinary incontinence (up to 35% of men) [11]. This is making the quest for alternative treatment options a hot topic in urology. Among the various alternatives, focal therapy is emerging as a less invasive and conservative technique to treat only the cancerous part of the prostate, while preserving healthy tissue and minimizing side effects. It can be performed using cryotherapy, laser, or high-intensity focused ultrasound (HIFU), which result in less pain and side effects, as well as shorter recovery times than traditional prostate cancer surgery. However, urologists are very concerned that focal therapies leave unnoticed lesions in the prostate that would eventually cause a cancer recurrence, which results in a very slow adoption rate of this approach (between 1–8% of the cases). On the other hand, the transition to focal therapy in replacement of radical surgery is now reality for breast, kidney and lung cancer, where the localization of the tumor and the positioning of the ablation tool is relatively easier to ensure that cancer cells are mostly eradicated.

From the technical point of view, all methods currently used to perform ablation in prostate cancer are limited by poor navigation, inadequacy of imaging to delineate tumor boundaries, and variable precision of tissue destruction, which leads to significant rate of cancer persistence within treatment zones (6–50%) and the presence of residual cancer within the prostate on re-biopsy (24–49%). In fact, the main challenges for a successful focal therapy are planning the procedure and precisely deploying multiple cryo-needles or the laser tip to form an ablation volume that adequately covers the target volume while sparing critical structure around it.

4.1 The Technical Solution

In PROFTH we aimed at addressing the technical shortcomings of focal therapies, by developing a standardized method to plan, execute and monitor the focal therapy. From an engineering point of view, this PoC aims at providing a prototype of focal therapy planning and monitoring software interoperable with the PROST robotic platform, which will allow urologists to carry out well planned, repeatable and comparable clinical trials. The novelty proposed is the shift from the focal therapy of a large portion of the prostate, i.e. the full or half gland, to the volume strictly necessary to kill cancerous cells, to ensure the proper safety margins and to spare delicate nervous structures. The PROFTH algorithms are computing the ablation volumes limited to cover only the prostate lesions, the minimum number of needles necessary to the procedure, the correct access direction and penetration depth. The focal therapy is supported by the PROST robotic device, and the pre-operative 3D model developed in PROFTH can be superimposed in real time to the 3D model acquired

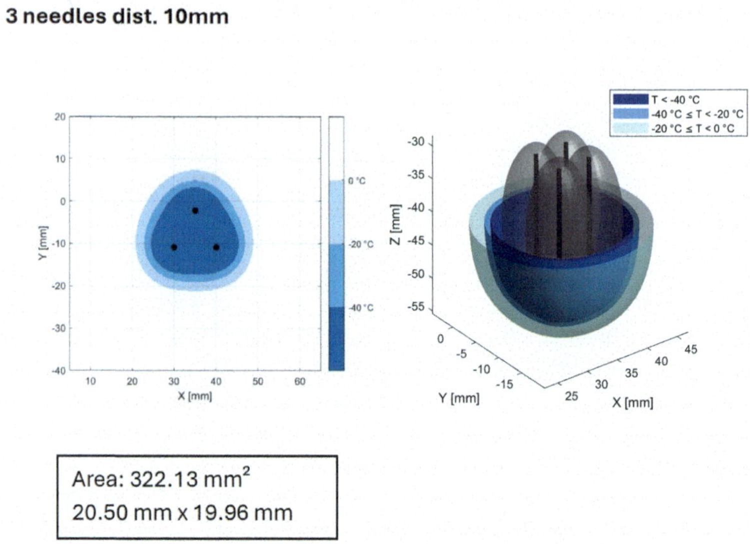

Fig. 8 The model of the temperature gradient during a cryo-ablation focal therapy

by ultrasound images, thus mapping the therapy plan to the current patient anatomy. Since the prostate tissue properties are not known in advance, the therapy must be monitored in real time by the analysis of the ultrasound images that will inform the physician when the ablation volume has reached the size needed for ablation.

The PROFTH project has been organized in three steps. The first phase focuses on the characterization of the ablation process and the identification of the main requirements to integrate existing ablation devices with the PROST technology. The second phase dealt with the realization of a biomechanical model of the prostate for the ablation procedure. We have been addressing the characterization of the ablation process in the context of prostate procedures, identifying the physical parameters of the process and developing a mathematical model of the freezing and thawing phases required for the PCa ablation. Finally, we have been working on the computation of the access directions to the PCa, by optimizing the volume coverage inside the prostate, minimizing the number of access paths and avoiding the critical structures of the area. The PROFTH algorithms will be validated in discussions with urologists expert of focal therapy, in laboratory tests with phantoms simulating the prostate tissue in which impurities of the size and type of PCa have been injected (Fig. 8).

To further connect the outcome of this PoC with the previous achievements of the team, the safety margins around the cancer focus could be analyzed by the PROCT sensor that will identify the micro extent of the lesion and provide signal attenuation indicating the presence of cancer.

5 The ROBIOPSY Project

The results achieved by the ARS grant and its spin-off projects may be lost if not translated into a commercial product. Therefore, in 2022 we founded the Needleye Robotics company to industrialize and certify the PROST prototype for robotic prostate biopsy. In 2023 Needleye Robotics received a grant (N. 101112739) from the EIC Transition program for the project ROBIOPSY (AI and Robotics for Prostate Biopsy) that will support the development of the product prototype and its pre-certification tests. In ARS, we have demonstrated autonomous surgical tasks, translated them into the PROST prototype and validated in pre-clinical tests, which are the starting point of ROBIOPSY.

Key feature of ROBIOPSY is the use of automatic procedures to ensure the effective integration of image fusion algorithms with a robotic device to overcome the cognitive and manual limitations of human operators. Figure 9 shows a comparison between the current manual biopsy procedure (left), and the ROBIOPSY approach (right). The cognitive and manual functions carried out by the physician are augmented by software algorithms (blue) and robotic motions (orange), but still all decisions are made by the physician. Software algorithms provide guidance for: (1) identification of the prostate boundaries and biopsy targets in the MRI images, (2) fusion of MRI and US images, (3) acquisition of the US images and (4) computation of the optimal needle trajectories. The orange phases are the robotic actions: (5) computation of the robot positions, (6) tracking of the needle by the US probe, (7) robot motion to the entry point, (8) adjustment of the US probe, and (9) needle insertion monitoring. This process is repeated until all targets have been reached.

The expected benefits for doctors, and consequently, for patients and healthcare services are:

- Reduced error in cancer diagnosis.
- Accurate monitoring of the disease course.
- Ambulatory use.

Although we will focus on prostate biopsy first, the developed robot-assisted technology has the potential to be used in other prostate-related applications, with low-dose brachytherapy, tumour ablation, gold marker implantation being the next logical steps. ROBIOPSY will enable the immediate ablation of the lesions with the available commercial products thus creating a *single-day* diagnosis and treatment for the early detection and cure of prostate cancer. Figure 10 shows the second PROST prototype on which usability tests were carried out and software was developed.

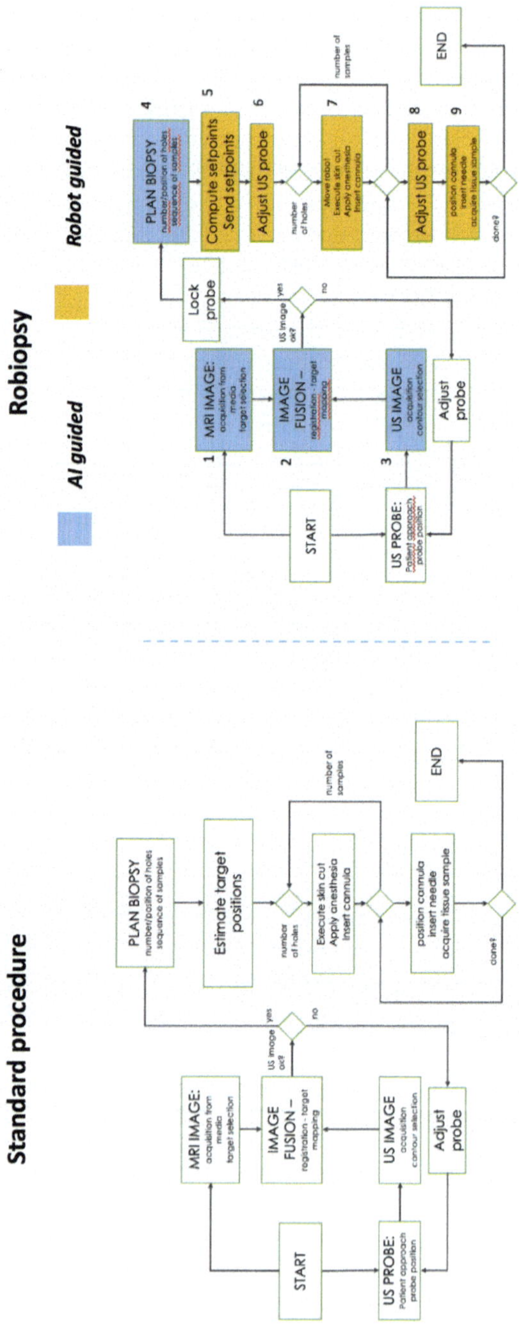

Fig. 9 Comparison between standard and robotized biopsy procedure

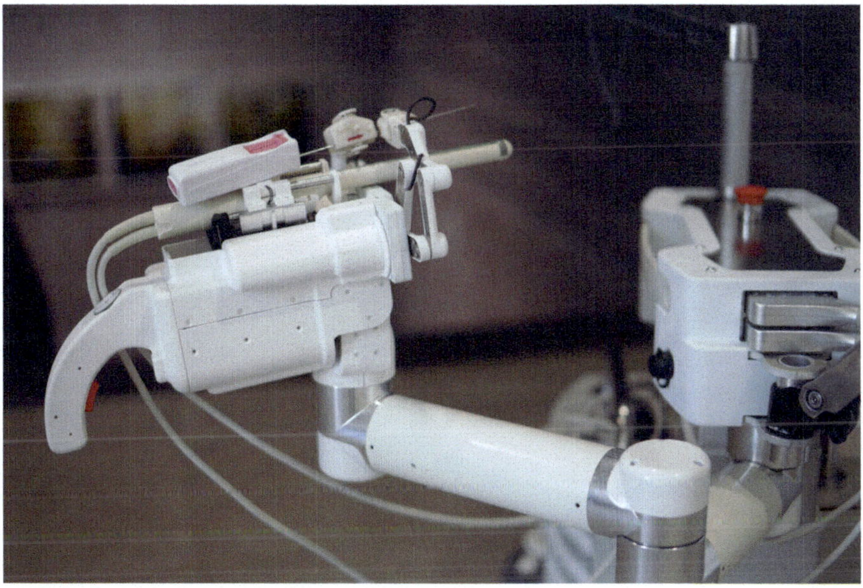

Fig. 10 The robotic head of the PROST2 prototype

References

1. P.C.S. World Cancer Research Fund, https://www.wcrf.org/preventing-cancer/cancer-statistics/prostate-cancer-statistics/
2. Taitt, H.E.: Global trends and prostate cancer: A review of incidence, detection, and mortality as influenced by race, ethnicity, and geographic location. Am. J. Mens Health **12**(6), 1807–1823 (2018)
3. JRC Publications, https://ec.europa.eu/jrc/en/publication/epidemiology-prostate-cancer-europe. Accessed: 2025-02-15
4. Merril, J.: Prostate cancer market snapshot: more than provenge. The Pink Sheet **12** (2010)
5. King, C.R., Long, J.P.: Prostate biopsy grading errors: a sampling problem? Int. J. Cancer (Radiat. Oncol. Invest) **90**, 326–330 (2000)
6. Maris, B., et al.: Toward autonomous robotic prostate biopsy: a pilot study. Int. J. Comput. Assist. Radiol. Surg. **16**(8), 1393–1401 (2021)
7. Maris, B., Palladino, L., Fiorini, P.: 3d slicer module for semantic segmentation of ultrasound images in prostate biopsy using deep learning techniques. Proc. CARS Comput. Assis. Radiol. Surg. 158–159 (2021)
8. Palladino, L., Maris, B., Antonelli, A., Fiorini, P.: Autonomy in robotic prostate biopsy through ai-assisted fusion. In: 2021 20th International Conference on Advanced Robotics (ICAR), pp. 142–147 (2021)
9. Margolis, D., Huang, J., Natarajan, S., Priester, A., Marks, L.: Prostate MRI and ultrasound with pathology and coordinates of tracked biopsy (prostate-MRI-U.S.-biopsy). Accessed: 2025-02-15
10. van den Bos, W., et al.: Focal therapy in primary localised prostate cancer: the European association of urology position in 2018. Eur. Urol. **74**(1), 84–91 (2018)
11. Alvarez, J., O'Neil, B., Koyama, T., et al.: The comparative harms of open and robotic prostatectomy in population based samples. J. Urol. **195**(2), 321–329 (2016)

Conclusions

Paolo Fiorini and Marco Bombieri

Abstract In this chapter we summarize the development and the findings of the project ARS, an ERC Advanced Grant funded by the European Union in 2017 for five years. Due to the COVID-19 pandemic, the project was extended to six years till September 30th 2023 allowing the completion of the experiments that were interrupted because of the pandemic. Section 1 summarizes the ARS objectives and points out some of the unexpected results that we have achieved, as it should happen in research. Section 2 summarizes the book organization in three Parts and sixteen chapters. In the first Part we include the (mostly) theoretical results, in the second Part we present the simulation and experimental validations of the results, and in the third Part of the book we describe the non-technical issues related to ethical and social aspects of robotic autonomy in surgery, to communicate our finding to different audiences, and to the exploitation of the ARS project results. Section 3 gives some indication on a few, among the many, open questions that researcher will have to solve to move forward in this field.

1 Project Objectives and Unexpected Findings

The goal of the project was to explore the technological needs, and the implication of embodied intelligence, i.e. what devices and algorithms should be developed to endow a physical agent of some level of autonomy and how such device would

P. Fiorini (✉)
Department of Engineering for Innovation Medicine, University of Verona, Verona, Italy
e-mail: paolo.fiorini@univr.it

M. Bombieri
Department of Computer Science, University of Verona, Verona, Italy

Department of Information Engineering and Computer Science, University of Trento, Trento, Italy

P. Fiorini (ed.), *Towards Autonomous Robotic Surgery*, Springer Tracts in Advanced Robotics 161, https://doi.org/10.1007/978-3-032-04247-7_16

be accepted by the public. Embodied intelligence has been a recurrent objective in robotics, even in its early days [1, 2], but the available technology was its strong limiting factor. The advent of powerful computers able to run complex machine learning and Large Models has made possible the implementation of autonomous capabilities.

We choose the domain of robot-assisted surgery because of its potential impact on health care, although our exploitation efforts are showing that such an impact is not immediate, because of many organizational and financial constraints. Surgical robotics is the most advanced field of service robotics, it is used in many hospitals worldwide and it is supported by many innovative companies and very skilled surgeons. Furthermore, Intuitive Surgical, the manufacturer of da Vinci Surgical System, has donated many dismissed da Vinci robots to robotics laboratory worldwide, supporting the development of the da Vinci Research Kits (dVRK), creating a network of dedicated researchers and a growing body of scientific and technical skills. The Altair Robotics Laboratory at the University of Verona is part of this network, and we were able to count on the competence and skills on many colleagues to overcome the difficulties of our project.

The availability of a dVRK and the support of a competent community was one of the factors motivating the ambitious goals of the ARS project to demonstrate the autonomous execution of relevant surgical tasks. This book aims at documenting the work carried out during the ARS project in a single and coherent narration, starting from the basic concepts of surgical knowledge to the development of a clinical prototype.

The project results closely match its initial objectives, but many unexpected findings were discovered by the researchers working on the project. The idea of deriving task knowledge *top-down* was part of the initial ARS plan. However, the derivation of the algorithmic representation of a surgical procedure from its description in the textbook was made possible by the availability of LLM's, which did not exist when the project was first conceived. These results are described in Chapter 2, they support the development of a pipeline from text to action that will permit also the autonomous acquisition of knowledge by a robot. In chapter "Surgical Task Planning and Learning" we showed that logical languages are a very good solution to represent long sequence of actions overcoming the difficulties of *explainbility* of deep networks. This was one of the original objectives of the project, but the integration of machine learning and logical representation permitted to improve the quality of the logic program and of its interface with the anatomical environment. The logical approach to task representation lead immediately to the integration of textual and logical task description as described in chapter "Towards Surgical Task Planning from Text". In the original ARS formulation, simulation methods were introduced to verify the quality of a task plan, but chapter "The Cognitive Architecture" presents the use of simulation as the background of task execution, to provide feedback to the robot about errors in the plan or in the environment model. *Bottom-up* learning, i.e. the acquisition of task structure from data was an aspect of knowledge representation described in the original ARS formulation. However, we discovered the power of Dynamic Motion Primitives (DMP) to integrate machine learning with analytical motion representation and to add further steps in the difficult quest of deriving task structure from clinical data, as described in chapter "Learning Surgical Gestures from Data". Finally, we improved the execution set-up by developing new methods for hand-eye calibration and for instrument localization that allowed safe instrument motions in the critical anatomical environments, as described in chapter "Situation Awareness in Autonomous Surgical Robots: Calibration and Medical SLAM".

As it should happen in successful research activities, many important results were not expected at the beginning of the project. It is because of the ingenuity and persistence of my former doctoral students that we were able to make this much longer than expected road of scientific achievements.

2 Book Organization

The book is organized in three parts and sixteen chapters. Part I addresses the issues related to knowledge extraction, representation and task planning, which are key element of robotic autonomy. An autonomous robot should be able to find the information needed to carry out a task without human intervention and organize it so that it can use it during task execution. To simplify this difficult task, we identified the knowledge sources (surgical textbooks), the steps needed to convert it into a sequence of actions (Natural Language Processing) and the structure to represent it (logical programming). Deep Learning and Large Language Models were tools used to analyze the surgical text, as discussed in chapter "Learning Surgical Procedures from Text". To ensure execution explainability plans were formed using the logical framework of Answer Set Programming (ASP) which also grounds the variables to the sensor readings, as discussed in chapter "Surgical Task Planning and Learning". Plans can also be derived directly from textual description further simplifying their explainability as discussed in chapter "Towards Surgical Task Planning from Text". Demonstration learning was used to define the robot control policies, as presented in chapter "Learning Surgical Gestures from Data", together with a first step to address the issue of tasks segmentation from clinical data, as described in chapter "Learning Surgical Gestures from Data", Sect. 2. Chapter "Simulation and Autonomy" motivates the importance of simulation as a tool for knowledge representation and task learning.

Part II addresses task execution, by discussing plan instantiation, simulation and execution, and by presenting how these concepts are integrated to demonstrate some basic robotic capabilities. The first chapter of this part is chapter "Situation Awareness in Autonomous Surgical Robots: Calibration and Medical SLAM". that describes how the plans are grounded in the current anatomical environment and how their execution is monitored with a new hand-eye calibration algorithm and the anatomical SLAM to accurately track the instrument positions in the deformable and dynamic anatomical environment. Chapter "The Cognitive Architecture" describes the software architecture proposed for the experiments in which the simulation is the real-time task supervisor. This architecture supports the experimental verification of autonomous tissue retraction described in chapters "Autonomous Tissue Retraction with DEFRAS" and "Learning Tissue Retraction in Simulation". In chapter "The Cognitive Architecture" we address also the issue of human interpretation of a task, introducing the need of common sense reasoning in surgical planning. Chapter "New Hardware: Design, Models and Analysis" describes the new hardware developed to overcome some of the limitations of current robotic systems. In particular, chapter "New Hardware: Design, Models and Analysis", Sect. 1 describes a model of needle deflection, chapter "New Hardware: Design, Models and Analysis", Sect. 2 describes a novel sensing approach based on electrical bio-impedance measuring, and chapter "New Hardware: Design, Models and Analysis", Sect. 3 describes a novel force and torque sensor for surgical instruments.

Part III summarizes some of the non-technical issues related to the introduction of robotic autonomy in the society. This part of the project was a research project in its own right, since it let us explore the ethical aspects of autonomy, carry out experiments of social interaction with our communication activities, and explore how autonomy can be transformed into a product with the project exploitation. Chapter "The Ethical and Social Aspects of Autonomy" addresses the concepts related to ethics of autonomous robots and the benefits that they could bring to people. Chapter "Automation on the Brink of Autonomy: Letting Go of Control" explores the evolving relationship between mankind and machines, its risks and potential benefits. Chapter "Communication Strategy of the ARS Project" describes the activities carried out during the whole project to define a communication strategy and to engage the different audiences of the ARS project. Chapter "The Exploitation of Results" describes the project funded to support the commercialization of a medical robot with a minimal set of autonomous features.

3 Discussion and Open Questions

The research described in this book only scratched the surface of robotic autonomy, which encompasses most scientific and technological fields, from material science to artificial intelligence, from control theory to modelling and simulation.

In this last section, we should indicate a couple of issues that were not addressed in the research presented here. A set of important considerations refer to the availability and analysis of clinical data. Unfortunately, data collected during robot-assisted procedures are, in most cases, not made available to the research community thus preventing the analysis of how real procedures are carried out. This prevents addressing the coherence between nominal and real procedures. By *nominal* procedure we refer to the description presented in the textbooks, whereas *real* procedures are what occurs in the operating room. An autonomous surgical robot should behave like a real surgeon and therefore react as an experienced surgeon to unexpected events.

Real procedures are affected by, at least, two elements altering the task sequence and execution. The first is mentioned in chapter "The Cognitive Architecture", Sect. 3

and refers to the *interpretation* that each surgeon gives to the surgical acts, depending on patient's anatomy and pathology status. This interpretation may include variations of each action parameters, e.g. cut depth or suture length, and may be effectively addressed by automatically learning how the patient's conditions affect each specific procedure action. This phase is the necessary *grounding* of the nominal procedure to the specific intervention.

However, a more difficult case may happen when the surgeon inserts a phase in the procedure that was not included in the nominal description. In this case, learning this variation can be particularly difficult. In fact, assuming the availability of clinical data, the data analysis must identify the new phase inserted in the procedure and the causes that prompted the variation from the nominal procedure. In this case, it would be very difficult to distinguish the new phase from the previous phase, that could have been longer than expected, and the insertion of the new phase in the nominal procedure would be particularly difficult.

An interview with the surgeon may clarify the motivation of inserting the new phase, and the task plan will need to be modified, and perhaps new variables inserted, to account for this change. This case is similar to the occurrence of phase replanning, but instead of being initiated by the robot and by following a known alternative, this change is initiated by the surgeon, and it may not be included in the possible alternatives known a priori.

The advent of LLMs and other multi-modal foundation models has the potential to open new horizons also for autonomy in robotic surgery. These massive models, pre-trained on huge and diverse datasets, have demonstrated good capabilities in reasoning, multi-modal understanding, and instruction-following that could also be leveraged for surgical contexts. In particular, LLMs and foundation models may enable richer semantic interpretation of surgical plans, higher-quality interpretation of surgical images and videos, assist in real-time decision-making through dialogue-based interfaces, and support the integration of symbolic and sub-symbolic knowledge, bridging the gap between formal task representations and the nuanced, often unstructured realities of real-world procedures. Their capacity to adapt to new instructions and interact using natural language could also facilitate better human-robot collaboration and explainability. However, incorporating such models into safety-critical domains like surgery presents significant challenges in terms of reliability, validation, and regulatory acceptance, which remain open research and policy questions.

Another critical, and more philosophical, issue is related to *knowledge generation*, or even the simpler *experience building*. One may think of a process of life-long learning by the robot, which continues to acquire new data to improve its reasoning capabilities. However, given the lack of transparency and explainability of current deep networks, it is impossible to trace the impact of new data on the overall network structure. One may ask the network to formalize its knowledge as a series of logical conditions, in which the new knowledge can be represented explicitly as new statements. This will represent an interesting integration of symbolic and sub-symbolic knowledge representations. Now however, life-long learning is not accepted by medical device regulations, which expect a medical device to be completely predictable. This is an interesting contradiction between human and machine behaviors: medical professionals are expected to learn from new results and devise new solutions, when necessary; machines instead are required to always repeat their behavior without adaptation.

When robots will achieve full autonomous capabilities these questions would have been solved and we will deal with a robotic surgeon, rather than a surgical robot.

References

1. Fiorini, P., Chang, J.: Autonomous organization of grasping tasks. In: SPIE Symposia on Aerospace Sensing, Artificial Intelligence VII, Orlando, FL, pp. 591–602, March 27–31 (1989)
2. Fiorini, P., Chang, J.: A procedure concept for local reflex control of grasping. In: NASA Conference on Space Telerobotics, Pasadena, CA, vol. 4, pp. 81–90, Jan 31–Feb 2 (1989)

Correction to: New Hardware: Design, Models and Analysis

Andrea Calanca, Zhuoqi Cheng, Diego Dall'Alba, Paolo Fiorini, Giovanni Gerardo Muscolo, and Chiara Zandoná

Correction to:
Chapter 11 in: P. Fiorini (ed.), *Towards Autonomous Robotic Surgery*, Springer Tracts in Advanced Robotics 161, https://doi.org/10.1007/978-3-032-04247-7_11

The original version of this chapter was inadvertently published with the incorrect affiliation "Department of Computer Science, University of Trento, Trento, Italy" which has now been removed from the author Giovanni Gerardo Muscolo. The chapter has been updated with the changes.

The updated version of this chapter can be found at
https://doi.org/10.1007/978-3-032-04247-7_11

P. Fiorini (ed.), *Towards Autonomous Robotic Surgery*, Springer Tracts in Advanced Robotics 161, https://doi.org/10.1007/978-3-032-04247-7_17

The manufacturer's authorised representative in the EU is Springer Nature Customer Service Centre GmbH, Europaplatz 3, 69115 Heidelberg, Germany. If you have any concerns regarding our products, please contact ProductSafety@springernature.com

Printed and bound by CPI Group (UK) Ltd, Croydon, CR0 4YY
21/09/2026
02220009-0007